Deep dyslexia

International Library of Psychology

General editor: Max Coltheart
Professor of Psychology, University of London

£17-50
9 . B 80

 E DS POLYT

Deep dyslexia

Edited by
**Max Coltheart, Karalyn Patterson and
John C. Marshall**

Routledge & Kegan Paul
London, Boston and Henley

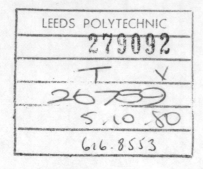
First published in 1980
by Routledge & Kegan Paul Ltd
39 Store Street, London WC1E 7DD,
9 Park Street, Boston, Mass. 02108, USA and
Broadway House, Newtown Road,
Henley-on-Thames, Oxon RG9 1EN
Set in 10/12pt Linocomp Baskerville by
Rowland Phototypesetting Ltd,
Bury St Edmunds, Suffolk
and printed in Great Britain by
Lowe & Brydone Printers Ltd
Thetford, Norfolk

British Library Cataloguing in Publication Data

Deep dyslexia. – (International library of
psychology).

1. Dyslexia
I. Coltheart, Max
II. Patterson, Karalyn
III. Marshall, John Charles
IV. Series
616.8'553   RC394.W6   80-40022

ISBN 0 7100 0456 7

Contents

Preface

In July 1977 a meeting of the International Neuropsychology Society was held in Oxford. The three editors and most of the contributing authors of this book happened to be present, and it therefore seemed highly appropriate that we should meet for an informal discussion of deep dyslexia, a topic to which all of us had devoted considerable time and energy. Although this was, of course, an excellent opportunity to inquire of each other about all the details of the patients that, typically, do *not* appear in published papers, we probably expected our little gathering to behave like the usual desultory academic discussion. But the excitement and productive interchange which transpired and which, moreover, continued unabated for more than three hours was a revelation to us all. We shouted and screamed at each other, noted new and surprising similarities and differences between our patients; we explored and made explicit some of the theoretical preconceptions we were bringing to the analysis of our data; we heard of new tests that one or the other of us had used and that the others might profitably try out on their subjects. 'That', we thought, 'is how conferences ought to be.' And so we decided to try it on a grander scale. The result was a four-day symposium on deep dyslexia, sponsored by the Medical Research Council, and held at Jesus College, Cambridge, in September 1978. This book represents the result, but certainly not the proceedings, of that symposium.

The topic might appear recondite – one particular pattern of impairment (among many), in one aspect of language facility (among several), investigated intensively in some dozen brain-damaged patients (among multitudes). Yet we would argue that the interest and significance of the topic ranges far beyond this specific description, in at least three respects. First, we believe that the study of deep dyslexia (and indeed many other pathologies) is germane to the ways in which we look at normal reading and language functions. Second, the condition seems quite crucial to the development of *theory* regarding these processes in both normal and impaired states. And third, deep dyslexia may provide an opening to more general techniques and paradigms for the investigation and interpretation of neuropsychological syndromes. In this last respect, we would like to think that the work reported here – preliminary and fragmentary as it is – constitutes a case study of what, even now, can be achieved by painstaking, extensive reports of individual patients, guided by an explicit commitment to seek explanatory theories of the behavioural consequences of brain-damage. We shall only progress beyond the classical 'diagram-makers' if we take as seriously as they did the requirement that our conjectures about disordered systems should be expressed sufficiently formally that counter-examples can be recognized as such.

The book addresses the putative syndrome from a variety of angles. Many of the chapters present data – old and new – from patients, together with theoretical accounts that attempt to make sense of the initially bewildering complexity of performance. Many chapters tie together the data from a variety of different types of acquired dyslexia with recent results from normal adults and children. We also include some more specifically neurological theorizing and observation, and set the whole within the historical context of early case-reports. Finally, there are two innovations that we consider important for future work of the sort considered here. The book includes cross-language comparisons of the symptom-complex. Brains may be similar from one culture to another but orthographies certainly are not. We can confidently predict that further insights will emerge from comparing the differential effects of similar lesions upon the ability to read orthographies as dissimilar as alphabets, syllabaries, and 'ideographic' scripts. The other innovation is that we have included quite a lot of *raw* data of one sort and another; the reader who wishes to construct his or her own picture of deep dyslexia, a picture uncontaminated by any of our own varied interpretations, should accordingly be able to do so. There is, however, some limit to this diversity of approach which reflects, no doubt, the fact that many of the contributors are experimental cognitive psychologists who share at least a common 'core' of methodology and theoretical stance.

On the basis of our claim of breadth – both in presentation of the symptom-complex and in its relevance to other matters – we have two hopes for the book: first, that readers may come to the book for different reasons and from different backgrounds and find something of use and interest; second, that the book will encourage detailed investigations of other neuropsychological syndromes which, like deep dyslexia, speak to many issues in cognitive neuroscience.

Acknowledgments

We are grateful to the following members of the Department of Neurological Surgery and Neurology, Addenbrooke's Hospital, Cambridge: Mr A. E. Holmes, for permission to publish neurological and psychological details of patient D.E.; Dr I. M. S. Wilkinson, for permission to report similar data for patient P.W.; and Mrs F. M. Hatfield, Chief Speech Therapist, for her continuous support and co-operation in the studies of these patients. Thanks are due also to Dr Yoko Fukusako, Head of Speech Pathology Services, Tokyo Metropolitan Geriatric Hospital, who provided access to the patients studied by Dr Sasanuma; and to the physicians and surgeons of the National Hospital, Queen Square, London, for providing facilities for the work of Dr Shallice and Dr Warrington. We also gratefully acknowledge the continued support and encouragement that the neurologists and neurosurgeons of the Department of Clinical Neurology and the Department of Neurological Surgery, Oxford, have afforded the work of Dr Newcombe and Dr Marshall.

We would also like to thank the Medical Research Council, and in particular Dr Bronwen Loder, for making it possible for the contributors to this volume to spend a most productive four days together in the pleasant surroundings of Jesus College, Cambridge; and to acknowledge the numerous forms of assistance provided by Patricia Caple.

Finally, we wish to acknowledge the assistance of the patients: D.E., K.F., G.R., V.S., P.W., Y.H., K.K., and others. Their willingness to co-operate in investigations of their imperfect reading abilities has, we believe, allowed significant advances to be made in our understanding of what normal reading is and of the ways in which it may be impaired.

1 The conceptual status of deep dyslexia: an historical perspective

John C. Marshall and Freda Newcombe

About GR + history (orig)

In our paper for the 1971 meeting of the International Neuro-psychology Society at Engelberg we insinuated the existence of a symptom-complex that we called deep dyslexia (Marshall and Newcombe, 1973). We say 'insinuated' rather than 'argued for' because our efforts there were restricted to bringing together a set of brain-injured patients under a common label which was really no more than a promissory note for the syndrome we were conjecturing. The most striking aspect of the behaviour of the patient that we studied (Marshall and Newcombe, 1966) was that he would produce surprising numbers of frank semantic errors when attempting to read aloud individual words (without context, time pressure, or stimulus degradation). Table 1.1 shows a representative sample of such errors from our subject, G.R., an intelligent and, prior to sustaining a left hemisphere injury, literate adult.

TABLE 1.1 *(G.R.) Semantic errors*

act	→ 'play'
close	→ 'shut'
dinner	→ 'food'
afternoon	→ 'tonight'
uncle	→ 'cousin'
tall	→ 'long'

In addition, G.R. would sometimes make derivational errors, mis-reading, for example, an adjective or verb as its related nominal (or vice versa). Errors of this nature (discussed in Marshall, Newcombe, and Marshall, 1970) are displayed in Table 1.2.

I

TABLE 1.2 *(G.R.) Derivational errors*

wise	→ 'wisdom'
strange	→ 'stranger'
entertain	→ 'entertainment'
pray	→ 'prayers'
truth	→ 'true'
birth	→ 'born'

Errors in which there was a clear visual (shape) similarity between stimulus and (the written form of) his (oral) response were also common (Table 1.3).

TABLE 1.3 *(G.R.) Visual errors*

stock	→ 'shock'
quiz	→ 'queue'
deuce	→ 'duel'
saucer	→ 'sausage'
crowd	→ 'crown'
crocus	→ 'crocodile'

A syntactic hierarchy could also be observed such that concrete nouns stood the best chance of being read correctly. Adjectives, verbs and abstract nouns were of intermediate difficulty, and function words were very rarely read correctly. G.R.'s most frequent response to presentation of a function word was 'Don't know!' Occasionally, however, his response would be rather more informative; a sample of his 'better' attempts at coping with the 'little words' (his phrase) is given in Table 1.4.

TABLE 1.4 *(G.R.) Function words*

for	→ 'and'
his	→ 'she'
the	→ 'yes'
in	→ 'those'
be	→ 'Small words are the worst'
some	→ 'One of them horrid words again'

Finally, we note that G.R. can never read aloud a non-word – an orthographically legal character string which happens not to have found a semantic niche in the English language. Once more, G.R.'s typical response upon being presented with a pronounceable non-word is to indicate that he simply cannot perform the task. Table 1.5, however, also includes some responses where the non-word has been read as if it were a visually similar real word.

Table 1.5 *(G.R.) Non-words*

wux	→	'don't know'
nol	→	'no idea'
zul	→	'zulu'
wep	→	'wet'
dup	→	'damp'
tud	→	'omo . . . tide'[a]

[a] Both responses are the names of common detergents. *Tud* is visually similar to *tide*; in addition, it is possible that *tud* was 'misread' as *sud*, an 'internal' response that was followed by an overt semantic error.

Let us surmise, then, that this particular cluster of error-types and differential difficulty in response to lexical formatives, grammatical formatives, and legal non-words does indeed constitute a symptom-complex in, at least, the minimal sense that if substantial numbers of semantic errors are present then the other four features will reliably co-occur. The logic of any more profound analysis of deep dyslexia as a symptom-complex would seem to presuppose some basic statistical regularity in the error-types which do (and do not) appear together. Thus, to pick a well known example of this kind of argumentation, the first line of attack upon the Gerstmann syndrome (Gerstmann, 1930) is to suggest that the four defining characteristics (finger agnosia, right–left confusion, agraphia, and acalculia) do not co-occur with any greater strength than any other collection of, in this case, parietal signs (Benton, 1961). Similarly for deep dyslexia: the notion would be considerably weakened if different numbers (from zero to *n*!) of error-types co-occurred with semantic errors in different patients. It is with the above 'null hypothesis' in mind that we now turn to review the (putative) cases of deep dyslexia (in alphabetically written languages) that were reported prior to our 1966 paper.

1 Franz (1930)

In his presidential address to the Western Psychological Association in July 1928, Shepherd Ivory Franz reported a patient who made frequent semantic errors to individual words and continued to do so despite intensive remedial practice and training in reading. The subject was a professional man (an architect), presumably middle-aged (he seems from Franz's description to have occupied a position of some seniority), and presumably right-handed (no indication is given to the contrary). He sustained a closed head injury, having 'been hit on the head by a brick which had fallen from the tenth storey of a building the construction of which he was supervising'. The man had a right-sided hemiplegia, but no information is given concerning visual functions (e.g. visual fields).

His spontaneous speech was very severely impaired: 'For a relatively long time he could use only two affirmative, one negative, and two affective expressions.' Although some improvement took place over the two years that Franz followed his progress, his (spontaneous) vocabulary remained very restricted: 'Under the older neurological classification, he would have been classed as a complete motor aphasic.' His comprehension of speech, however, seems to have been remarkably good, extending to the appreciation of jokes. He seems to have had no difficulty in repeating individual words; no information is given concerning memory span, object-naming or colour-naming. Some general ability was preserved, at least to the extent that the patient could play dominoes (both fairly and with cheating).

When asked to read individually presented words, the subject made such responses as *hen* → 'egg' or *cat* → 'mice'. Errors of this nature persisted despite Franz's showing the card, pronouncing the correct response himself, and having the patient repeat it thirty or forty times. Little or no improvement took place over a period of two years post-injury. Sometimes quite long sequences of semantic errors (single words) were given to a particular stimulus, and Franz had the impression that the patient recognized (in some cases at least) that his response was wrong, and that he was attempting to correct himself. Very occasionally the patient would produce a neologistic response but in all cases they could plausibly be interpreted as inaccurate vocalizations of a real word, e.g. *lost* → 'sol' (= soul), or *hand* → 'chiff' (= handkerchief). There was one such instance that Franz regarded as a derivational error, *push* → 'pudden' (= pushing, or pulling). No other error-types were mentioned, although it is reported that the patient would sometimes recognize and call attention to familiar names in the newspaper. Writing ability (with the left hand) was essentially non-existent; the patient could write his signature, albeit very badly. The ability to produce complex architectural drawings and plans was, however, extremely well preserved. When Franz thought he detected an error in such sketches it always turned out finally that the patient was right and Franz wrong.

Franz interpreted the semantic errors in reading as a disorder of association – 'a dissociation of ideas and reactions'. He emphasized the fluctuations in performance and drew a partial analogy with semantic errors in second language learning. Franz conducted a number of 'free-association' tests (orally) with the patient, and although his responses were sometimes rather bizarre ('blind' → 'good', 'cellar' → 'sweet'), Franz emphasized that under these conditions the patient's expressive vocabulary was much larger than was apparent during spontaneous speech. Verbs, adjectives, adverbs, and abstract nouns were all elicited in association tests. Many of the patient's associations appear to be 'mediate', and Franz seemed to think that the reading problem arose from a similar disorder of selection; too many responses are potentially available and the subject cannot 'pick' the correct one when reading. Although some of the patient's associations are 'fixed' (e.g. 'up' → 'down', 'east' → 'west', 'cup' → 'saucer'), it is the variation in response from trial to trial (in both reading and association) that Franz stressed.

While the paradigm for interpretation that Franz used is perfectly clear, he emphasized that he had not provided an *explanation* for the phenomena:

Brain destruction may be an important incident in making speech associations difficult, but at the present time the brain destruction is neither explanatory of the associative losses nor can it be definitely classificatory until we further investigate speech from the standpoint of abilities and disabilities of association.

Franz's challenge still stands.

2 Beringer and Stein (1930)

Our next putative example was reported by Kurt Beringer and Johannes Stein at a joint conference of the Swiss Association for Psychiatry and the South West German Psychiatrists' Group in Basle in October 1929. Their patient was a woman, aged 64, educational level unspecified, and (presumably) right-handed. She had sustained an embolism of one branch of the left posterior cerebral artery. She had a right homonymous hemianopia, and 'a tendency to tire abnormally quickly in the apparently intact field of vision'. No information is given concerning the state of the motor system.

Beringer and Stein report the case as an example of 'pure alexia', for it would seem that her spontaneous speech, comprehension of speech, and repetition ability were unimpaired, as was her spontaneous writing. Kleist, Goldstein, and Minkowski were in the audience and joined in the discussion which followed the lecture. Minkowski, for one, was clearly absolutely amazed that a patient could make outright semantic errors in reading without the presence of associated language deficit: he asked, in an obviously rhetorical tone of voice, whether

a patient who was observed and examined in such detail was really totally free from aphasic disturbances, whether she did not suffer some damage, in part at least, in vocabulary or in grammatical constructions with respect to the smaller language units, as is often the case not only with the restitution of motor aphasia but also with other aphasic types.

We have been unable to locate any published answer to Minkowski's question.

Beringer and Stein described the woman's alexia as 'characterized by agnosia for letters and words', and as uninfluenced by the form of the input (handwriting, Gothic, or Roman type). Errors on word-reading were, however, frequently drawn from the same 'sphere of meaning' as the stimulus item; examples include *Reichstag* (Parliament) → 'Berlin' (Berlin), *Indien* (India) → 'Elefant' (elephant), and *Fuchs* (fox) → 'Hase' (hare). Her performance was dramatically improved by being given (semantic) cues to the sense of the stimuli: 'She was completely puzzled by the word "sixteen", and was unable to recognize either the whole word or the individual letters, but she read it at once on being told that it was a number.' She was asked to read out the animals, or the musical instruments from a (semantically) mixed list of fifteen words – 'she succeeded, although she had previously been alectic for these very words, such as cello, and horse.' Similarly, if presented with a list of words all drawn from the same category, she was initially quite unable to read any of them. But told that they were all, for example, tools, she succeeded in reading eleven out of twelve correctly. Similar results are reported for lists of virtues, crimes, and temporal expressions, although occasional derivational errors were made (e.g. *mercy* → 'merciful'). Beringer and Stein report that she could cope with abstract words just as well (or as badly) as with concrete words, but there does seem to be a syntactic hierarchy in her performance. She continued to try to read the newspaper following her embolism, and would sometimes succeed in reading out correctly a whole series of words, 'especially *nouns*'. In all conditions of testing, however, function words (*is, and, although, would,* etc.) were read particularly badly. She would sometimes attempt to spell out the sequence of letter names in the stimulus, either before or after trying to read the word as a whole, but numerous errors were made. The patient was quite uncertain as to the correct spelling, and even in cases where she had got it right she 'would abandon her own correct spelling when a false one was suggested to her'.

The patient made numerous mistakes when copying letters and geometric designs. However, she 'succeeded readily with spontaneous writing' although she could not (after a delay) read back what she herself had written.

Beringer and Stein provide two inter-related explanations for the nature of the reading deficit. In the first place they draw attention to the restricted, labile, fluctuating, and easily fatigued state of the patient's visual performance. Perimetric investigation showed various departures from normality in the apparently 'intact' visual field. The limits of the field seemed to vary more than in normal subjects as a function of size, intensity, and duration of stimulation. Likewise, the discrepancy between perception of moving versus static stimuli was outside the normal range. The just noticeable difference for a light-stimulus that gradually increased in intensity was also abnormal. Furthermore, the perception of movement was disturbed:

very rapid movements were not recognised. When watching a cartoon film she did not notice, for instance, the leap of an animal from one side of the picture to the other when this happened very quickly. The patient was aware only that the animal was suddenly there, or that it had been at one side and was now at the other. On one occasion she deduced from this that the animal had jumped. On another she drew from the false perception the conclusion that there were two animals.

Other investigations are reported from which it appears that the subject's ability to recognize 'poorly illuminated geometrical shapes in a darkened room' was weaker than normal. The relevance of 'visual fatigue' to reading performance was pointed out by the subject herself who stated: 'If I want to read the paper, I must often wait for a moment and look away, then I can read again.' Beringer and Stein attempt to check this by getting the patient to relax in a darkened room and then putting the light on:

> She was asked to read immediately after this relaxation, and at once read the first three words correctly, then her performance became uncertain and incorrect. After another period of darkness she again read correctly at first then wrongly, and she repeated this several times.

Now, this 'instability' of vision does not, of course, in itself serve to explain the occurrence of semantic errors in reading. Accordingly, Beringer and Stein suggest that although the fluctuating visual image of the word is not sufficient to determine directly and uniquely a (correct) vocal output it does suffice to evoke the appropriate 'sphere of meaning'. This notion is reminiscent of the two-threshold logogen model that Morton (1968) proposed in explanation of our own early results (Marshall and Newcombe, 1966), with the following difference: the *form* of representation that Beringer and Stein implied for the 'sphere of meaning' was in part at least, imagistic. They seem to be suggesting (or more accurately their patient suggests) that the word conjures up an appropriate visual image, which is in turn responded to as in an object- or scene-naming task. Thus the patient read *Reichstag* as 'Berlin' and then explained: 'I had the impression of somewhere I had been, where there was so much to see and to look at, you just had to sit

down on a park bench and then look at it all, the whole picture.'
Although such commentaries are interesting, it is, of course, not
required that one takes them as veridical accounts of the actual
process that was involved in the production of the overt response
'Berlin'. (Pylyshyn, 1973, and Nisbett and Wilson, 1977, discuss
some of the more general theoretical issues that are at stake.) As
Minkowski remarks: 'the associative connection is obvious and
intelligible without any further consideration'. None the less, the
notion needs airing for the idea of 'picturability' will turn up again
in the later history of our topic (e.g. in Faust, 1955).

3 Low (1931)

The next case was seen by A. A. Low in Chicago in 1929. The
patient, a man of 38, education and handedness unspecified, was
admitted to hospital following, we presume, a left-hemisphere
stroke. His vision appears to have been normal, but there was a
complete right-sided hemiplegia and 'the tongue protruded toward
the right side and showed a slight tremor'.

When the patient was admitted in July he seems to have suffered a
total loss of speech; by September he had 'a partial motor aphasia
and expressed himself with difficulty. He could name objects and
was able to carry out simple commands but was unable to carry out
complicated orders or to name the use of objects.' Further restitution
of function is observed and by the middle of November

the patient had a fair ability to use spontaneous speech. He
spoke in well-formed sentences, though with some difficulty in
finding words. No agrammatism was noted in spontaneous
speech. He was well able to point to objects named verbally or
in print, to name the objects indicated by the examiner and to
designate the use of objects.

Immediate repetition was essentially without error for both words
and nonsense words, irrespective of number of syllables. The patient
had thus made a remarkably good recovery in his oral language
abilities (albeit with some residual aphasic signs) by the time that
the investigations of visual language processing were launched. In
contrast, writing to dictation was very poorly performed, although

copying (with the left hand) of both print and cursive handwriting was quite good.

At this time the patient's 'reading aloud was fair for most words.' However, 'when given a sentence or paragraph to read, he left out many words and combinations of words, giving a distinct impression of agrammatical reading.' As Low writes, 'The agrammatical disturbance being confined to reading aloud only, the case represented a rare instance of an agrammatical disturbance in an isolated faculty of speech and called for detailed study.' Over the next few months Low devised and administered an astonishing number and variety of reading (and other) tests to his patient. Although Low's taxonomy of errors differs from our own it is clear from his examples that *all* the features we discussed in relation to G.R. are to be found in the performance of Low's patient. The patient makes semantic errors (*dad* → 'father', *child* → 'girl', *vice* → 'wicked'), derivational errors (*goes* → 'go', *reinstatement* → 'instate', *fleeing* → 'flee'), and visual errors (*life* → 'wife', *sword* → 'words', *shirt* → 'skirt'). Of all parts of speech the patient experienced the greatest difficulty when attempting to read (short) 'particles' (pronouns, articles, prepositions, conjunctions, adverbs, and auxiliary verbs). The patient also conspicuously failed to read pronounceable nonsense syllables, and would frequently 'infuse meaning into the material' (*sto* → 'story', *jun* → 'jump', *lom* → 'lemon'). A similar 'tendency toward supplementing meaning was again in evidence' when the patient was asked to read isolated letters or abbreviations (*J* → 'John', *A.A. Low, M.D.* → 'Low, doctor medicine').

Low is particularly careful in his attempts to isolate the exact nature of the patient's errors. The following quotation illustrates the type of argument that Low uses to support the claim that some errors are indeed visual:

Mistakes like 'wife' for 'life', 'space' for 'pace' referred to a substitution of words which both look and sound alike. From such errors it is impossible to infer whether the patient read primarily with the aid of visual or of auditory images. But if he misread 'words' for 'sword', it was obvious that what he substituted was two words that merely looked alike. This mistake was obviously made because of a misapprehension of the visual images. A mistake which would have pointed definitely to a misapprehension of the auditory image, like 'tree' for 'key' was never made, although the tests provided ample opportunity for such errors.

With respect to the distinction between grammatical and lexical formatives, Low notes that while the patient 'simplified' complex words by dropping prefixes and suffixes (re-, de-, -ment, -s, -ing), he did *not* typically simplify compound nouns (e.g. armchair, doghouse, songbird, farmhand) in which both elements have full semantic value. Such compounds are read as easily as 'their isolated components'. Some of the derivational errors can be eliminated by context. Low tested the patient three times on sixty 'determined plurals' (e.g. *many houses, much money*) where 'after the patient reads "many" no choice is left him but to follow up with a plural formation. Similarly, after the pronunciation of the word "much" no room is left but for a succeeding singular.' Low continues:

The fact that in three separate performances not one confusion of plural and singular occurred was taken as undisputable evidence that the patient had a considerable facility for handling singular and plural, and that the mistakes observed in the preceding tests referred to a tendency to leave out affixes, not to an ignorance of 'grammar'.

Low is careful, wherever possible, to check that his syntactic interpretations of error rates are valid. Thus having observed that the patient is particularly poor at reading 'short' particles (*at, from, to, as*, etc.) he rules out the possibility that 'shortness' (rather than grammatical function) is responsible for the deficit by noting that the patient is good at reading short (three-letter) nouns and adjectives.

Low concludes:

All the defects of the various functions were reduced to a relative inefficiency to analyse parts out of a whole, on the one hand, and to a relative preference for synthesizing parts into a whole, on the other hand. All the symptoms were thus traced to one unifying lesion.

This vague theoretical account does not, of course, specify a psychological mechanism responsible for the 'analytic' impairment.

None the less, Low's strategy is obviously sensible; one should consider the strongest possible claim – a unitary source for the observed symptoms – in order to facilitate its refutation. (We have not discussed here the many other psycholinguistic tests – including sentence and paragraph reading – that were administered. We would simply urge anyone interested in the psychology of language to read Low's descriptive masterpiece for themselves.)

4 Goldstein (1948)

We have previously mentioned that Kurt Goldstein was in the audience for Beringer and Stein's presentation in 1929. Finally, with Marianne Simmel, he observed a similar case of his own.* The patient (case 23) was a young man of 26, who had sustained a gunshot injury leading to 'occlusion of left carotid artery with cerebral infarction.' The bullet, it seems, 'went out at the base of the skull without apparently injuring actual brain matter.' The man was left-handed and his 'formal' education was rather limited. He was, however, an avid reader and had an extensive knowledge of Shakespeare and of Voltaire and Rousseau (the latter two in translation). He had also picked up 'a not inconsiderable amount of Greek' whilst in reformatory or jail. Visual functions seem to have been normal (although no formal testing is reported) as were motor functions with the exception of 'tactile agnosia' in the right hand.

The man had a severe expressive aphasia, and indeed 'spoke very little spontaneously'. What he did say was restricted to nouns and verbs (with very clear pronunciation). Speech in response to questions was somewhat better in terms of vocabulary size although here too he would produce one-word sentences and 'occasionally a noun and verb or adjective together, but never the article'. Some stock phrases might also be uttered ('pretty good', 'I know', 'I'm lost', 'I don't mind'). His comprehension was not good. Simple commands (sit down) would be understood but 'he failed whenever such a request contained more than one concrete item, e.g. "stand up and close your eyes".' Immediate repetition was good for single words, with the exception of function words, but very poor for short sentences. Digit span was restricted to one or two items. Spon-

* Some of the data reported in this section were very kindly supplied by Professor Simmel.

taneous writing was poor and writing to dictation very bad, although copying was unimpaired.

When attempting to read aloud individual words numerous semantic errors were made (e.g. *era* → 'time', *tide* → 'water', *down* → 'up', *low* → 'small', *big* → 'little', *draw* → 'paint'). Similar semantic errors were found in tests of object-naming (*pipe* → 'cigar', *toaster* → 'eat', *lamp* → 'table'). Derivational (*lived* → 'live') and visual (*puddle* → 'puppy') errors also occurred in reading. Function words (*in, on, of, the*) were never read correctly; the most frequent response to them was no response, although sometimes they were misread as content words (e.g. *but* → 'button'). Goldstein checked that the function word phenomenon was not a purely output deficit. The patient could read *inn* but not *in, four* but not *for, two* but not *to*.

Reading of nonsense syllables was not investigated, although a (perhaps) related condition of testing is reported, namely the reading of 'mutilated words'. The patient would, for example, read *hsptl* as 'hospital' or *gradn* as 'garden'. Presented with mixed lists of correctly spelt words and their respective 'mutilated' forms he could pick out the correct form; this could be regarded as a forerunner of the lexical decision paradigm.

In his discussion of the case, Goldstein naturally stresses the role of comprehension in determining the patient's reading performance: 'Whenever the patient was able to read a word . . . there was never *any question as to his understanding* of the word. He *never*, as far as could be determined, *was able to read a word which he did not understand*, while at the same time he seemed to recognize a number of words and understand them without being able to read them correctly.'

The patient could 'recognize instantly' (both in free vision and with very short tachistoscopic exposure) '*a great number of words*, mostly nouns and verbs, but also a few adjectives, especially color names.' However, if the patient '*did not recognize a word instantly, no matter how much time he was given, he could not read it.*'

Goldstein accordingly regards the patient as reading by a holistic rather than a sequential strategy: '*Reading as a process starting from left to right was something completely alien to him.*' He could not, in other words, 'read by reading syllable after syllable.' Goldstein explains whatever success the patient did have in reading by invoking his '*extraordinary capacity of visual memory and imagery.*' Thus 'his visual memory made it possible for him to "read" a great number of words by simple recognition of the visual form.'

Given the patient's performance with stimuli such as *gradn* one might wonder exactly what is the form of this visual form. And one might also note that such an explanation of *correct* responses does not help us to understand the source of the *semantic* errors. Goldstein refers to the deficit as an 'impairment of abstraction and abnormal concreteness' but it is hard to see how one could cast these notions in the shape of an explicit information-processing model.

5 Simmel and Goldschmidt (1953)

A few years later, in 1950, Marianne Simmel was to observe another case whose reading disability was quite similar to that shown by the patient she investigated with Goldstein. The new patient was a left-handed woman of 24 who left school in order to get married after three years of high school. She is reported to have been an intelligent girl who did well in school. Seven years prior to the investigation, she had a child. 'A day or so before the baby's birth the patient began to have convulsions . . . she had 14 more convulsions after delivery by forceps, and was in a coma for several days.' For some time after she came out of coma the patient appears to have been severely agnostic, aphasic, and amnesic.

Seven years later the patient had made substantial recovery although numerous residual deficits were still in evidence. Ophthalmological and neurological findings, however, were within normal limits, with the exception of a marked reduction in visual flicker fusion frequency. No motor deficits were observed, including no 'primary dysarthria'.

The patient's spontaneous speech was 'on the whole very good', although some word-finding difficulties were noted. Verbal paraphasias did occur, albeit infrequently; literal paraphasias occurred very infrequently. Mistakes were occasionally made with function words (paragrammatism) but it is stressed that the patient did *not* speak in telegram style. 'Reactive' speech was much poorer: there were difficulties in remembering the question, and verbal paraphasias were frequent. In general, comprehension was only fair. Simple sentences were understood and simple instructions followed, but 'more complicated instructions or explanations which involved the simultaneous presentation of several factors seemed to present almost insurmountable obstacles to her.'

Oral repetition was well preserved for sentences, words, and nonsense syllables, but object-naming was grossly impaired. Numerous semantic paraphasias and considerable circumlocution were observed.

Writing, either spontaneously or to dictation was impossible, with the exception of the alphabet, the number series, and the patient's own name. Copying was 'generally poor and very laborious'. Although the patient could eventually copy letters and words 'the unit of her procedure was not the letter, but the single stroke, which gave rise to occasional constructive malformations.'

Reading 'consisted only of the recognition of individual words, primarily nouns, adjectives, and verbs. There was no reading of sentences, although she would occasionally read a "phrase" – a response similar to her spontaneous use of such automatic phrases.' Both visual (*chairman* → 'airmail', *shell* → 'tell') and semantic errors (*cents* → 'pennies', *blades* → 'razor') were frequently observed in single word reading. Function words were almost never read correctly (*not* → 'stop'); short (three-letter) nouns and verbs also occasioned great difficulty. Errors often had 'a similar letter configuration' to the correct response, e.g. *on* → 'no', *of* → 'for', *and* → 'can', *that* → 'plant', *but* → 'put', *shall* → 'tell'. Derivational errors are not reported and it seems that the reading of nonsense syllables was not tested.

Simmel and Goldschmidt discuss the patient's level of awareness of her errors. On some trials there was 'real "guessing"', of which she was perfectly conscious.' On the majority of trials which produced 'verbal paraphasias', however, 'she seemed satisfied with her performance; but when asked whether she was sure of the correctness of her productions, she usually said, "I don't know" or "You tell me".' (It is not reported whether the patient's confidence in her responses differed as a consequence of whether the error was visual or semantic.) When the patient failed to recognize a word, she occasionally 'started spelling the word, i.e. reading the single letters, more or less correctly. This procedure did not, however, help her in finding the word.'

No general interpretation of the patient's pattern of loss and preservation is given, although an impairment of the 'abstract attitude' is implied: 'on the Goldstein Block Design test, the Weigl test and object-sorting tests the patient's performance was extremely "concrete".'

6 Faust (1955)

It is not really clear that we should include Faust's patient (W.E.) in our survey, but for the sake of completeness we will give a brief description of the case. The patient was a partially left-handed man (age and education unspecified) who sustained a left parietal gunshot injury in the Second World War. A bullet was removed at operation two days later. He had a right-sided spastic paralysis and initially was totally unable to speak.

Capacity for speech slowly returned although there were considerable residual aphasic signs. Spontaneous speech was poorly articulated with long pauses and occasional word-finding difficulties. He did, however, have 'enough circumlocutions at his disposal to make himself understood'. Repetition of number and letter series was also impaired and the patient would often stop halfway through a series and after some time return to the beginning. No information is given about the patient's comprehension or ability to repeat. Colour-naming was severely impaired; the deficit was associated with perceptual disturbance – the patient's discrimination and sorting of colours was quite poor.

The patient's writing to dictation was fair and he was hesitant with longer words. Performance was improved when the examiner articulated the syllables of multisyllabic words separately, and this strategy was employed with some success by the patient himself. When asked to write isolated nouns he would often add the article. In copying written material, the patient would 'draw a copy of the shape of the letter, without any understanding of it'.

Reading performance was very poor, even for material that the patient had himself written earlier: 'Single words were very seldom read correctly. If a word was not grasped at once, further reading was impossible.'

It is not entirely clear from Faust's report whether or not the patient made *outright* semantic errors that he thought were (or might have been) correct responses. The patient did, however, show by description and circumlocution that he had at least partial comprehension of the words that he could not read aloud. Thus given *table, chair,* and *cupboard,* the patient, although unable to read the words individually, remarked 'I know that, those are all furniture.' Similarly, given *Hans, Andreas,* and *Martin,* the patient could indicate that the words were all forenames (although again he could not read them aloud). The patient was quite unable to cope with reading function words such as articles or prepositions.

When he could not read a word the patient essayed the strategy of reading the initial letters:

> He only succeeded in doing this when the rest of the word was covered up. He could not analyse the whole word (into its letters). If he covered up a part of the word, then he could read the initial letter correctly. However, it was impossible for him to combine with this the letter which followed and so read the first and second letters together.

No information is given concerning the other error-types that are pertinent to our proposed symptom-complex.

Faust stresses the role of an unfolding 'sphere of meaning' in determining the patient's performance, and he refers back to Beringer and Stein's case as showing a similar impairment. He notes that the patient did sometimes understand words with a 'concrete meaning' and that 'the further the meaning of a word is from the concrete, the more strongly marked is the impairment to recognition.' Words with an 'abstract meaning' (such as articles, prepositions, and some verbs) are thus 'the most difficult to read'. Faust summarizes this point by remarking that 'it is not the length of the word which is crucial for recognition of it, but rather its relation to concrete objects and to what is visually-picturable.' Faust's interpretation is thus related both to the *imageability hypothesis* and to the *operativity hypothesis* of Gardner (1973).

Preliminary discussion

A summary of the six cases is given in Table 1.6. This table cites examples of the pattern of reading impairment of these subjects as it relates to the initial conjecture: that deep dyslexia is indeed a symptom-complex. On the whole, there is some support for our suggestion that semantic errors occur in the context of derivational and visual errors, and that impairment is maximal when attempting to read function words or nonsense syllables. At very least, there are no counter-examples in the cases we have reviewed. The table, however, contains too many question marks (where information is simply not available) to permit the making of very strong claims.

It would seem that the syndrome (if such it be) is specific to reading performance in the following sense: although the majority of the patients reported do have additional aphasic symptoms neither the nature nor the severity of the associated impairment is (even approximately) constant. Spontaneous speech may be grossly non-fluent (and agrammatic) or fluent paraphasic, or anomic. If we are to believe Beringer and Stein's claim, speech may be quite un-impaired. Comprehension deficits are usually in evidence, but again they may range from severe to quite mild. The nature (and perhaps even the primary locus) of the brain injury (and the associated neurological disturbances) is likewise variable. The patient popu-

TABLE 1.6

Study	Semantic errors	Derivational errors	Visual errors	Function words	Nonsense syllables
Franz (1930)	*cat* → 'mice'	*push* → 'pudden'	?	?	?
Beringer & Stein (1930)	*Reichstag* → 'Berlin'	*mercy* → 'merciful'	?	very poor	?
Low (1931)	*child* → 'girl'	*goes* → 'go'	*sword* → 'words'	very poor	*jun* → 'jump'
Goldstein (1948)	*draw* → 'paint'	*lived* → 'live'	*puddle* → 'puppy'	very poor	*gradn* → 'garden'
Simmel & Gold-schmidt (1953)	*cents* → 'pennies'	?	*top* → 'put'	very poor	?
Faust (1955)	semantic descriptions	?	?	very poor	?

lation is itself heterogenous – men and women, old and young, left-handed and right-handed. The patients, prior to sustaining brain injury, were neither unintelligent nor poor readers. Indeed, if anything they appear to have had an above average interest and competence in reading. We have no information about how they were taught to read or what strategies they adopted as mature readers prior to injury. A reasonable guess would be that they had been 'chinese' rather than 'phoenician' readers (Baron and Straw-son, 1976). The reading problem does seem to co-occur with a writing deficit, which is often more severe than the disturbance of reading. (In some cases spontaneous and dictated writing is abolished.) Even this deficit does not, however, seem to be an invariant concomitant of deep dyslexia. Spontaneous writing seems to have been preserved in Beringer and Stein's case (and in Faust's patient writing performance was far superior to reading).

The evidence so far assembled does not, then, enable us (yet) to reject the hypothesis that deep dyslexia is indeed a functional, dynamic deficit of the *reading* system (or at least of one sub-type of possible reading systems). Despite the involvement of semantic and syntactic variables in determining performance the condition does not seem to be secondary to a more widespread (multi- or supra-modal) disturbance of linguistic ability. That is, theoretical in-terpretations of the condition may not need to make specific reference to the associated aphasic deficits that are found in the majority of the patients who have thus far been studied. It may be that no particular constellation of aphasic signs constitute necessary and sufficient conditions for the emergence of deep dyslexia. But all of this leaves us more or less where we started – in search of a psychological explanation (an information-processing model con-sistent with linguistic descriptions of the condition, and with available neurological constraints) for a uniquely perplexing dis-order.

Three very general questions thus arise. First, to what extent can we interpret deep dyslexia as a structured breakdown in the (or a) primary reading mechanism employed by the normal, fluent adult reader (Ellis and Marshall, 1978; Holmes, Marshall and New-combe, 1971)? Second, if real insight is not forthcoming by adoption of the first viewpoint, can we achieve a new synthesis by conjec-turing that the responsible lesions have uncovered and allowed to emerge overtly an intact but subsidiary reading system, the neuro-logical substrate for which is perhaps to be found in the right hemisphere (Coltheart, 1977)? Third, can we begin to discover universal and specific constraints upon reading mechanisms by comparing dyslexic breakdown across a variety of script-types, in particular by investigating languages written in non-alphabetic orthographies (Marshall, 1976)?

Finally, we wish to emphasize yet again the importance of attempts to falsify the claim that deep dyslexia is a real syndrome. Any valid taxonomic classification presupposes a functional unity in the pattern of impaired and preserved abilities within and between classes. The effects of a chance constellation of lesions, however often observed, or even of a single lesion that for purely topological reasons (Brain, 1964) impairs a variety of independent systems, are unlikely to be theoretically revealing. Our own preference is that there is indeed a disruption of a single underlying mechanism which shows itself in a meaningful cluster of surface manifestations. But we must not ignore the possibility that we are studying an accident of anatomy or sampling, whose consequences have misled us by their tantalizing appearance of order. In short, deep dyslexia will not exist unless or until it finds a place within a credible neurolinguistic theory.

References

Baron, J. and Strawson, C. (1976) Use of orthographic and word-specific knowledge in reading words aloud. *Journal of Experimental Psychology, Human Perception and Performance, 2,* 386–93.

Benton, A. L. (1961) The fiction of the 'Gerstmann Syndrome'. *Journal of Neurology, Neurosurgery and Psychiatry, 24,* 176–81.

Beringer, K. and Stein, J. (1930) Analyse eines Falles von 'Reiner' Alexie. *Zeitschrift für die Gesamte Neurologie und Psychiatrie, 123,* 473–8.

Brain, Lord (1964) Statement of the problem. In A. V. D. de Reuck and M. O'Connor (eds), *Disorders of Language.* London: Churchill.

Coltheart, M. (1977) Phonemic dyslexia: some comments on its interpretation and its implications for the study of normal reading. Paper presented at the International Neuropsychology Society Meeting, Oxford.

Ellis, A. W. and Marshall, J. C. (1978) Semantic errors or statistical flukes? A note on Allport's 'On knowing the meaning of words we are unable to report'. *Quarterly Journal of Experimental Psychology, 30,* 569–75.

Faust, C. (1955) *Die zerebralen Herdstörungen bei Hinterhauptsverletzungen und ihr Beurteilung.* Stuttgart: Thieme.

Franz, S. I. (1930) The relations of aphasia. *Journal of General Psychology, 3,* 401–11.

Gardner, H. (1973) The contribution of operativity to naming capacity in aphasic patients. *Neuropsychologia, 11,* 213–20.

Gerstmann, J. (1930) Zur Symptomatologie der Hirnläsionen im Übergangsgebiet der unteren Parietal – und mittleren Occipitalwindung. *Nervenartzt, 3,* 691–5.

Goldstein, K. (1948) *Language and Language Disturbances.* New York: Grune & Stratton.

Holmes, J. M., Marshall, J. C. and Newcombe, F. (1971) Syntactic class as a determinant of word-retrieval in normal and dyslexic subjects. *Nature, 234,* 416.

Low, A. A. (1931) A case of agrammatism in the English language. *Archives of Neurology and Psychiatry, 25,* 556–97.

Marshall, J. C. (1976) Neuropsychological aspects of orthographic representation. In R. J. Wales and E. Walker (eds), *New Approaches to Language Mechanisms*. Amsterdam: North Holland.

Marshall, J. C. and Newcombe, F. (1966) Syntactic and semantic errors in paralexia. *Neuropsychologia, 4*, 169–76.

Marshall, J. C. and Newcombe, F. (1973) Patterns of paralexia. *Journal of Psycholinguistic Research, 2*, 175–99.

Marshall, M., Newcombe, F. and Marshall, J. C. (1970) The microstructure of word-finding difficulties in a dysphasic subject. In G. B. Flores d'Arcais and W. J. M. Levelt (eds), *Advances in Psycholinguistics*. Amsterdam: North Holland.

Morton, J. (1968) Grammar and computation in language behavior. *Progress Report No. 6*, Center for Research in Language and Language Behavior, University of Michigan.

Nisbett, R. E. and Wilson, T. D. (1977) Telling more than we can know: verbal reports on mental processes. *Psychological Review, 84*, 231–59.

Pylyshyn, Z. W. (1973) What the mind's eye tells the mind's brain: a critique of mental imagery. *Psychological Bulletin, 80*, 1–24.

Simmel, M. L. and Goldschmidt, K. H. (1953) Prolonged posteclamptic aphasia: report of a case. *A.M.A. Archives of Neurology and Psychiatry, 69*, 80–3.

2 Deep dyslexia: a review of the syndrome

Max Coltheart

In the preceding chapter, Marshall and Newcombe elaborate a proposal which they first put forward in 1971: that one can identify a particular form of acquired dyslexia, *deep dyslexia*, and that this disorder is a symptom-complex in the sense that it consists of a set of symptoms which regularly co-occur.

Although there are several symptoms closely associated with deep dyslexia – these are discussed in Marshall and Newcombe's chapter and also in this chapter – one symptom is of central importance: the *semantic error*. The patient is asked to read a single printed word, and produces a response which, although incorrect in the sense that it is not identical to the stimulus, nevertheless is semantically related to that stimulus. Marshall and Newcombe's patient, for example, when asked to read aloud the word *gnome*, said 'pixie'.

Semantic errors have been observed in other linguistic activities such as object-naming, speech repetition, or spontaneous speech, but these errors have not attracted much theoretical attention. As far as semantic errors in the oral reading of patients with acquired dyslexias are concerned, they are mentioned sporadically in the neuropsychological literature up to 1966, and these early reports are discussed in the previous chapter. As Marshall and Newcombe point out in that chapter, many of the earlier reports provide frustratingly few details concerning the characteristics of patients and their reading abilities. Fortunately, Marshall and Newcombe's initial study of deep dyslexia, published in 1966, has been followed by a number of detailed investigations of deep dyslexic patients, and this recent work has provided, and continues to provide, a great deal of information about the syndrome.

My aim in this chapter is to review this work in detail, in an attempt to answer the following question: if a patient makes semantic errors in reading aloud, are there other symptoms which such a patient will invariably display? If deep dyslexia is defined by the occurrence of semantic errors, and is in addition a symptom-*complex*, then it must be possible to identify a collection of symptoms which are consistently associated with the occurrence of semantic errors. The symptom-complex may turn out to have a different logical structure: for example, it may turn out to be necessary to define deep dyslexia in terms of two necessary symptoms, whose *joint* occurrence is always associated with the remaining symptoms of the symptom-complex. Another possibility is that the symptom-complex has no such logical structure: that it consists of *n* symptoms and that these are all of equal status as far as the definition of deep dyslexia is concerned. A detailed examination of the symptoms displayed by deep dyslexic patients will permit adjudication between these various possibilities.

Case studies have been selected according to two criteria. First of all, the patient must have made semantic errors in reading aloud. Second, a reasonable amount of detail about the patient's other symptoms must be available from the published report or, in the case of recent studies, from the investigators themselves. Cases about which very little is known are obviously of little use when one is attempting to discover what other symptoms are displayed by patients who make semantic errors. It should be noted, however, that none of the cases which are neglected here because too little detail is available have any features which conflict with the characterization of deep dyslexia developed in this chapter.

Applying these two criteria to the neuropsychological literature in English results in the identification of twenty-two patients: sixteen were readers of English and six readers of Japanese. Doubtless there are case studies published in other languages, especially French, German or Russian; but to the best of my knowledge these twenty-two patients are the only ones described in English who made semantic errors in reading aloud and about whom fairly detailed information is available.

Table 2.1 lists these twenty-two cases and the sources of information about them. In the remainder of this chapter, the patients will be identified by their numbers as given in this table.

So far, the only symptom these patients have in common is the semantic error; that, after all, is how they qualified for inclusion in

Table 2.1. But if deep dyslexia is a symptom-*complex*, then there must be other symptoms which all of these patients display; and a list of these symptoms would be a characterization of deep dyslexia.

TABLE 2.1 *Twenty-two cases of patients who made semantic errors in reading aloud*

Case no.	Sources of information
1	Low (1931)
2	Goldstein (1948): Case 23
3	Marshall and Newcombe (1966): G.R.
4	Brown (1972)
5	Shallice and Warrington (1975): K.F.
6	Andreewsky and Seron (1975)
7	Marin, Saffran and Schwartz (1975); Saffran, Schwartz and Marin (1976); Schwartz, Saffran Marin (1977): H.T.
8	Marin *et al.* (1975); Saffran *et al.* (1976); Schwartz *et al.* (1977); Saffran and Marin (1977): V.S.
9	Schwartz *et al.* (1977): W.S.
10	Schwartz *et al.* (1977): B.L.
11	Saffran (personal communication): J.R.
12	Patterson and Marcel (1977); Patterson (1978); Patterson (1979): D.E.
13	*ibid.*: P.W.
14	Whitaker (1976): H.C.E.M.
15	Kapur and Perl (1978): P.D.
16	Warrington and Shallice (1979): A.R.
Japanese cases	
17	Kotani (1935) – see Sasanuma (this volume)
18	Sakamoto (1940) – see Sasanuma (this volume)
19	Ohashi (1965) – see Yamadori (1975) and Sasanuma (this volume)
20	Sasanuma (1974)
21	Yamadori (1975)
22	Niki and Ueda (1977) – see Sasanuma (this volume)

Thus the next step is to consider what other symptoms occurred with these patients.

When one sets out to do this, it is immediately obvious that some symptoms are irrelevant as far as the search for a symptom-complex is concerned, because, although clearly present in some patients, they are clearly absent in others. Right hemiplegia and right hemianopia are two examples. All of these patients had left-hemisphere damage, and in some this had produced a right hemiplegia and/or hemianopia; but not in all. Patients 2, 5, 8, 11, 19 and 21 were not hemiplegic. Patients 1, 2, 5, 7, 8, 12, 13, 19 and 21 were not hemianopic. Thus the symptom complex does not include hemiplegia or hemianopia, even though some deep dyslexics suffer from one or other or both of these symptoms.

Symptoms whose occurrence is very obviously inconsistent in this way will thus not be considered further. A few symptoms mentioned in some of the case studies will be neglected for a different reason, namely, because information about the presence or absence of the symptoms is available for only a very few of the twenty-two cases.

What remains after this weeding-out is the collection of symptoms listed in Tables 2.2 to 2.5. In these tables, each symptom is described at the head of the appropriate *column*, and each *row* corresponds to one of the twenty-two cases. A + sign at the intersection of a column and a row means that this symptom was present in this patient; a − sign means it was absent; no symbol means that no information is available about the presence or absence of this symptom in this patient.

If there were no empty spaces in these tables, it would be relatively simple to assemble a list of those symptoms which are consistently present in deep dyslexia: one would simply delete from the set of symptoms used in these tables those which occur inconsistently. The only problem then would be an inductive one: a patient might turn up tomorrow who failed to show a symptom which all twenty-two of the cases considered so far did show, and so revision of the symptom list would be required.

However, there *are* empty spaces in Tables 2.2 to 2.5, and there are some other complications too, which need to be considered. Consequently, some discussion of these tables is required. One immediately apparent complication is case 16, patient A.R. (Warrington and Shallice, 1979). The most cursory inspection of these tables indicates that A.R. stands out from the remaining patients in a number of ways. He is the only one who was not selectively impaired at reading function words aloud; the only one who read adjectives better than nouns; the only one whose lexical decision performance was poor; and the only one who could read aloud pronounceable non-words with any degree of success (25 per cent and 28 per cent, on two separate occasions).

This particular patient will be considered individually later in the chapter. For the moment, consideration of Tables 2.2 to 2.5 will proceed without taking case 16 into account: thus the data base will consist of twenty-one patients, not twenty-two.

TABLE 2.2 *Error types in deep dyslexia*

Case no.	Semantic errors	Visual errors	Function-word substitutions	Derivational errors
1	+	+		+
2	+	+		
3	+	+	+	+
4	+			
5	+	+	+[a]	+
6	+	+[a]	+[a]	+
7	+	+	+[a]	+
8	+	+	+	+
9	+	+	+[a]	+
10	+	+	+[a]	+
11	+[a]	+[a]	+[a]	+[a]
12	+	+	+	+
13	+	+	+	+
14	+	+		+
15	+	+	+[a]	+
16	+	+	+[a]	+
17	+			
18	+			
19	+			
20	+	+		
21	+			
22	+	+		+

[a] Personal communication.

Error types

As indicated in Table 2.2, these patients' incorrect responses are of several kinds. They do not only make semantic errors; as pointed out in Chapter 1, they make three other basic kinds of errors in reading aloud too. Sometimes the response will resemble the stimulus visually but in no other way: *gallant* → 'gallon' or *perform* → 'perfume'. It appears that these are visual and *not* phonological errors, since responses which are phonologically but not visually similar (e.g. *freeze* → 'phrase') do not occur. Sometimes the only similarity between stimulus and response is that both are function words. Case 3, for example, read *for, me, before, up* and *other* all as

TABLE 2.3 *Inability to derive phonology from print*

Case no.	Inability to pronounce printed non-words correctly	Inability to judge whether printed words rhyme, except visually	Lexical decisions not affected by pseudo-homophony	Kana worse than kanji
1	+			
2				
3	+[a]			
4				
5				
6	+			
7	+[a]	+	+[a]	
8	+	+	+[a]	
9	+[a]	+	+[a]	
10	+[a]	+	+[a]	
11	+[a]	+[a]	+[a]	
12	+		+	
13	+		+	
14				
15				
16				
17				+
18				+
19				+
20				+
21				+
22				+

[a] Personal communication.

'and'; this kind of error will be referred to as a function-word substitution. Sometimes the relationship of stimulus to response is grammatically derivational: the two words have the same free morpheme but different bound morphemes, e.g. *sickness* → 'sick', *wrestle* → 'wrestler', and *marriage* → 'married'.

Inspection of Table 2.2 provides convincing evidence for the claim that, at least for patients reading English, any patient who makes semantic errors will also make visual errors, derivational errors, and function-word substitutions. There are no counter-examples to this claim, and very few blank cells which might have provided counter-examples.

TABLE 2.4 *Word-property effects*

Case no.	Reading aloud is better for concrete/ high imagery words than abstract/low-imagery words	Content words read aloud better than function words	Nouns read aloud better than adjectives; adjectives better than verbs
1		+	+
2		+	?
3	+	+	+
4		+	
5	+	+	+
6		+	+
7	+[a]	+	+
8	+[a]	+	+
9	+[a]	+	+
10	+[a]	+	+
11	+[a]	+[a]	+[a]
12	+	+	+
13	+	+	+
14			
15		+[a]	
16	+	−	−
17			
18			
19			
20			
21			
22	+		

[a] Personal communication.

The classification of errors

Several problems crop up when one is attempting to classify a set of error responses in terms of this fourfold error classification, and a

TABLE 2.5 *Miscellaneous symptoms in deep dyslexia*

Case no.	Comprehension with inability to pronounce	Copying is preserved	Agrammatism of speech	Object-naming is preserved	Auditory STM is impaired	Writing impairment (spontaneous or dictated)	Lexical decision surprisingly good	Printed context affects ability to pronounce
1	+	+	–	+	+	+	+	+
2	+	+	+	–		+	+	
3	+	+	+	fair	+	+	+[a]	+
4			–	+		+[a]		+
5	+				+			
6	+	+[a]	+	+[a]		+	+[a]	+
7	+	+[a]	+	+[a]	+[a]	writing fairly well-preserved	+[a]	+
8	+		+	+[a]	+[a]			+
9	+[a]	+[a]	–	+[a]	fair span[a]	+[a]	+[a]	
10	+[a]	+[a]	+	+[a]	+[a]	+[a]	+[a]	
11	+[a]	+[a]	+[a]	–[a]	+[a]	+[a]	–[a]	
12	+	+[a]	+	+	+[a]	+[a]	+	
13	+	+[a]	+	+	+[a]	+	+	
14		–	+ no spontaneous speech	–	+			
15	+	+	+			some[a]		
16	+?		–	–	–[a]		–	
17	+	impaired	+	difficult		+		
18	+	fair	–	impaired				
19			–	some difficulty		+		
20			–	slow		+		
21		+	?–	mild impairment		+		
22	–		–			+		

[a] Personal communication.

29

brief digression will now be made so as to discuss these problems. The first problem is *circumlocution*. Sometimes the patient will produce a phrase or sentence when trying to read a single word aloud. Examples include:

agent	→ 'not a spy, a firm's . . .'	(3)
trip	→ 'tight, as in tightrope'	(5)
impossibility	→ 'perhaps, not'	(13)
living-room	→ 'Oh, I know what that is, it is the place we go after dinner to watch TV.' (Benson and Geschwind, 1969)	
Holland	→ 'It's a country, not Europe . . . no . . . not Germany . . . it's small . . . it was captured . . . Belgium! That's it, Belgium.' (Luria, 1970)	

These circumlocutory responses correspond to semantic errors in the sense that the patient has obviously obtained some semantic information about the stimulus and is using this for generating his response. They differ from semantic errors in that the patient does not select a single-word response on the basis of this semantic information. Eventually, some theoretical account of circumlocutory responses will be required, and in particular an account of how they are related to semantic errors. At present, the usual practice is to consign them to the category of 'other responses' or 'unclassified responses'.

A second problem is *self-correction*. Patients will sometimes produce a response and then indicate that they consider it to be an error. For example, case 5 'was sometimes aware that he had made a semantic error and would delete it by saying "no"' (Shallice and Warrington, 1975, p. 196). Another example is *while* → 'white, but no' (12). Since Patterson (1978) has shown that patients give lower confidence ratings to incorrect responses when they are semantic errors than when they are visual or derivational errors, it is clear that self-corrections would be more common with semantic errors than with visual or derivational errors. Different investigators have adopted different practices with self-corrections: Shallice and Warrington (1975) classified them as omissions (non-responses).

A third problem is *multiple response*. Patients will sometimes produce several different words when trying to read one word aloud:

protocol → 'high person, NATO, queen' (13) or *as* → 'at, ass, the butt' (9).

These three problems deserve attention, and need eventual resolution, but are not especially serious, because circumlocutions, self-corrections, and multiple responses do not occur with great frequency. A difficulty which is somewhat more serious is the overlap between the four categories of error given in Table 2.2. To take an extreme example: suppose a patient produced the response *her* → 'she'; which error category does it belong to? The two words are semantically related; they are visually similar; they are both function words; and they have a common free morpheme whilst differing in inflectional morpheme. Therefore, one could assign this response to any one of the four error categories.

There is no complete solution to this problem, but the introduction of a fifth error category, the visual and/or semantic error, helps. This category is for any response which is both visually *and* semantically related to its stimulus: *lose* → 'stole', *trust* → 'truth', *pond* → 'pool', or *last* → 'late' are examples. A common practice is to classify stimulus and response as visually similar if at least 50 per cent of the letters in the response are also in the stimulus: thus any response satisfying this criterion is a visual error, or, if there is also a semantic relationship, a visual and/or semantic error. The term 'and/or' is used because a response such as *pond* → 'pool' could be just a visual error, just a semantic error, or the result of joint action of the processes producing visual and semantic errors (see Shallice and McGill, 1978, for an analysis of the third of these possibilities).

A sixth error category is also needed, because of the error-type first noticed by Marshall and Newcombe (1966). Their patient read *sympathy* as 'orchestra'; Marshall and Newcombe suggested that this was a visual error (converting *sympathy* to symphony) followed by a semantic error (converting symphony to 'orchestra'). As Table 2.6 indicates, these compound errors have since been observed in other patients: they might be termed visual-then-semantic errors.

These issues concerning the extension of error classification were dealt with by Marshall and Newcombe (1966) and particularly by Shallice and Warrington (1975), and the sixfold classification stated and illustrated in Table 2.6 stems, with minor differences, from the classifications they proposed.

The problem of overlap is greatly ameliorated by the use of this sixfold classification, but it is not eliminated. The assignment of the

TABLE 2.6 *Sixfold classification of deep-dyslexic oral reading errors, with examples*

Case No.	1	2	3	4	5
Visual	life → 'wife' pace → 'space' sword → 'words'	liver → 'live' flow → 'flower' but → 'button'	thin → 'think' bad → 'bed' deep → 'deer' wide → 'wisdom' shallow → 'sparrow'		fixed → 'mixed' bow → 'bowl' charm → 'chair'
Semantic	dad → 'father' child → 'girl' vice → 'wicked'	wed → 'marry' draw → 'paint' era → 'time' security → 'loan' 'money', 'safe' Penn station → 'New York'	liberty → 'freedom' ancient → 'historic' bush → 'tree' antique → 'vase' uncle → 'nephew'	zebra → 'giraffe' play → 'ball'	air → 'fly' hurt → 'injure' found → 'lost' little → 'small' listen → 'quiet'
Visual and/ or semantic	shirt → 'skirt'	pen → 'pencil'	sad → 'sack' next → 'exit' low → 'shallow' young → 'strong' brass → 'band'		last → 'late' trust → 'truth' raise → 'rise' pale → 'ale' evil → 'devil'
Visual then semantic			sympathy → 'orchestra' earl → 'deaf'		coward → 'place in the Isle of Wight'
Function-word substitution		down → 'up'	for → 'and' me → 'and' her → 'she' other → 'and' his → 'she'		her → 'she' him → 'his' my → 'by' out → 'in'
Derivational	graves → 'grave' card → 'cards' fleeing → 'flee' registered → 'register' goes → 'go'	lived → 'live'	beg → 'beggar' length → 'long' political → 'politician' heat → 'hot' entertain → 'entertained'		baker → 'bakery' sit → 'sat' am → 'be' jealousy → 'jealous' heroic → 'hero'

Case No.	6	7	8	9	10
Visual	venu → 'veau' assez → 'assis'	bane → 'bananas' earn → 'learn' proof → 'roof'	must → 'mustard' pipe → 'pine' near → 'year' wife → 'white'	flow → 'flower' come → 'comb' soul → 'soup' selfish → 'fishes'	pure → 'purple' keep → 'knee' but → 'button' thick → 'chicks'
Semantic	or → 'diamant' vas → 'parti' est → 'nord' insulte → 'frapper' instruit → 'etudier'	merry → 'Christmas' gray → 'red' carpenter → 'nails' grass → 'lawn' May → 'January'	tulip → 'crocus' march → 'August' robin → 'bird' comfort → 'blanket' bush → 'grass'	dark → 'shadow' fighter → 'boxing' cane → 'crutch' earth → 'world' rust → 'dull'	child → 'girl' gift → 'bring' big → 'tall' flesh → 'fat' read → 'book'
Visual and/or semantic	mars → 'mai . . . mars' mardi → 'lundi . . . mardi'	bake → 'cake' broil → 'boil' four → 'fourteen' clues → 'cue'	broil → 'boil' fifteen → 'five'	bad → 'sad' bake → 'cake' seek → 'seeing' air → 'airplane'	broil → 'brown' sad → 'mad'
Visual then semantic		stream → 'train' praise → 'like the sun'	overturn → 'music'	jig → 'peanut butter and jelly'[a] hurry → 'something about the bees'	
Function-word substitution	mieux → 'plus' très → 'non' là-bas → 'parce'	about → 'how' as → 'he'	me → 'him' on → 'it' how → 'where'	you → 'why' for → 'we' by → 'me' in → 'he'	in → 'the' our → 'the' or → 'the' by → 'the' this → 'down'
Derivational	accelere → 'acceleration' art → 'artiste'	loving → 'love' wanted → 'wanting' sits → 'sitting'	child → 'children'	teach → 'teacher' paint → 'painter' child → 'children' older → 'oldest' knew → 'knows'	teach → 'teacher' singer → 'sung' eat → 'eating' dine → 'diner'

[a] From JIF, a brand of peanut butter.

TABLE 2.6 Continued

Case No.	11	12	13	14	15
Visual	but → 'butter' wire → 'wine' ambulance → 'umbrella'	hovering → 'Hoover' crag → 'crab' idiot → 'idol' origin → 'organ' scandal → 'sandals'	bush → 'brush' crab → 'crag' bead → 'bread' signal → 'single' picking → 'pickles'	error → 'terror' prosper → 'proper' alter → 'actor' confiscate → 'Confucius' variety → 'verify'	chapter → 'chaplain' patent → 'patient' custom → 'custody' hug → 'rug' mature → 'mate'
Semantic	cow → 'donkey' stove → 'dinner' wash → 'scrubbing' chimney → 'furnace'	girl → 'boy' tartan → 'kilt' excavations → 'digging' ideal → 'milk' Thermos → 'flask'	postage → 'stamps' stage → 'coach' sepulchre → 'tomb' negative → 'minus' gable → 'eaves'	permit → 'ask' reception → 'visitors' production → 'play' amusement → 'ticket' entertainment → 'card'	blossom → 'bud' story → 'books' income → 'tax' elevator → 'lift' short → 'walk'
Visual and/ or semantic	sailboat → 'boat'	amount → 'account' incident → 'accident' fragment → 'fracture' judge → 'jury' shade → 'shadow'	brass → 'band' incident → 'accident' submerge → 'submarine' trouble → 'terrible' fragment → 'segment'	memorable → 'memorial' inaccurate → 'incorrect'	breast → 'chest' justice → 'judge' pond → 'pool' secret → 'silent' penalty → 'guilty'
Visual then semantic	butterfly → 'good, bacon . . . no' when → 'chicken' hond → 'motorcycle'	charter → 'map' favour → 'taste' pivot → 'airplane' glem → 'jewel'	brought → 'buying' copious → 'carbon' rud → 'naughty'		decent → 'ascension, up'
Function-word substitution	an → 'you' their → 'you' him → 'me'	where → 'now' this → 'is' off → 'from' both → 'another'	to → 'which' where → 'because' or → 'with' and → 'of' to → 'it'		me → 'him'
Derivational	wrote → 'write' fish → 'fishing' shoe → 'shoes'	coil → 'coiled' hovering → 'hover' directing → 'direction' death → 'dead' signal → 'sign'	length → 'long' ride → 'rider' grown → 'growing' bedevilled → 'devils' mercantile → 'merchant'	punishment → 'punish' revise → 'revision' prove → 'proof' wise → 'wisdom' impure → 'pure'	alone → 'lonely' clothes → 'clothing' fear → 'afraid' stolen → 'steal' truth → 'true'

her → 'she' error, for example, remains arbitrary. A policy which would dispose of the remaining difficulties, but which might perhaps be regarded as dangerously restrictive, would be to categorize errors according to the following scheme:

(1)   If stimulus and response have a common free morpheme but different bound morphemes, this is always a derivational error.
(2)   Otherwise, if stimulus and response are both function words, this is always a function-word substitution.

All remaining errors can then be unambiguously assigned to one of the remaining four categories or to the category 'Unclassifiable responses'.

It should be noted that the use of a sixfold error classification does not commit one to the empirical claim that there are really six different types of error. It might turn out, for example, that derivational errors are really only visual errors (or semantic errors). Until one can demonstrate that this is so, however, it is clearly essential to retain separate categories, just in case these really are different kinds of error. As a matter of fact, evidence is accumulating (e.g. Patterson, 1978) that derivational errors may not be reducible simply to visual or to semantic errors.

Agrammatism in speech?

So far, this chapter has provided evidence that patients who make semantic errors also always make visual errors, derivational errors and function-word substitutions. The next symptom to be considered is agrammatism in speech. A number of the patients listed in Table 2.1 were not only aphasic, but quite clearly were classifiable as Broca's aphasics. One symptom of Broca's aphasia, possessed by these patients, is agrammatism of speech: function words and inflections are selectively absent from speech which is still relatively meaningful and communicative. Since these patients also had difficulty with function words and inflections in reading aloud, it is obviously natural to conclude that their speech disorder and their reading disorder have a common cause, and hence to conclude that deep dyslexia is not specifically a disorder of *reading*, but a general linguistic disorder manifesting itself not only in print comprehension but also in speech production. However, it is clear that this conclusion is incorrect, because although many of the patients who made semantic errors in reading aloud also exhibited agrammatism of speech, some definitely did not. The speech of these patients was not completely intact, but speech defects were minimal, and certainly did not suggest agrammatism, as the quotations below will demonstrate.

Case 1, although described in a paper entitled 'A case of agrammatism in the English language' was not agrammatic in speech, only in reading:

He has a partial motor aphasia and expresses himself with difficulty . . . [he] had a fair ability to use spontaneous speech. He spoke in well-defined sentences, though with some difficulty in finding words. No agrammatism was noted in spontaneous speech . . . The agrammatical disturbance being confined to reading aloud only, the case represented a rare instance of an agrammatical disturbance in an isolated faculty of speech. (Low, 1931, p. 558)

Case 5 also failed to show agrammatism of speech:

His expressive speech was somewhat hesitant and halting, but not to the extent that he was unable to converse coherently. His grammatical ability did not appear to be qualitatively worse than his word-finding abilities and he was able to use appropriately both abstract and function words as well as concrete ones. (Shallice and Warrington, 1975, p. 188)

Further information about the speech of this patient is given by Warrington, Logue and Pratt (1971), Warrington and Shallice (1969) and Shallice and Butterworth (1977). These sources confirm that case 5's speech was not agrammatic.

For case 9, Schwartz, Saffran and Marin (1977) present a profile using the Goodglass and Kaplan aphasia diagnosis battery. They note that it does not correspond at all to a Broca-type profile and comment that 'speech . . . consisted of syntactically well-formed although simple sentences'.

Furthermore, the patients of Beringer and Stein (1930) and

Simmel and Goldschmidt (1953) had fairly normal, and certainly grammatical, speech, although they made semantic errors in reading aloud. Further information about these patients is given in Chapter 1.

Finally, in only one of the six Japanese cases (17 to 22) was there any clear evidence of agrammatism of speech; and in fact in four of these six cases speech was reported to be grammatically correct.

Consequently, we must conclude that agrammatism of speech is *not* one of the symptoms of deep dyslexia since, although many deep dyslexics have agrammatic speech, some do not. Patients can be agrammatic in their reading without being agrammatic in their speech.

Derivation of phonology from print

As discussed in chapters 4, 8 and 10, there are in principle at least two ways in which a reader might derive a word's phonology from its printed form. One way is *lexical*: a lexical entry for the orthographic stimulus is looked up, and the phonological representation of that orthographic stimulus retrieved from its lexical entry. The other way is *non-lexical*: grapheme-phoneme correspondence rules are applied to the orthographic stimulus.

The lexical method cannot be used for non-words, since non-words do not have lexical entries. The non-lexical method cannot be used for irregular words such as *yacht* or *sword*, since these do not conform to grapheme-phoneme correspondence rules.

These issues are discussed in more detail by Coltheart (1978). They are clearly of relevance to the neuropsychology of reading, since, as noted in chapters 5 and 12, there exist patients who can read regular words with more success than irregular words, which indicates a dissociability between mechanisms which use grapheme-phoneme correspondence rules and mechanisms which do not. The latter are impaired in these patients, and it is only the latter which can deal with irregular words.

If a patient cannot read a simple regularly spelled function word such as 'and' aloud, it might be argued that this demonstrates a lack of both the lexical *and* the non-lexical routes from print to phonology, since either route should suffice for this reading task. However, this argument is not entirely secure, since it could be that some sort of syntactic filter is actively preventing the emission of the response 'and'. Such ideas have been proposed by Andreewsky and Seron (1975). Given this, additional methods for investigating the non-lexical derivation of phonology from print are desirable. Some appropriate methods are:

(a)   Reading non-words aloud;

(b)   Judging whether or not two printed non-words rhyme, when visual judgments are precluded by controlling for visual similarity;

(c)   Judging whether or not a printed non-word is a pseudo-homophone, i.e. is pronounced exactly like some English word (e.g. shert).

Some of these tasks have been used with many of the patients under consideration (see Table 2.3). The results have been uniform: in all cases, patients have been entirely unable to derive phonology from print non-lexically.

If non-lexical phonology is abolished, this would not prevent patients from doing phonological tasks with *words*, such as reading words aloud; since these cannot be performed perfectly, there must also be impairment (though not abolition) of the *lexical* derivation of phonology from print, in deep dyslexia.

In the case of Japanese, every patient who made semantic errors in reading aloud showed very severe impairment in dealing with words written in the kana script, with relative preservation of the ability to deal with words written in the kanji script (see Chapter 3). The kana script consists of symbols representing individual syllables, with an invariant and one-to-one relationship of symbol to syllable. This would make reading based upon intermediate non-lexical conversion of print to phonology as simple as it could be. If kana is in fact read using an intermediate phonological code, whilst kanji is read by direct visual access, abolition of non-lexical phonology would selectively impair kana relative to kanji.

One may argue, then, from the data given in Table 2.3, that any patient who makes semantic errors will also show a complete inability to derive phonology from print by any non-lexical method, together with some impairment in the lexical derivation of phonology from print.

Word-property effects: syntactic category and imageability

As Table 2.4 shows, two properties of a word strongly affect the likelihood that a deep dyslexic will be able to read it aloud. The first is the word's syntactic category. Nouns are easiest; then adjectives; then verbs. Function words are especially difficult. The second property is the degree to which the word is concrete or imageable: concrete or easily imageable words can be read aloud with a greater degree of success than abstract or difficult-to-image words. Since the imageability of a word is highly correlated with its concreteness it is difficult to decide which is the relevant variable; Patterson and Marcel (1977) provided evidence that the relevant variable is imageability rather than concreteness. Since there is a correlation between syntactic category and imageability, some or all of the syntactic category effect could actually be due to imageability. Shallice and Warrington (1975), however, have provided evidence that not all of the part-of-speech effect can be reduced to imageability effects.

Table 2.4 indicates, then, that any patient who makes semantic errors in reading aloud will in addition show an imageability effect (he will have more success in reading aloud high-imageable words than low-imageable words) and a syntactic-category effect (content words will be much easier than function words; amongst content words, nouns are easier than adjectives, and adjectives than verbs). As noted earlier, patient 16, to be discussed individually later in this chapter, did not show this syntactic-category effect.

Context effects

These are intriguing but have not received much systematic study. However, it has been shown in a variety of ways that whether or not one of these patients will be able to read a printed word aloud can be influenced by including this word in a printed context. Low (1931, p. 504) noted that his patient, who frequently omitted the terminal -*s* from plural nouns or added it to singular nouns when reading aloud, *never* made such errors if the noun were preceded by an adjective specifying the noun's number (*many houses, much money, six brothers*, etc.). He also noted (p. 566) that the ability to pronounce printed function words was improved when they were part of stock phrases such as *from Heaven, beyond repair, what price glory, off guard, clear as mud*, etc.; and (p. 572) that function words could be volunteered for the gaps in such sentences as *spitting — floor — prohibited*.

Marin, Saffran and Schwartz (1975) found that cases 7 and 8 did not omit the terminal *-s* when reading aloud such nouns as *trousers, clothes, news* and *suds*, though they often did for nouns where removal of the *-s* produced a commonly used singular form. In addition, these patients could read a word which could be a noun or a verb (e.g. *sleeping, fighting, fight*, or *fly*) more often when it was in a sentence in which it acted as a noun than in a sentence in which it acted as a verb. Very similar results are described for case 6 by Andreewsky and Seron (1975). For example, in the printed sentence *Le car ralentit car le moteur chauffe*, the patient could pronounce the first *car* (a noun) but not the second (a conjunction), and in the pseudo-sentence *Le train ralentit mer le moteur chauffe*, the high frequency concrete noun *mer*, easily pronounced when in isolation, could not be pronounced in the pseudo-sentence context.

Saffran, Schwartz and Marin (1976), studying cases 7 and 8, found that the incidence of semantic errors to such words as *robin, May, baron*, and *grass* was considerably reduced when these words were used as people's names, as in *Robin Kelly, May Johnson, John Baron* and *Helen Grass*. Embedding words in phrases had a similar effect.

These results indicate that the patients may treat multi-word sequences as single linguistic units, and conversely can perform appropriate syntactic analyses of sentences, phrases, or even in-dividual words (discovering that the *-s* in *news* is not the plural morpheme). Much more work along these lines is needed if we are to understand how such linguistic syntheses and analyses are achieved.

Other symptoms

Object-naming difficulties were severe in some of these patients but, as Table 2.5 indicates, not in all of them. The occurrence of deep dyslexia without severe anomia is important. Suppose one argued that when phonological processing of printed words is impaired words lose the characteristic that distinguishes them from other visual stimuli such as objects or pictures, namely, that words carry phonological information and objects and pictures do not. If so, the response *crocus* → 'tulip' would be equivalent to calling a real crocus or a picture of a crocus 'a tulip', a response which might occur in anomia. However, one can rule out such theorizing about the semantic error since it occurs when the naming of objects and pictures is far superior to reading aloud.

Table 2.5 indicates that some degree of impairment of writing always accompanies deep dyslexia, whilst copying (even from print to cursive) is intact. Patient 14, who could not copy, is not an exception to this since she was a very severe case of presenile dementia who had numerous additional deficits (for example, no spontaneous speech at all).

In various ways with various patients, it has been shown that, on some of the occasions when a word cannot be read aloud correctly, it can nevertheless be comprehended.

Finally, deep dyslexics show some degree of impairment of short-term memory for spoken words. This symptom has been rather neglected in previous discussions of deep dyslexia, perhaps because it is not mentioned in most of the published reports: much of the information about short-term memory in Table 2.5 was obtained by personal communication. This is the only symptom of those consistently associated with the semantic error which has nothing to do with print, and it is not easy to think of theories of deep dyslexia which can explain why a defect of auditory-verbal short-term memory is a constant symptom. One possibility is this: if a person is about to produce a semantic error, but his non-lexical system for deriving phonology from print is intact, his knowledge of the phonology of the word he is looking at will allow him to reject the semantic error response since it does not match the stimulus phonologically. Therefore, a prerequisite for the occurrence of semantic errors is abolition of the system or systems responsible for non-lexical phonology. If these phonological systems are also used for auditory-verbal short-term memory tasks, then semantic errors can only occur when there are also defects in auditory-verbal short-term memory. The claim that deriving phonology from print and remembering spoken words use some common cognitive sub-system is a strong one; if it can be refuted, then the co-occurrence of the semantic error and defective auditory-verbal short-term memory remains a puzzle.

The symptom-complex

Having analysed Tables 2.2 to 2.5 in some detail, it is now possible to attempt to assemble a list of all those symptoms which occur consistently in these deep dyslexic patients. Some of the symptoms which have been discussed so far are preservations, not impairments: preservation of lexical decision ability, for example, or preservation of copying. These clearly must be considered, since it is valuable to know that one can be a deep dyslexic and yet still be able to copy or make lexical decisions. However, if what is meant by the term symptom-complex is a set of symptoms which define a syndrome, one cannot include preservations amongst such a set; they must all be impairments. Copying will be used to illustrate this point. Since all deep dyslexics so far studied can copy, the form of damage to the brain which produces deep dyslexia must be different from the form of damage to the brain which produces impaired copying. However, there is no reason why a patient might not have *both* forms of damage to the brain: this would produce a deep dyslexic who cannot copy. Thus one cannot say that preservation of copying is a symptom of deep dyslexia, because it must be *possible* for deep dyslexics who cannot copy to exist. This applies to any symptom which is not an impairment. Thus the symptom-complex we are seeking must consist of a list of impairments.

The question asked at the beginning of this chapter was: if semantic errors occur, what other symptoms are also certain to occur? This list of symptoms constitutes the symptom-complex of deep dyslexia; and as far as the twenty-one patients being discussed here are concerned, the list is as follows:

1   Semantic errors.
2   Visual errors.
3   Function-word substitutions.
4   Derivational errors.
5   Non-lexical derivation of phonology from print impossible.
6   Lexical derivation of phonology from print impaired.
7   Low-imageability words harder to read aloud than high-imageability words.
8   Verbs harder than adjectives which are harder than nouns in reading aloud.
9   Function words harder than content words in reading aloud.

10 Writing, spontaneously or to dictation, is impaired.
11 Auditory-verbal short-term memory is impaired.
12 Whether a word can be read aloud at all depends on its context.

As discussed at the beginning of this chapter, symptom-complexes can have various internal logical structures. Given a set of n symptoms, some of the possibilities are:

(a) A patient can have any subset of these symptoms but only patients with all n symptoms belong to the syndrome;
(b) A patient with any subset of m symptoms $(m<n)$ counts as belonging to the syndrome;
(c) The possession of a specific subset of the symptoms guarantees that the remaining symptoms will occur, so that the syndrome is defined as the occurrence of this specific subset.

At present, it appears that deep dyslexia takes the (c) form, with a critical subset of symptoms consisting solely of one symptom, the semantic error, since as far as can be ascertained with these twenty-one patients, the occurrence of the semantic error guarantees that the other eleven symptoms will occur. If this is so, these other symptoms are redundant as far as the definition and identification of deep dyslexia are concerned.

Apart from this claim that symptom 1 implies all other symptoms, there appear to be no other known logical implications between these symptoms. For example, 5 can occur without 1 (see the discussion in Chapter 5); 2 can occur without 1 (Kinsbourne and Warrington, 1962); 6 can occur without 1 (Chapter 12); 10 can occur without 1 in alexia with agraphia; and so on. Symptom 1 is thus the linchpin; without it, the co-occurrence of the other symptoms no longer holds.

This analysis of the twenty-one cases has revealed that the disorder from which they suffer, deep dyslexia, possesses a uniformity and homogeneity which makes it unique amongst neurolinguistic syndromes. No other neurolinguistic syndrome has been characterized in such detail; nor can it be said of any other syndrome: 'All and only those patients displaying symptom X_1 represent instances of this syndrome; in addition, these patients will also always display symptoms X_2, X_3, ... X_n'.

It is unfortunate that this appealing state of affairs has been achieved only by so far overlooking one patient, case 16 (Warrington and Shallice, 1979). The chapter, therefore, concludes with some suggestions about this patient.

Postscript: case 16 (A.R.)

Over a number of sessions, this patient was given approximately 2000 single words to read. He misread 409 of these, and of his errors 5 per cent were semantic and not visual (e.g. *month* → 'week'). Thus, like the other twenty-one cases discussed in this chapter, A.R. made semantic errors. However, A.R. was quite unlike the other twenty-one cases, in at least four ways:

1   His reading aloud of non-words was not entirely abolished (25 per cent and 28 per cent on two occasions).
2   His reading aloud was no worse for function words than content words.
3   He read adjectives no worse than nouns.
4   His performance on lexical decision tasks with printed stimuli was very poor.

If one wishes to argue not only that deep dyslexia exists, but that it is as uniform and homogeneous a syndrome as it appears to be when one does not consider A.R., then one is compelled to claim A.R. was not a deep dyslexic. This claim is inconsistent with the principle that deep dyslexia is defined by a single symptom, the semantic error, because, according to that principle, A.R. was a deep dyslexic, since he did make semantic errors. This contradiction demands resolution.

There appear to be two possible ways in which resolution might be achieved. The first way is to note that the percentage of A.R.'s errors which were semantic errors is very low (5 per cent). Semantic-error percentages are normally much higher than this (see Table 5.3). Thus, if one proposed that deep dyslexia is defined by the occurrence of semantic errors *as a reasonably large proportion of all errors*, one could exclude A.R. However, this is unsatisfactory for at least two reasons: first, the arbitrariness of the term 'a reasonably large proportion', and second, the existence of case 5, whose semantic-error percentage was very similar to that of A.R. Since case 5 displayed symptoms just like those of other deep dyslexics, one would not want to exclude him from this category.

A second way of resolving the difficulties engendered by A.R. is to propose that deep dyslexia must be defined by the joint occurrence of more than one symptom – the semantic error plus something else. The problem here is to choose the 'something else' in some principled manner. The second symptom could be complete inability to read non-words, or selective difficulty with function words, or the part-of-speech effect (nouns better than adjectives better than verbs). Any one of these three symptoms, conjoined with the semantic error, produces a symptom pair which is evident in all the cases of Table 2.1 except A.R., and therefore sets A.R. apart from all the other cases. But there is no obvious way in which to decide which of these three symptoms should be used if deep dyslexia is to be defined in terms of the semantic error plus a second symptom.

These are two ways in which one might attempt to defend the purity of the syndrome. An alternative is to acknowledge that the syndrome is not so pure, and that isolated cases of deep dyslexia which depart somewhat from the standard can crop up. As an illustration, consider the theory that deep dyslexia arises when access from print to left-hemisphere reading systems is entirely abolished, a theory discussed in Chapters 16 and 17. On this theory, the deep dyslexic is reading with the right hemisphere. Since there is evidence that the right hemisphere entirely lacks the ability to derive phonology from print (see Chapter 16) the deep dyslexic lacks this ability too. However, language lateralization varies in the degree to which it is complete. Suppose that in some people there is some ability of the right hemisphere to derive phonology from print. If one such person suffered the form of left-hemisphere damage which produces deep dyslexia, he would be a deep dyslexic with some residual ability to read non-words aloud. On some theories of the semantic error, this residual ability would reduce the rate of semantic errors: if the patient is unsure whether to read *bush* as 'bush' or 'tree', even a limited amount of phonological information from the printed word would allow him to rule out 'tree' as a possible response. Since function words are in general shorter and phonologically simpler than content words, residual phonological ability might selectively favour function words, thus closing the gap which normally exists between the two types of words in deep dyslexia. Thus some kind of account of the aberrant symptoms displayed by

A.R. might be given if one assumed that his right hemisphere possessed some rudimentary ability to derive phonology from print – except that his very poor performance on the lexical decision task would remain unexplained.

These are questions which can only be elucidated by further studies of patients who make semantic errors in reading aloud.

References

Andreewsky, E. and Seron, X. (1975) Implicit processing of grammatical rules in a case of agrammatism. *Cortex, 11*, 379–90.

Benson, D. F. and Geschwind, N. (1969) In P. J. Vinken and G. W. Bruyn (eds), *Handbook of Clinical Neurology*, vol. 4. Amsterdam: North Holland.

Beringer, K. and Stein, J. (1930) Analyse eines Falles von 'Reiner' Alexie. *Zeitschrift für die Gesamte Neurologie und Psychiatrie, 123*, 473–8.

Brown, J. S. (1972) *Aphasia, Apraxia, Agnosia*. Springfield, Ohio: Thomas.

Coltheart, M. (1978) Lexical access in simple reading tasks. In G. Underwood (ed.), *Strategies of Information Processing*. London: Academic Press.

Goldstein, K. (1948) *Language and Language Disturbances*. New York: Grune & Stratton.

Kapur, N. and Perl, N. T. (1978) Recognition reading in paralexia. *Cortex, 14*, 439–43.

Kinsbourne, M. and Warrington, E. K. (1962) A variety of reading disability associated with right hemisphere lesions. *Journal of Neurology, Neurosurgery and Psychiatry, 25*, 339–44.

Low, A. A. (1931) A case of agrammatism in the English language. *Archives of Neurology and Psychiatry, 25*, 555–97.

Luria, A. S. (1970) *Traumatic Aphasia*. The Hague: Mouton.

Marin, O. S. M., Saffran, E. M. and Schwartz, M. F. (1975) Dissociations of language in aphasia: implications for normal function. *Annals of the New York Academy of Science, 280*, 868–84.

Marshall, J. C. and Newcombe, F. (1966) Syntactic and semantic errors in paralexia. *Neuropsychologia, 4*, 169–76.

Patterson, K. (1978) Phonemic dyslexia: errors of meaning and the meaning of errors. *Quarterly Journal of Experimental Psychology, 30*, 587–601.

Patterson, K. (1979). What is right with 'deep' dyslexics? *Brain and Language, 8*, 111–29.

Patterson, K. E. and Marcel, A. J. (1977) Aphasia, dyslexia and phonological coding of written words. *Quarterly Journal of Experimental Psychology, 29*, 307–18.

Saffran, E. M. and Marin, O. S. M. (1977) Reading without phonology: evidence from aphasia. *Quarterly Journal of Experimental Psychology, 29*, 515–25.

Saffran, E. M., Schwartz, M. F. and Marin, O. S. M. (1976) Semantic mechanisms in paralexia. *Brain and Language, 3*, 255–65.

Sasanuma, S. (1974) Kanji vs. kana processing in alexia with transient agraphia: a case report. *Cortex, 10*, 89–97.

Schwartz, M. F., Saffran, E. M. and Marin, O. S. M. (1977) An analysis of agrammatic reading in aphasia. Presented at International Neuropsychological Society meeting, Santa Fe.

Shallice, T. and Butterworth, B. (1977) Short-term memory impairment and spontaneous speech. *Neuropsychologia, 15*, 729–35.

Shallice, T. and McGill, J. (1978) On the origin of mixed errors. In J. Requin (ed.), *Attention and Performance*, VII. Hillsdale: Lawrence Erlbaum.

Shallice, T. and Warrington, E. K. (1975) Word recognition in a phonemic dyslexic patient. *Quarterly Journal of Experimental Psychology, 27*, 187–99.

Simmel, M. L. and Goldschmidt, K. H. (1953) Prolonged posteclamptic aphasia: report of a case. *A.M.A. Archives of Neurology and Psychiatry, 69*, 80–3.

Warrington, E. K., Logue, V. and Pratt, R. C. T. (1971) The anatomical localization of selective impairment of auditory-verbal short-term memory. *Neuropsychologia, 9*, 377–87.

Warrington, E. K. and Shallice, T. (1969) The selective impairment of auditory-verbal short-term memory. *Brain, 92*, 885–96.

Warrington, E. K. and Shallice, T. (1979) Semantic access dyslexia. *Brain, 102*, 43–63.

Whitaker, H. (1976) A case of the isolation of the language function. In H. Whitaker and H. A. Whitaker (eds), *Studies in Neurolinguistics*, Vol. 2. New York: Academic Press.

Yamadori, A. (1975) Ideogram reading in alexia. *Brain, 98*, 231–8.

3 Acquired dyslexia in Japanese: clinical features and underlying mechanisms

Sumiko Sasanuma

The Japanese orthography is unique in that two types of non-alphabetical symbols, kana (phonetic symbols for syllables) and kanji (essentially nonphonetic, logographic symbols representing lexical morphemes), are used in combination. As a result of the dual nature of this orthography, we often see various types of dissociations, in brain-damaged subjects, between the ability for kana versus kanji processing and/or differential strategies for processing these two types of written symbols (Asayama, 1912, 1914; Kotani, 1935; Sakamoto, 1940; Imura, 1943; Sasanuma and Fujimura, 1971, 1972; Sasanuma, 1974; Sasanuma and Monoi, 1975; Yamadori, 1975; Yamadori and Ikumura, 1975; Niki and Ueda, 1977).

Clinical studies of aphasic patients have shown that there is a sizeable number of patients who exhibit a selective impairment of kana processing, where their ability to process kanji is relatively well preserved or almost intact in contrast to a severe impairment in kana. On the other hand, there are some rare patients who show a selective impairment of kanji processing with a remarkable preservation of kana processing (Imura, 1943; Sasanuma and Monoi, 1975). It has also been observed that even in patients with global aphasia (severe impairment of all language modalities including reading and writing) the ability to match some high frequency kanji words to corresponding pictures is sometimes retained. Furthermore, analyses of errors in kana and kanji processing in these and other types of patients (e.g. alexic patients) have often disclosed that the strategies used for decoding the two types of symbols are different, i.e. a visual (or a direct grapheme-meaning) processing for kanji in contrast to a phonological (or an indirect grapheme-phoneme-meaning) processing for kana (Sasanuma, 1974).

Introspection by normal adults provides another source of data with respect to the differential processing of kana and kanji characters. It has been reported that there are many adult readers who claim to be 'visual' readers of kanji characters in the sense that they extract the semantic properties of lexical items written in kanji directly from the graphic symbols without any phonological mediation (Suzuki, 1963).

Thus, there seems to be converging evidence suggesting that kana and kanji processings represent distinct modes of linguistic behavior which call for different types of cognitive strategies.

The purpose of this paper is to review some selected cases of acquired dyslexia in Japanese, as well as to present some new data obtained with our own cases, in order to see whether the 'dual-coding' hypothesis of reading (Allport, 1977; Coltheart, Chapter 10 this volume; Marcel and Patterson, 1978; Marshall, 1976; Morton and Patterson, Chapter 4 this volume; Shallice and Warrington, 1975)[1] applies in the case of the Japanese orthography. Since this hypothesis was based on studies of users of alphabetical orthography, normal as well as pathological cases, it is of theoretical interest to determine the extent to which it can take account of a different set of orthographic principles, such as those found in Japanese.

A brief introduction to the kana and kanji systems

Table 3.1 shows a sample of words in kana and kanji, and a sentence in which kana and kanji are used in combination according to standard principles. It can be seen that kanji characters are much more complex in configuration than kana characters, although there are certain structural regularities in the way the component elements of kanji (strokes) are combined (Fujimura and Kagaya, 1969). The base form of lexical formatives such as nouns, verbs and adjectives is usually represented by kanji (although they can always be represented phonetically in kana also) while all the grammatical morphemes (such as the inflectional endings of verbs and adjectives, as well as various kinds of function words) are written only in kana. In other words, kanji characters represent the semantic building blocks in the sentence and stand out as bold figures against the background of kana symbols. One of the important elements of kanji characters is the 'radical,' or semantic marker. As is shown in Table

3.2, radicals, such as 木 (tree) and 言 (speech or language), are component parts of a number of kanji that have meanings associated with a given radical. In fact, in the standard dictionary for kanji, characters are arranged in terms of their radicals.

TABLE 3.1 *Examples of words (in kana and kanji) and a sentence in Japanese*

Nouns	kana	ねこ	しんぶん
	kanji	猫	新聞
		/neko/	/shiNbuN/
		(cat)	(newspaper)
Verbs	kana	ねむる	よむ
	kanji	眠る	讀む
		/nemuru/	/yomu/
		(to sleep)	(to read)
Adjectives	kana	くろい	ふるい
	kanji	黒い	古い
		/kuroi/	/furui/
		(black)	(old)
Sentence		黒い猫が[a] 眠っている[b]	
		kuroi neko ga nemut-te-i-ru	
		A black cat is sleeping	

[a] A case particle for subject.
[b] An auxiliary verb for present progressive.

There are two sets of kana (having 69 symbols each), *hiragana* (cursive kana) and *katakana* (square kana), representing 69 moraic units (consonant-vowel syllables of equal temporal duration).[2] Both varieties derive from a 'simplified' version of kanji characters and are equivalent to one another (somewhat as the upper and lower case letters of an alphabet are equivalent), although the *katakana* syllabary is used primarily for representing loanwords and in other contexts where one might use italics in English.

TABLE 3.2 *Examples of kanji characters with radicals:*
木 *(tree) and* 言 *(speech, language)*

木		言	
机	(desk)	話	(story)
杖	(cane)	詩	(poetry)
材	(timber)	語	(word)
村	(village)	評	(criticism)
枝	(twig)	訂	(correction)
板	(board)	証	(evidence)
松	(pine)	訳	(translation)
檜	(cypress)	誤	(error)

Children learn to handle these two sets of kana signs first, mastering the grapheme-syllable correspondence rules for each kana quite early (usually by the end of the first grade) and then start learning kanji.

Unlike kana characters, each of which has a one-to-one correspondence with a syllable, most kanji characters have several alternative readings, i.e. both an *on*-reading (Sino-Japanese reading derived from the Chinese pronunciation of the characters at the time of borrowing) and a *kun*-reading (a native Japanese reading), or more than one of either kind. These different readings take place in different semantic and/or morphological contexts. Table 3.3 shows some examples where a given kanji is a part of compound words expressing different meanings and is thus given different pronunciations. In other words, the phonological reading of a kanji character is determined by the meaning of the character (singly or in compounds) in a given context, and this meaning must be understood in some basic way before a notion of the correct reading (or the way it might be written phonetically in kana) can be formulated.

TABLE 3.3 *Examples of* on- *and* kun-*readings for kanji characters*

	目 (eye)	花 (flower)	波 (wave)
kun-reading	/me/:/medama/ 目 玉 (eyeball)	/hana/:/hanaya/ 花 屋 (florist)	/nami/:/tsunami/ 津 波 (tidal wave)
on-reading	/moku/:/mokuteki/ˑ 目 的 (purpose)	/ka/:/kabiN/ 花 瓶 (vase)	/ha/:/bōhatei/ 防 波 堤 (breakwater)

As a corollary, there are many sets of kanji characters which are homophonous, or share the same phonological form, usually in *on*, as illustrated in Table 3.4. All the characters in the top column are read /ka/ despite the fact that each has a different meaning. Likewise, all the characters in the lower column are read /shi/ despite their different meanings. Faced with this abundance of homophones in a conversational situation, we often try to 'evoke the visual image' of a given homophone by asking the speaker which kanji character(s) corresponds to the meaning of the word said.

By the end of high school most children can read and write the minimal set of 1850 kanji characters that has been adopted for standard use by the Ministry of Education. As a matter of fact, however, one needs to know as many as 3000 kanji characters in

TABLE 3.4 *Examples of homophonous kanji characters*

	/ka/
(flower)	花
(scent)	香
(section)	課
(course)	科
(load)	荷
(mosquito)	蚊
	/shi/
(teacher)	師
(city)	市
(history)	史
(poetry)	詩
(death)	死
(resources)	資

order fully to understand a newspaper or a monthly magazine. Of note here is that in the use of these 3000 characters the number of different words is far larger, because each character can combine with one or two other characters to form compound words.

Due to the large number of characters and words, the number of years of education significantly influences the degree of proficiency in handling kanji. It is not unusual, for instance, for even a highly educated person to sometimes be unable to pronounce some low-frequency kanji words although the same person could usually recognize or figure out the meaning of these words. It is even less unusual to be unable to write (or to recall the precise visual form of) a low-frequency kanji word, and to represent it in kana instead. However, the reverse situation never happens with normal literate adults. That is, they have no difficulty in reading aloud or transcribing any Japanese words in kana as long as they know the phonetic forms of the words, because there is a highly consistent one-to-one correspondence between each kana character and the syllable it stands for, and because the overall number of such characters is fairly small.

Different patterns of dyslexia in Japanese: a review of some cases in the literature

In 1912, a Japanese neurologist, T. Asayama, first reported the case of an aphasic patient who exhibited a disproportionately greater difficulty in processing kana compared to kanji. Two years later (1914), the same case was reported in German by the same author. During the period of some six decades that followed, a number of similar cases were reported, as well as some rare cases in which the impairment pattern was in the opposite direction; i.e. kana ability was preserved disproportionately better than that for kanji.

Out of these cases I have selected a few in which the description of the linguistic impairment, and in particular the reading impairment, is in fair detail. The following are brief summaries of these cases:

Case 1 (T.S.) (Kotani, 1935)

The patient was a 28-year-old ex-serviceman, who sustained a severe penetrating bullet wound in the left temporo-parietal region involving the angular gyrus and supramarginal gyrus. A neurological examination at three months after the injury revealed a right mild facial weakness of the upper motor neuron type, a mild right hemiparesis and hypoesthesia. Visual acuity was normal in both eyes but a complete right homonymous hemianopia was disclosed.

The salient features of the patient's language and speech included an overall reduction in spontaneous speech with a conspicuous word finding/naming difficulty (50 per cent correct responses on confrontation naming of daily objects, and a complete failure to name familiar colors, which he could recognize with a success rate of 100 per cent when spoken by the examiner); a mild to moderate comprehension difficulty for spoken language; and a severe impairment of reading and writing abilities. His speech tended to become halting and explosive whenever he was unable to get the word he wanted, but no articulatory or prosodic abnormalities were recognized.

There was a clear-cut dissociation between his reading comprehension and oral reading for kanji. His reading comprehension of concrete nouns and color names written in kanji (matching of kanji with objects and colors) was only mildly impaired (90 per cent and 70 per cent correct responses, respectively). On the other hand he had great difficulty in reading them aloud (30 per cent and 20 per cent correct responses, respectively). Another dissociation was observed between the comprehension of *kun*-readings and *on*-readings for kanji. On a task of auditory comprehension for a set of kanji characters (pointing to kanji read aloud by the examiner), his performance was significantly better when a *kun*-reading was used (90 per cent correct) than when an *on*-reading was used (20–30 per cent correct). However, when these *on*-readings were used in compound words, then his reading comprehension improved a great deal (95 per cent correct responses).

In contrast to his fairly well-retained ability in comprehending kanji characters, his kana processing ability was profoundly impaired. He was unable to read aloud or comprehend at all even a single word in kana out of the same sets of words used for the kanji task, although his auditory recognition for the same words was somewhat better. His oral reading of isolated kana characters was also severely impaired. Furthermore, even when he was able to recognize a given kana word on rare occasions, he was unable auditorily to single out each component kana syllable of the recognized word from its context.

Among his error responses, 'don't know' responses predominated. In the auditory recognition of kana and kanji words, however, he made a few semantic and visual/semantic errors for kanji (e.g. 村 village → 森 forest, 鍵 key → 鋏 scissors), as well as for kana (e.g. あめ rain → そら sky).

To summarize, this is a case of dyslexia accompanied by a moderate to severe aphasia of Broca's type. Prominent features of the dyslexia included a marked dissociation between kana and kanji processing, with an almost total disability to read aloud or comprehend words in kana; a better performance on the comprehension than on the oral reading of words in kanji; and a superior comprehension of words in kanji when read aloud with a *kun*-reading rather than with an *on*-reading. This pattern of performance seems to reflect a severe impairment in the phonological processing of written words, on the one hand, and a relatively well preserved non-phonological, or direct, access to the lexical/semantic system, on the other.

Case 2 (S.N.) (Sakamoto, 1940)

This patient was a 50-year-old right-handed ex-serviceman with a one-month history of gradually progressive forgetfulness and difficulty in reading and writing. On neurological examination, a right-sided homonymous hemianopia was disclosed. There was no indication of object or simultaneous agnosia, color agnosia, right-and-left disorientation, autotopagnosia or apraxia.

S.N.'s spontaneous speech was fluent and grammatical, but a marked word-finding difficulty was noted. A naming difficulty for daily objects was also present, with occasional circumlocutions. Repetition was intact, as was the comprehension of spoken language. However, a marked difficulty in both written and mental mathematical calculation was present.

Both S.N.'s reading and writing abilities were severely impaired. He was totally unable to write in kana or kanji spontaneously, except for the signing of his own name. His reading performance disclosed a clear-cut dissociation between kana and kanji. He had an almost total inability to read aloud isolated kana characters, and great difficulty in both the oral reading and comprehension of words in kana (e.g. concrete nouns such as ハタ flag and タコ kite).

The types of paralexic errors made by S.N. consisted of visual errors (e.g., ね → わ, ク → タ), phonological errors (e.g., る /ru/ → り /ri/), and errors of perseveration. There was no difference in performance between *katakana* and *hiragana*. Of note was the fact that S.N. was always uncertain about his responses and was not sure even when his response was correct.

In contrast to his kana ability, S.N.'s reading ability for kanji was well preserved, i.e. he could read aloud about half of the 250 characters tested and could comprehend many more, indicating a dissociation between his oral reading and comprehension. (He used to comment 'I can't say it aloud although it's on the tip of my tongue. But if I see the character I can understand immediately what it means.') Of note was a tendency for his performance to be affected by the configurational complexity of kanji characters, i.e. simple characters with a small number of strokes (e.g. 木 tree, 人 man) were more difficult for him than complex characters with a greater number of strokes (e.g. 湖 lake, 熊 bear).[3] Another observation of note was that compound words tended to be easier for him than single-character words, e.g. he was able to read aloud 乗馬隊 cavalry, and yet was unable to read each component character 乗 to ride, 馬 horse, 隊 corps, when presented individually.

The majority of S.N.'s paralexic errors with kanji were semantic in nature, or circumlocutions (e.g. wolf: 'It's a fierce animal living in the woods.'; cherry tree: 'It's a tree which bears blossoms.').

In summary, this is a case of so called 'alexia with agraphia' with almost intact oral language, except for a moderate impairment in word-recall and object-naming. The salient feature of S.N.'s dyslexia was a disproportionately greater impairment for kana than for kanji, with the different types of strategies used to cope with each impairment giving rise to different types of errors.

Case 3 (O.S.) (Niki and Ueda, 1977)

This patient was a 67-year-old, highly intelligent woman who had been involved in various community activities. She sustained a cerebrovascular accident four months prior to the examination and found herself unable to read. The neurological examination disclosed a mild right hemiparesis, slight reduction of muscle tonus, and mild to moderate hypoesthesia, but no abnormal reflexes. Motor co-ordination was somewhat impaired on the right with intensional tremor. Cerebral nerve involvement included a mild reduction of visual acuity and right homonymous hemianopia. A recent CT scan (November, 1977) indicated a circumscribed low-density area in the left lingual gyrus extending to the left posterior horn, with some adjacent ventricular dilatation.

On neuropsychological examination, conducted at four months post-onset, her oral language was fluent and grammatical except for a mild naming difficulty for daily objects, and a somewhat greater difficulty for naming familiar colors. Comprehension of spoken language was intact.

Her reading ability, on the other hand, was severely impaired, with her writing ability being mildly impaired also. She was able to read aloud correctly only 30 per cent of a list of kana characters presented individually. Her performance improved somewhat (50 per cent correct responses), however, when two or more kana characters were combined to make up concrete kana words such as とり bird, はな flower, and くり chestnut. 'I don't know' responses constituted the majority of her errors followed by visual errors ね→ぬ. Sporadic phonological errors were also observed.

Of note was that tracing a character with a finger, or the use of kinesthetic facilitation, had a marked de-blocking effect, enabling her to achieve a correct reading of most kana characters.

In reading kanji aloud, a clear-cut dissociation between concrete and abstract words became apparent. She was able to read in-stantaneously all concrete words presented (e.g. 鳥 bird, 花 flower, 栗 chestnut, 椅子 chair, 電燈 lamp), whereas she was unable to read any of the abstract words presented (e.g. 愛 love, 心 mind, 悪 evil). (Whether she exhibited a similar concrete/abstract dissociation in kana reading is not reported.)

Of note, however, was that her oral reading was significantly better on those abstract compound words consisting of two or more characters (37 per cent correct responses), e.g. 心境 mental state, 悪役 villain's part. Similarly, she had a marked tendency to try to read aloud a single kanji word by means of combining it with another kanji character, producing a semantically related nominal compound, e.g. 電 /den/ electricity → 電気の電 /denki no den/, which means something like '/denki/ (an electric light, electricity) . . . , it's /den/ in /denki/'. Her performance tended to be better also on those abstract words which had a high familiarity for her, e.g. 活動 activities (25 per cent correct responses). On color names she achieved 40 per cent correct responses; if told beforehand that they would be names of colors, then her performance jumped to 70 per cent correct responses.

This patient's error types for kanji included, besides 'don't know' responses and visual errors (e.g. 百 → 白, 勢 → 熱), a great deal of 'semantic errors', e.g. 心 mind → 情 'isn't it emotion?'; 悪 evil → 敵 'enemy?'; 宣伝 propaganda → 編集 'editorial?'.

She was unable to read at all any short phrases or sentences made up of kana and kanji combinations. Her reading ability for numbers, however, was retained fairly well from the time of the onset of her CVA. No clear-cut dissociation was observed between reading aloud and comprehension.

In summary, the dyslexic impairment shown by O.S., a highly skilled reader premorbidly, is a case of 'pure alexia' in the context of minimal aphasia. Characteristic features of her reading impairment included not only visual errors but semantic errors for kanji, a concrete/abstract word effect, a word frequency effect, and a compound formation tendency in the oral reading of single kanji. These include some characteristic features of 'visual dyslexia', but also some cardinal features of 'deep dyslexia'. Unlike the previous cases, however, no dissociation was observed between oral reading and comprehension.

Case 4 (M.U.) (Sasanuma and Monoi, 1975)

This patient was a 29-year-old right-handed cabaret manager who sustained a severe head injury which was followed by intracerebral hemorrhage producing an enlarging hematoma in the left infra-sylvian region. Left frontotemporal craniotomy was performed immediately but left him with symptoms of severe aphasia and right hemiparesis. Neuro-ophthalmologic examination showed no abnormalities and full visual fields. No parietal lobe signs were elicited.

A linguistic examination performed at three-and-a-half months after onset disclosed a typical pattern of *Gogi* (word-meaning) aphasia, which was first described by Imura in 1943 as being a unique syndrome characterized by a selective impairment of kanji processing, but which shares some features in common with the mixed form of Goldstein's Transcortical Aphasia (Goldstein, 1917).

M.U.'s characteristic symptoms included severe difficulties in semantic comprehension and in the retrieval of content words, whether in spoken or written form, as well as a selective impairment of kanji processing. At the same time, there was a marked preservation of phonological functions as reflected in such abilities as fluent oral repetition, reading words and sentences of considerable complexity aloud if written in kana, and writing words and sentences in kana to dictation, all with little or no accompanying comprehension.

The reading comprehension of patients with Gogi aphasia is usually markedly impaired even at the level of isolated words, whether in kanji or kana, and M.U. was no exception. With respect to the comprehension of written sentences in which both kanji (content words) and kana (function words) were used in standard combination, his performance was a total failure. When M.U. was asked to read words and sentences aloud, a dissociation of kanji and kana processing became apparent. He read 8 of 10 kana words aloud with ease and fluency but with little comprehension of their meaning. In contrast, he could read aloud correctly (but without comprehension) only 4 of the same 10 words written in kanji. He completely failed at reading sentences aloud because of his specific inability to read the kanji words in the sentences.

The types of error responses exhibited by M.U. include a great deal of verbal paralexias (substitutions of irrelevant words), neologisms, and a small number of semantic errors (e.g. 机 desk → 椅子 chair, 煙草 cigarette → 灰皿 ashtray). In addition, however, there were two other error types of particular interest. One was a confusion between the *on*-reading and *kun*-reading of some kanji characters when reading them aloud, which can be interpreted as another manifestation of a lack of comprehension of word-meaning. The other interesting type of error was M.U.'s tendency to place pauses (i.e. breath-group boundaries) at wrong loci when reading a sentence in kana aloud (e.g. in the very middle of a lexical morpheme, breaking it into two). A written text in Japanese typically has no regular spacing between words, although the alternation of kana and kanji serves to indicate word boundaries to a certain extent, along with some punctuation marks (such as commas and periods). As the proportion of kana characters used in a text increases, the physical cues for the identification of word boundaries tend to diminish. Hence, in order to be able to find correct word boundaries (which is a prerequisite for intelligible reading) one has to rely increasingly on the comprehension of the meaning of the text as a whole. M.U.'s pause errors, therefore, reflect a lack of comprehension of the message.

To summarize, the pattern of dyslexia exhibited by M.U. is in harmony with the syndrome of *Gogi* aphasia, which seems to reflect a gross impairment of the lexical/semantic processing of words and sentences, coupled with a marked preservation of non-lexical phonology. The selective impairment of kanji processing and the error types manifested by M.U. seem to be in accord with such an underlying defect.

Summary and comments on the four cases

Since the above four cases have been reported by different authors, there is a considerable variability in the methods and types of examinations used, criteria for the evaluation of impairment, etc., and certain aspects of the symptom patterns crucial for interpreting the nature of the impairments are sometimes missing. With these limitations in mind, one can still extract some important information from these reports.

The pattern of dyslexia exhibited by T.S. (case 1), who had a severe aphasia of Broca's type, can be categorized as being a variant of 'deep dyslexia' as it is described by several authors (e.g. Marshall and Newcombe, 1973, 1977; Patterson and Marcel, 1977; Saffran and Marin, 1977; Shallice and Warrington, 1975).[4] Some salient features observed in T.S. include a selective impairment of kana processing with a considerable preservation of kanji processing and a significantly better comprehension than oral reading of words in kanji, especially for *kun*-readings. According to the standard model, this symptom pattern is suggestive of an almost total inability to convert a kana-grapheme to a phonological code, and to gain access to the internal lexicon via this code, coupled with a relatively well preserved direct (visual) access from kanji to the lexical/semantic system followed by considerable difficulty in gaining access to output phonology.

The dyslexia shown by S.N. (case 2), an example of 'alexia with agraphia' in the context of fluent and grammatical oral language, can be considered to represent another variant of deep dyslexia. The pattern of his dyslexia is similar to that manifested by T.S., except for a lesser degree of overall impairment, indicating the impairment of similar underlying mechanisms.

The dyslexia exhibited by O.S. (case 3) can be categorized as 'pure alexia', with an almost intact oral language and only a slight impairment in writing. Her dyslexic symptoms, however, included most of the features observed in T.S. and S.N., e.g. a greater impairment of kana than kanji processing and semantic errors for kanji, a concrete/abstract word effect, and a word frequency effect. This pattern of symptoms suggests again the impairment of similar underlying mechanisms, although the nature of her semantic errors coupled with the absence of any dissociation between comprehension and oral reading abilities would seem to indicate that her major difficulty is in gaining access to the semantic system via the visual code (Warrington and Shallice, 1979), rather than in retrieving post-lexical phonology.

The pattern of dyslexia shown by the last case, M.U. (case 4), with '*Gogi* aphasia', on the other hand, is quite different from the preceding three cases, i.e. the selective impairment of kanji processing accompanied by peculiar error types, as contrasted with a marked preservation for kana processing, indicating a great difficulty in retrieving lexical/semantic information for written words. The underlying deficit suggested by this performance pattern would be a gross impairment not only in gaining access from the written word to the lexical/semantic system, but also in processing within the system itself, coupled with a well retained ability for phonological coding without reference to the lexicon. This impairment pattern is quite different from that of deep dyslexia, but can be considered to be a variant of the 'surface' dyslexia described by Marshall and

Newcombe (1973) in that the patient has to rely solely on phonological reading due to deficits in the direct route.

Taken together, these studies indicate that there are some similarities, as well as differences, in the dyslexic patterns of these patients as compared to the patterns observed for brain-damaged users of alphabetical orthography. In terms of similarities, almost all types of paralexic errors (visual, phonological and semantic errors) are seen in these patients. In terms of differences, on the other hand, despite the fact that the degree and the nature of the linguistic involvement are widely different from one case to another, there is a common trend toward a dissociation between kana and kanji processing abilities in the direction of a significantly greater impairment for kana than for kanji in all of the cases but M.U. There was also a notable trend in the distributional pattern of the error types, i.e. semantic errors tended to occur with kanji words and phonological errors with kana, while visual errors were seen in both kana and kanji. In addition, there was a tendency for compound-kanji words to be more easily recognized (case 1) or to be read aloud (case 2) than single-kanji words, and a related tendency for the patients to respond with semantically related compound-kanji nouns for single-kanji targets (case 3).

In order to elaborate on the above findings, I would like to present, in the following sections, some of our own data obtained with two of our dyslexic cases. In particular, we have attempted to explore those aspects which have been major topics of interest in the Indo-European literature in recent years but have been dealt with only insufficiently in the Japanese literature thus far.

Some test findings with two aphasic dyslexics

Two aphasic adults, each with a specific type of dyslexia, were given a series of tests designed to investigate the patterns of their impairment in processing individual written words and to determine the underlying mechanisms of their impairment. The nature of these tests and procedures used with the two patients have been geared to those developed and used by other investigators for the study of dyslexic patterns in users of alphabetical orthography in such a way that a useful comparison can be made between their data and Japanese data.

Description of patients and control subjects

The two patients, Y.H. and K.K., were enrolled in the Speech Pathology Service, Tokyo Metropolitan Geriatric Hospital (TMGH), throughout the period of the present study.[5]

Y.H. is a right-handed 57-year-old housewife with eleven years of education. She has had an eight-year history of aphasia and right hemiplegia due to sub-arachnoid hemorrhage (ruptured aneurysm) in the region of the left middle cerebral artery. On neurological examination at the TMGH in March 1978, an additional mild hypoesthesia in the right extremities was disclosed.

When she was first referred to the Speech Pathology Service, TMGH, in April 1978, the overall pattern of her linguistic impairment indicated a severe aphasia of Broca's type. Her oral expression was extremely limited and agrammatic with considerable word-finding/naming difficulties (63/100 correct responses on confrontation naming of daily objects), and slow, short-phrased (mostly one-word) utterances, although no specific articulatory abnormalities were observed.

Her auditory comprehension was much less impaired than her expressive aspects, i.e. showing good performance on high frequency words and short familiar expressions but falling off for sentences of increasing length and complexity.

In her reading and writing, a clear-cut dissociation between kana and kanji processing was observed; her performance on words in kanji being fairly well-preserved in contrast to a severe impairment in processing words in kana. She failed completely on matching individual kana characters with spoken syllables as well as on writing individual kana characters to dictation. Her reading and writing of longer and more complex material, such as sentences, was almost nil.

A recent CT scan (May, 1978) indicated a massive low density area in the temporo-parietal region of the left hemisphere with a marked enlargement of the left lateral ventricle.

The other patient, K.K., is a right-handed 51-year-old government official with fourteen years of education. Three months prior to his referral to the Speech Pathology Service, TMGH, he sustained a post-operative aphasia following the surgical removal of an intra-cerebral hematoma due to aneurysm in the region of the left posterior temporal lobe. The neurological examination disclosed a slight right hemiparesis and a right homonymous hemianopia.

The results of a linguistic evaluation disclosed an overall pattern of Wernicke's aphasia characterized by fluent but paraphasic speech (22/100 correct responses on confrontation naming of daily objects). He showed a moderate to severe impairment in his auditory comprehension, exhibiting some errors even at the level of individual words and a considerable difficulty in comprehending longer and more complex sentences.

K.K.'s reading and writing were impaired also; kana being preserved much better than kanji. In fact he performed perfectly both on matching individual kana characters with spoken syllables and on writing individual kana characters to dictation. He showed an increasing difficulty, however, in reading and writing longer and more complex sentences.

A recent CT scan of K.K. (June, 1978) indicated a well-defined low density area in the region of the left posterior temporal lobe with a moderate enlargement of the left lateral ventricle.

Control subjects. Three normal adults with no history of brain damage served as control subjects for selected subtests given to Y.H. and K.K. Two of the three subjects (one male and one female) were employees of the TMGH and the remaining one (female) was a spouse of a patient at the TMGH. They were matched with Y.H. and K.K. in terms of age and education.

Tests

Each patient was given the following tests grouped into four broad categories (parts).

I *Oral reading of individual words*
1 Reading aloud concrete nouns and abstract nouns in kanji and kana.
2 Reading aloud verbs and adjectives in kanji and kana.
3 Reading aloud function words in kana.

II *Grapheme-phoneme correspondence*
1 Reading aloud nonsense words in kana.
2 Rhyming task: 'Do these two kana characters rhyme with each other?'

III *Lexical decision*
1   Words and nonwords in kanji.
2   Words and nonwords in kana.

IV *Modified Peabody*
1   Matching 50 written words in kanji and kana with pictures.
2   Reading aloud the same 50 words in kanji and kana.
3   Matching the same 50 spoken words with pictures.

All these tests were administered under no time pressure, with one
or two test sessions per week, spread over two (for K.K.) and three
(for Y.H.) months. The order of the administration of these tests was
from part I to part IV, and from test 1 to 3 (or test 2) within each
part.

Part I Oral reading of individual words

It seemed necessary, first of all, to obtain data on the overall pattern
and degree of the oral reading impairment in each patient. For this
purpose, the patients were given the following tests requiring the
processing of written words in various syntactic classes: concrete
and abstract nouns, verbs, adjectives and function words.

I.1 Reading aloud concrete nouns and abstract nouns in kanji and kana[6]
For the kanji, we used a set of 40 single-character 'concrete' words
and another set of 40 single-character 'abstract' words taken from
Kitao's list of the 881 *kyoiku* kanji characters rated by 1000 college
students in terms of concreteness (C), hieroglyphicity (H), and
familiarity (F) (Kitao, Hatta, Ishida, Babazono and Kondo, 1977);
the concrete words were those 40 kanji with the highest C-values in
the list, while the abstract words were those 40 with the lowest
C-values. The two lists of abstract and concrete words were
equivalent in terms of their F-values.

   The kana version of the concrete and abstract lists consisted of 2-
to 3-kana-character words equivalent to the kanji version in terms of
concreteness/abstractness values and controlled for frequency of
usage.

I.2 Reading aloud verbs and adjectives in kanji and kana
A set of 19 single-kanji, high-frequency verbs with inflectional endings in kana and a set of 21 single-kanji, high-frequency adjectives also with inflectional endings in kana were used[7] together with a kana version of the same sets with items consisting of 2 to 3 characters.

I.3 Reading aloud 'function'[8] words in kana
A set of 39 function words in kana, 2 to 3 characters in length, were used, comprising conjunctions (7), interrogative words and particles (6), demonstratives (7), and other types of particles (14).

TABLE 3.5 *Performance of Y.H. and K.K. on the oral reading of single words*

| | Y.H. | | | | K.K. | | | |
| | Kanji | | Kana | | Kanji | | Kana | |
	%[a]	Sec[b]	%	Sec	%	Sec	%	Sec
Concrete nouns	37.5	(3.3)	5.3	(0.6)	50.0	(1.5)	94.7	(1.1)
Abstract nouns	0	(2.0)	0	(N.R.)	40.0	(1.9)	95.0	(1.4)
Verbs	26.3	(6.2)	0	(5.7)	5.3	(5.5)	100.0	(1.1)
Adjectives	0	(4.0)	0	(N.R.)	42.9	(3.5)	95.2	(1.5)
Function words	–		0	(N.R.)	–		92.3	(1.1)

[a] Per cent of correct responses over the total number of stimuli.
[b] The median value of the response latencies in seconds.

Table 3.5 summarizes the performance of Y.H. and K.K. on these tests, which will be examined in terms of the following five aspects: overall performance, kanji/kana processing, syntactic class effect, concreteness/abstractness effect and paralexic errors.

Overall performance. From Table 3.5, it can be seen that the overall performance level is more impaired in Y.H. than in K.K. Y.H. was able to read aloud only 37.5 per cent of the concrete nouns and 26.3 per cent of the verbs in kanji, and 5.3 per cent of the concrete nouns in kana; 'I can't' or 'I don't know' (categorized as 'no response') being her most prevalent responses for the rest of the test items.

K.K., on the other hand, did much better, showing performance levels ranging from 5.3 per cent to 100 per cent on these tests.

Kanji/kana processing. Both Y.H. and K.K. showed a clear dissociation between kanji and kana processing but in the opposite direction. That is, Y.H. showed a more severe impairment in kana than in kanji, whereas K.K. showed a selective impairment of kanji with a relatively good performance in kana.

Concreteness/abstractness effect. Y.H. showed a large effect on this dimension, with no correct responses on abstract nouns in either kanji or kana, while performing 37.5 per cent correctly on concrete nouns in kanji, and 5.3 per cent on concrete nouns in kana. For K.K., on the other hand, a smaller difference was observed between concrete and abstract words in kanji (50 and 40 per cent on concrete and abstract nouns, respectively), and no effect was observed between the two corresponding sets of words in kana (94.7 and 95 per cent respectively).

Syntactic class effects. Y.H.'s performance on (concrete) nouns, verbs, and adjectives in kanji were 37.5, 26.3 and 0 per cent respectively, showing the expected tendency for nouns to be facilitated among these different syntactic classes. On the corresponding words in kana, she performed correctly only on 5.3 per cent of the (concrete) nouns and on 0 per cent of the verbs, adjectives and function words. For K.K., the syntactic hierarchy was seen only with words in kanji, i.e. 50 per cent on (concrete) nouns, 42.9 per cent on adjectives, and 5.3 per cent on verbs, indicating that he did significantly worse on verbs than on adjectives. This is in contrast to the order shown by Y.H., whose performance was significantly worse on adjectives than on verbs, a fact which we cannot adequately explain at this moment. No systematic trend in K.K.'s performance was observed on words in kana, (concrete) nouns (94.7 per cent), verbs (100 per cent), adjectives (92.7 per cent), and function words (92.3 per cent).

Types of paralexic errors. Table 3.6 summarizes the various types of paralexic errors Y.H. and K.K. made on these tests. An examination of the table shows that the distributional patterns of error types for Y.H. and for K.K. are quite different.

For Y.H., the total number of paralexic errors across different syntactic classes was 28, i.e. 25 with kanji and 3 with kana words, which is only 12.9 per cent of her total errors (217), 'no response' (don't know) predominating among the rest of the errors. Of these

TABLE 3.6 Types of errors for Y.H. and K.K. in the oral reading of individual words

	Kanji					Kana						
	Concrete nouns n=40	Abstract nouns n=40	Verbs [+kana endings] n=19	Adjectives [+kana endings] n=21	Total n=120	Concrete nouns n=19	Abstract nouns n=20	Verbs n=19	Adjectives n=21	Function words n=39	Total n=118	Grand total n=238
Y.H.												
Paralexic errors	14	1	7	3	25			1		2	3	28
Visual errors	(14)	(1)	(7)	(3)	(25)							(25)
Phonological errors								(1)		(2)	(3)	(3)
Semantic errors												
Others												
No response	11	39	7	18	75	18	20	18	21	37	114	189
Total errors	25	40	14	21	100	18	20	19	21	39	117	217
K.K.												
Paralexic errors	20	24	18	12	74	3	1		1	3	8	82
Visual errors						(3)	(1)		(1)	(1)	(6)	(6)
Phonological errors	(1)				(1)					(2)	(2)	(3)
Semantic errors	(4)			(1)	(5)							(5)
Others	(15)	(24)	(18)	(11)	(68)							(68)
No response												
Total errors	20	24	18	12	74	3	1		1	3	8	82

69

28 paralexic errors, 25 (all of the errors with kanji) were semantically similar to the stimulus words (e.g. 目 eye → 口 mouth, 山 mountain → 森 forest), the remaining 3 (made with kana) being visually and/or semantically similar nouns, substituted for 2 function words and 1 verb (ぐらい about → さくら cherry blossoms; きり only → のり seaweed; ひらく to open → さくら cherry blossoms). Of the 25 semantic errors, 22 were semantically related nouns comprising all of the paralexic responses to the noun stimuli (15) and verb stimuli (7) (e.g. 飲む to drink → 水 water, 聞く to listen → 耳 ear, 寝る to sleep → 昼寝 nap). Of these 22, 11 were semantically related noun compounds (e.g. 体 body → 体操 gymnastics, 歯 teeth → 歯科 dentist, 湯 hot water → 銭湯 public bath). There were no instances of unambiguously phonological paralexias.

The number of paralexic errors for K.K. was 74 with kanji and 8 with kana, which occupied 100 per cent of his total errors because he never failed to respond. Of these 74 paralexic errors with kanji, the majority (68) were of a type unrelated in any way to the target, 53 of these 68 being neologisms, with one visual error (湯 hot water → 場 place) and 5 semantic errors (犬 dog → 馬 horse, 島 island → 海 sea). Of K.K.'s paralexic errors in kana, 6 were phonological and 2 were visual or visual/phonological (つもり tsumari → つまり tsumori; ほそい hosoi → おそい, osoi).

To summarize, an analysis of the oral reading performance of Y.H. and K.K. on single words of various categories reveals that the patterns of impairment in these two patients are markedly different from each other.

The oral reading of Y.H. was severely impaired, particularly with words in kana and words with a low concreteness value, and with words belonging to a syntactic class other than concrete nouns, i.e. verbs, adjectives and function words. In terms of error types, a large majority of her paralexic errors (in fact, all of her paralexias with kanji were semantic in nature and showed a strong noun facilitation tendency (22/25 or 88 per cent). This pattern of impairment seems to be consonant with 'deep' dyslexia as it has been described in the Indo-European literature. A central factor producing this syndrome has been suggested to be a special kind of phonological disability where the patient is unable to gain access to the phonological representation of printed letter strings, words or nonwords, with only the nonphonological (direct) pathway being spared for the processing of written words, although this pathway is not without flaw, either.

The pattern of the impairment for K.K. was in sharp contrast to that for Y.H. His ability to read kana words aloud, including function words, was remarkably intact, no concreteness/abstractness effect or syntactic class effect being observed. His ability to process kanji words, on the other hand, was clearly impaired, exhibiting a syntactic as well as a weak concreteness/abstractness effect. In terms of his error types, the majority in kanji were paralexic errors which were unrelated to the target, with only a small number of visual and semantic errors. In the case of kana words, on the other hand, phonological errors predominated, followed by visual errors. The picture emerging from this pattern of deficits is clearly dissimilar to that of deep dyslexia, and is closer to 'surface' dyslexia as described by Marshall and Newcombe (1973), the underlying mechanisms of which they have suggested as being an impaired direct route to the lexicon, coupled with a partial disfunctioning of pre-lexical phonology.

Part II Grapheme-phoneme correspondence

In the previous section it was suggested that the pre-lexical phonological recoding of written words, or the knowledge of grapheme-phoneme correspondence, might be severely impaired in Y.H., while being preserved relatively well in K.K. In order to explore this point further, however, it was necessary to examine their phonological coding in a context in which the possible effects of the lexical-semantic system had been eliminated. Each patient, therefore, was given a test of reading aloud orthographically regular nonwords in kana as well as a test of recognizing the presence or absence of rhyme in a pair of kana characters.

II.1 Reading aloud nonsense words in kana

A set of 30 non-words were constructed by means of changing the sequential order of the characters, or replacing one kana character with another character, in each of 20 2-character and 10 3-character high frequency real words.

II.2 Recognition of rhyming in kana: 'Do these two kana characters rhyme with each other?'

The subject was presented with a set of 20 pairs of single kana characters, half of which rhymed (had the same vowel) and the other half of which did not (had different vowels), and was asked to judge whether each pair rhymed or not.

TABLE 3.7 *Performance of Y.H. and K.K. on the oral reading of nonsense words in kana and on a rhyming test with kana*

	Y.H.		K.K.		Controls	
	%	Sec	%	Sec	%	Sec
Oral reading						
2-character						
strings	0		90.0	(1.3)	100.0	(1.0)
(n=20)						
3-character						
strings	0		70.0	(1.5)	100.0	(1.1)
(n=10)						
Rhyming						
(n=20)	55.0[a]	(9.7)	85.0[a]	(2.8)	89.7[a]	(2.5)
					(R:85.0-100.0)	

[a]Chance level = 50.0 per cent.

The performance of Y.H. and K.K. and the mean performance of the control subjects on these tests are presented in Table 3.7. It can be seen that Y.H. failed completely ('Don't know' or 'I can't' responded to all items) on the oral reading of non-words in kana, and performed at a chance level on the rhyming test, supporting the notion that her ability to derive a pre-lexical phonological code from the written word is almost completely disrupted.

K.K., on the other hand, performed rather well, even close to normal, on the oral reading of nonsense kana strings, and showed a within-normal range performance on the rhyming test, indicating that his pre-lexical phonology is preserved relatively well. The fact that he performed significantly worse on the oral reading of longer (3-character) than shorter (2-character) non-words, however, may indicate that his difficulty is not in grapheme-phoneme conversion itself but in transmitting the result of the rule application to the output system (Morton and Patterson, Chapter 4 this volume).

In summary, these test results indeed seem to indicate that pre-lexical phonology in Y.H. is almost completely disrupted, while it is relatively spared in K.K.

Part III Lexical decision tasks

Previous research on lexical decision tasks with deep dyslexic patients (Patterson, 1979; Patterson and Marcel, 1977) have shown that these patients in general have no difficulty in judging whether letter strings are real words or not. This finding has been interpreted as indicating that the nonphonological, or direct route, from the printed word form to the internal lexicon is essentially intact in deep dyslexic patients. It seemed necessary, therefore, to examine the extent to which this direct access to the internal lexicon is functioning in Y.H. and K.K. using lexical decision tasks in Japanese.

We have devised kana and kanji versions of the lexical decision test. The kana version consisted of 40 3-character strings, i.e. 20 high frequency real words and 20 non-word kana strings. The latter were constructed by transposing the pair of characters in each item of a list of real words. The kanji version of the test consisted of 40 2-character strings, i.e. 20 high frequency compound words and 20 non-words. The latter were constructed by combining pairs of high frequency kanji characters in such a way that no meaning could be derived from the compound thus synthesized.[9]

The results are summarized in Table 3.8 with separate entries for words and non-words. It can be seen from the table that for Y.H. there is a dissociation in performance between kanji and kana, i.e. a significantly above chance performance (70 per cent) for kanji (although this is clearly below the control subjects' range), and a significantly below-chance performance for kana (12.5 per cent), the latter being due to the fact that she responded with 'don't know's' to all of the non-words in kana and the majority of words in kana. For K.K., on the other hand, both kanji and kana (words and non-words combined) were well above the chance level, i.e. 87.5 per cent for kanji, which was within the normal range, and 70 per cent for kana, respectively.

These patterns of performance can be interpreted as indicating that both Y.H. and K.K. are able to discriminate words in kanji from non-words in kanji, i.e. they can recognize some kanji strings as real words while rejecting others as non-words, far more accurately than they can read these real words aloud. This suggests that these patients have a fairly good access from the printed kanji strings to the internal lexicon. It is also likely that this access is achieved chiefly through the nonphonological direct pathway because 1) kanji characters, as logographs (with only very weak, if any, relationship with the phonological code), are best suited for direct access; and 2) even Y.H., whose phonological pathway is essentially nonfunctional, achieved a significantly higher than chance performance on the kanji tasks.

TABLE 3.8 *Performance of Y.H. and K.K. on the lexical decision test*

	Y.H. Kanji % Sec	Y.H. Kana % Sec	K.K. Kanji % Sec	K.K. Kana % Sec	Controls Kanji % Sec	Controls Kana % Sec
Words n=20	70.0 (3.9)	25.0 (2.5)	75.0 (2.1)	90.0 (2.3)	100.0 (0.7)	100.0 (1.2)
Non-words n=20	70.0 (4.4)	0 (N.R.)	100.0 (2.0)	50.0 (8.5)	86.7 (2.0)	96.7 (1.4)
Total n=40	70.0 (4.2)	12.5 (2.5)	87.5 (2.0)	70.0 (4.7)	93.3 (1.4) (R:80.0-100.0)	98.3 (1.3) (R:97.5-100.0)

Chance level = 50.0 per cent.

In the case of kana sequences, on the other hand, the picture is quite different. For Y.H. it was extremely difficult to discriminate words in kana from non-words in kana, indicating that Y.H.'s non-phonological direct route is extremely inefficient for this type of task, resulting in a hit rate of 1 in 8 for gaining access from kana strings to the lexicon. These data might also be interpreted as suggesting that lexical access for kana strings in Japanese may be partially dependent on the functional integrity of pre-lexical phonology, at least in some individuals. A further possibility is that there is a separate lexicon for words in kana, the access to this lexicon being gained mainly through a pre-lexical phonological code.

K.K.'s above chance performance on the kana task (especially his high performance for real words, i.e. 90 per cent), on the other hand, may indicate that he has an almost normal access from kana sequences to the lexicon. We are not sure, however, how he achieves this access, whether through the phonological or the non-phonological route, or a combination of both routes. There are two observations, however, which suggest that he uses a combination of both routes: 1) K.K.'s percentage of correct 'yes' responses with kana words is higher than with kanji words, which may reflect the facilitating effect of phonological processing on direct processing in kana; and 2) K.K.'s chance performance of 50 per cent and unusually long mean response latency of 8.5 sec. on non-words may indicate that when non-words are unavailable to him through the visual route, the phonological route comes into play, thus requiring the extra processing time. The outcome of this extra processing is not quite successful, though, because of K.K.'s partial difficulty in transmitting the result of a phonological analysis to some central system (e.g. the kana lexicon), so as to make a judgment about 'wordness'.

In the next section, I would like to discuss to what extent these kana and kanji strings recognized as words can be comprehended or matched with their semantic representation.

Part IV Comprehension of single words: written word/picture matching test adapted from the Peabody Picture Vocabulary Test (PPVT)

We modified the Peabody Picture Vocabulary Test (Dunn, 1965) in such a way that the patients were required to match words written in kanji or kana (instead of spoken words) to a picture. In addition, in order to avoid fatigue on the part of the patients, the test was compressed into one third of the original length (i.e. 50 words instead of 150), in such a way that the whole span of difficulty levels covered in the original were represented by 50 words of increasing difficulty. For the purpose of comparison, the patients' oral reading and auditory comprehension of the same set of words were also tested.

The results are summarized in Table 3.9 together with the performance of the control subjects on the same tests. It can be seen that the performance patterns for kanji of Y.H. and K.K. are quite similar, i.e. both Y.H. and K.K. achieved 72 per cent correct responses on the visual comprehension of kanji words. This performance level is clearly inferior to the normal level of performance, but markedly superior to the patient's oral reading performance on the same set of words, 12 per cent for Y.H. and 4 per cent for K.K. (second row of Table 3.9), indicating a conspicuous dissociation between comprehension and oral production.

TABLE 3.9 *Performance of Y.H. and K.K. on the reading comprehension of words on a modified Peabody test in relation to their oral reading of the same words*

	Y.H. Kanji %	Sec	Kana %	Sec	K.K. Kanji %	Sec	Kana %	Sec	Controls Kanji %	Sec	Kana %	Sec
Comprehension	72.0[a]	(6.1)	8.0[a]	(12.8)	74.0[a]	(6.4)	66.0[a]	(13.0)	100.0[a]	(1.5)	98.3[a] (R:95.0–100.0)	(1.3)
Oral reading	12.0	(4.7)	2.0	(11.5)	4.0	(14.4)	82.0	(2.0)	97.3 (R:92.0–100.0)	(0.9)	100.0	(1.0)
Correct both on comprehension and reading	12.0		2.0		4.0		56.0					
Correct only on comprehension	60.0		6.0		70.0		10.0					
Correct only on reading	0		0		0		26.0					
Errors both on comprehension and reading	28.0		92.0		26.0		8.0					
Auditory comprehension	86.0[a]	(3.0)			86.0[a]	(3.4)			100.0[a]	(0.7)		
Correct only on auditory comprehension	22.0		78.0		14.0		8.0					

[a] Chance level = 25.0 per cent.

Analyses of their comprehension errors revealed that out of 14 (28 per cent) errors, Y.H. made 2 (4 per cent) semantic errors (e.g. 峡谷 gorge → 滝 waterfall), all of the rest being 'don't know's', while K.K. made 4 (8 per cent) semantic errors (e.g. 弓 bow → 矢 arrow), all of the rest being irrelevant errors. These results indicate that in both Y.H. and K.K. the semantic access for some kanji words is partial or incomplete in the sense that they can retrieve a word meaning only within a broad semantic sphere.

Of note is the finding that all the 6 kanji words that Y.H. was able to read aloud correctly, as well as the 2 words that K.K. read correctly, were those that had been comprehended by the respective patients, suggesting that the access to the output phonology for these words is preceded by a retrieval of its full semantic representation. In other words, the phonological coding for kanji words is post-lexical. What happens, then, for those words which were comprehended correctly and yet failed to be read aloud correctly, i.e. 30/50 (60 per cent) for Y.H. and 35/50 (70 per cent) for K.K. (fourth row of Table 3.9)? A disfunction of some sort in post-lexical phonology may be responsible for both cases, although there is a qualitative difference in the nature of the error responses between Y.H. and K.K. That is to say, all of Y.H.'s paralexic errors (18/30, or 60 per cent) were semantic in nature (e.g. 演奏 musical performance → 音楽会 concert; 下降 descent → 階段 staircase; 肥満 obesity → 肥満児 a heavy child), the rest of her errors (12/30, or 40 per cent) being 'no response'. On the other hand, all of K.K.'s errors were paralexias which were semantically irrelevant to the stimulus words, as was the case with K.K.'s results for test 1.

Of interest is the fact that K.K.'s paralexias, although grossly irrelevant to the stimulus words, were not completely random. That is, he seemed to retain some knowledge of the durational aspect of the kanji stimuli (as is reflected in the fact that he differentiated between 1-character and 2- or 3-character words and accordingly varied the number of syllables he uttered as he read them), and even some fragmental knowledge of one or more of the readings of some kanji (as is reflected in his *kun-on* confusions and in his partially correct readings of some compounds). He used this knowledge (of suprasegmental, and sometimes segmental, phonology) as a strategy for reading kanji words aloud, but he did so without reference to the lexicon.

This difference in the nature of the error responses between Y.H. and K.K. no doubt reflects the basic difference in the nature of their impairment, and hence the types of strategies adopted by each patient, i.e. a lexical strategy for Y.H. and a non-lexical phonological strategy for K.K. It is possible, further, that this difference in the nature of their impairment might be due, at least in part, to a different organization of semantic memory in these two patients. As a preliminary look into this aspect, we devised a categorization test, similar to the one reported by Warrington and Shallice (1979), in which each subject was asked to classify a total of 75 words in kanji (each printed on an index card) according to their superordinate categories (animals, plants, food, body parts, and daily objects). K.K. was able to classify correctly only 37 of the 75 items (49 per cent with chance level = 20 per cent), while Y.H. did so for 69 of the 75 items (92 per cent, which is almost within the range of normal subjects), suggesting that the internal organization of semantic memory in K.K. is, in fact, not quite normal.

With regard to the comprehension of kana words, the performance levels for Y.H. and K.K. were quite different again. Y.H. showed an extremely limited comprehension (a significantly below chance performance of 8 per cent, again indicating her refusal to respond to the majority of kana words). This is a significant dissociation from her comprehension of the same words in kanji, as was the case with her kana/kanji performance pattern on the lexical decision task. K.K., on the other hand, showed a better performance of 66 per cent correct responses with kana words, although this is clearly below the range of the control subjects, and even below his comprehension of kanji (72 per cent). The latter finding indicates that lexical/semantic access for kana is harder than for kanji for K.K.

As for the oral reading of kana words, Y.H. read aloud only one word correctly. The fact that this one word was one of the 4 which she had comprehended may indicate that she uses a direct route for the reading, as well as for the comprehension, of the kana words. K.K., on the other hand, read aloud 41 of the 50 kana words (82 per cent) correctly. This performance was significantly superior to his comprehension of the same words (66 per cent), on the one hand, and markedly superior to his oral reading of the same words in kanji (4 per cent), on the other. The former observation indicates that the strategy adopted by K.K. in reading kana words was again mostly non-lexical, i.e. applying grapheme-phoneme correspondence rules without reference to the lexicon. The latter observation of a marked dissociation in K.K.'s oral production of kanji and kana is of special note in that it illustrates the interaction that takes place between the formal nature of each code (kanji and kana) and the type of strategy used by the subject. That is to say, the strategy of non-lexical phonology that K.K. relied on was quite efficient when applied to kana but it was almost totally inadequate when used with kanji, giving rise to a marked dissociation.

Auditory comprehension of the same set of words was quite good for both Y.H. and K.K. (86 per cent correct for each), indicating that their auditory route for the processing of individual words was spared much more than, as well as relatively independent of, their visual route for the processing of written words.

Further comments on the findings with Y.H. and K.K.

The above findings on the reading performance of Y.H. and K.K. have generally confirmed and extended the previous findings reported in the literature on some features of dyslexic impairment among users of Japanese orthography.

The constellation of symptoms exhibited by Y.H. can be thought of as representing a Japanese version of deep dyslexia in the sense that she displayed almost all of the features of this syndrome (as exhibited by brain-damaged users of alphabetical orthography) in the form which is most compatible with the nature of Japanese orthography. K.K., whose symptom pattern is diametrically opposed to that of Y.H., likewise represents a Japanese version of 'surface' dyslexia.

The foregoing test data have also disclosed that the underlying deficits for the syndrome of deep dyslexia exhibited by Y.H. probably comprise at least the following: 1) a complete destruction of pre-lexical phonology; 2) a somewhat below normal direct access to the lexical/semantic system for kanji; 3) a severely impaired direct access to the lexical/semantic system for kana; and 4) a severe impairment of post-lexical phonology, or unavailability of output logogen (Morton and Patterson, Chapter 4 of this volume). That is to say, in order to give an adequate account of the constellation of symptoms exhibited by Y.H., one needs to postulate all of the above components, indicating that the underlying components producing the syndrome of deep dyslexia in Y.H. are indeed multiple (Shallice and Warrington, Chapter 5 this volume).

Likewise, it has been shown that the underlying deficits for the dyslexic syndrome exhibited by K.K. are also multiple: 1) a somewhat below normal direct access to the lexical/semantic system for both kanji and kana; 2) a partial impairment of pre-lexical phonology, or, rather, a below normal access to the lexical/semantic system via non-lexical phonological codes for kana words; and 3) a severe impairment of post-lexical phonology (or the unavailability of output logogen) for kanji, indicating again that the symptom complex called 'surface' dyslexia in K.K. is also a multiple-component syndrome.

General discussion

The above findings obtained with six Japanese dyslexics (the four previously reported cases and the two new cases) appear to indicate that the overall patterns of dyslexia exhibited by these patients are basically similar to those found among users of alphabetical orthography, suggesting that the neuropsychological mechanisms underlying the symptoms are essentially universal.

Superimposed on these similarities, however, there are some fine differences which seem to be uniquely related to the specific nature of the Japanese orthography. Of particular note would be 1) kana/kanji dissociations of various kinds and degrees at different levels of processing; 2) script-specific errors, i.e. a strong association of semantic paralexias with kanji and phonological errors with kana, occurring irrespective of the type of dyslexia; and 3) a tendency of compound formation in the oral reading of single-kanji words.

1 Kana/kanji dissociations

As already mentioned, kana and kanji represent two distinct graphemic codes, requiring different types of linguistic operations for their processing. It is no wonder, then, that various types of kana/kanji dissociations constitute one of the most prominent features of Japanese dyslexic symptomatology.

Examination of the test results obtained from Y.H. and K.K., as well as a careful look at the symptom patterns shown by the four reported cases (T.S., S.N., O.S., and M.U.), indicate that the kana/kanji dissociations exhibited by these patients can be interpreted as the products of an interaction among at least the following factors:

1) the nature of the orthographic code; 2) the nature of the task demands; and 3) the specific strategies available to (or left unimpaired for) the patient. A case in point would be the kana/kanji dissociation exhibited by Y.H., a deep dyslexic patient, on the task of word recognition/comprehension, i.e. an almost complete inability for kana to gain direct access to the lexical/semantic system, in contrast to a fair success for kanji. In terms of the three-factor-interaction framework above, this particular dissociation can be accounted for as a consequence of Y.H.'s sole dependence on the direct visual strategy, because of her total inability to use a phonological strategy, i.e. to derive a pre-lexical phonological code from the written word (1), for the processing of kana (2), in the task of gaining lexical access or word recognition (3). In other words, the direct visual strategy used by Y.H. was quite adequate for the lexical access for kanji but was wholly inadequate for kana. A similar dissociation exhibited by T.S. and S.N. with deep dyslexia could also be accounted for in terms of the same type of underlying mechanisms described above.

Another example is the double dissociation exhibited by K.K., a patient with surface dyslexia, between the oral reading versus the comprehension of kanji, on the one hand, and between the oral reading of kanji and kana, on the other, i.e. an almost complete unavailability of output phonology for kanji that had achieved semantic access, in contrast to a near normal processing for kana. This can again be interpreted as representing an example of the three-factor-interaction, where a predominant use is made of a non-lexical phonological strategy (1), for the processing of kanji (2), on the task of retrieving output phonology (3). That is to say, the non-lexical strategy used by K.K. on the oral reading task has proved to be grossly inadequate with kanji, while the same strategy is quite efficient for the oral reading of kana. Of interest is the fact that K.K. must have used a direct visual strategy for the recognition/comprehension of kanji resulting in a fairly good performance, but for the oral reading of the same words he seemed to have applied a strategy of non-lexical phonology for the most part, or he may have switched to it after his unsuccessful attempt at using the direct strategy. The latter interpretation may be supported by a markedly long mean response latency (14.4 sec., Table 3.9) for his oral reading of kanji. At any rate, K.K.'s choice of strategy among those available to him (since his impairment in either direct visual coding or in pre-lexical phonological coding is not complete, he still can make use of either of these two strategies to some extent) does seem to be influenced not only by the type of script but also by the nature of the task demands.

In other words, it appears that each script, kana and kanji, calls for the application of a specific strategy which is most suitable for its efficient processing in a particular task condition (Marshall, 1977), i.e. a direct visual strategy, or a strategy of script-to-meaning (to phonology, when demanded by the task such as an oral reading task) for kanji; and a phonologically mediated strategy, or a strategy of script-to-phonology (and then to meaning, as in a comprehension task) for kana. If one or the other of these strategies becomes partially or completely unavailable due to pathology, then, different types of kana/kanji dissociations will emerge (as well as the script-specific paralexias to be discussed below).

In the reading behavior of a normal individual, it will obviously be difficult to identify or separate out the operation of each of these strategies, because of a high degree of integration and flexibility with which different strategies are called into play in different proportions suitable to the demands of each reading situation.

In pathology, however, the redundancy of strategies, as well as flexibility of their use (which characterize normal reading behavior) may be drastically reduced with only very restricted options available to the patient depending upon the type and extent of the impairment incurred in each case. The kana/kanji dissociations described above may constitute an example of this sort, providing a unique opportunity of studying these reading processes (and strategies) in isolation.

2 *Script-specific paralexias*

Another feature of dyslexic symptomatology in the Japanese dual orthography is a high incidence of script-specific paralexic errors. That is, semantic errors tend to be produced with words in kanji, and phonological errors with words in kana, both types of errors being exhibited in varying proportions by practically all dyslexic patients irrespective of their type and degree of impairment.

In Y.H., a deep dyslexic patient, for example, all (100 per cent) of her paralexias on the oral reading of kanji words (nouns, verbs and adjectives included) were semantically similar to the target words. A somewhat smaller number of semantic errors on kanji words were also observed in the other deep dyslexic patients (T.S., S.N., and O.S.) discussed above. In addition, the tendency for semantic errors to occur with kanji was also observed, though much less frequently, in K.K. and M.U., whose symptom patterns represent variants of surface (rather than deep) dyslexia, indicating that the clear association between kanji and semantic paralexias transcends different types and degrees of dyslexia.

Likewise, a tendency for phonological paralexias to occur with kana words was observed in K.K. and M.U. (with surface dyslexia), and even in some deep dyslexic patients, e.g. S.N. and O.S., indicating a close association between kana and phonological errors.

What are the possible underlying mechanisms for this script-specificity for paralexias in Japanese patients? An obvious one would be the basic difference between the nature of the two linguistic codes, kana and kanji.

Kana are phonetic symbols, with a highly consistent one-to-one correspondence with syllables (morae), making them particularly suitable for the phonologically mediated non-lexical strategy, and are thus likely to be associated with phonological paralexias.

Kanji, on the other hand, are a logographic code, and are closely associated with a lexical/semantic representation, whereas their association with a phonological representation is minimal, thus making them highly suitable for the direct, lexical strategy, which in turn tends to yield semantic paralexias. In other words, the semantic (word meaning) information contained in the lexicon for kanji may prevail over the phonological information, and this semantic information may play a predominant role all through the recoding processes from lexical access through the retrieval of the output logogen, with minimum (non-lexical) phonological information to constrain the output, thus leading to a high incidence of semantic paralexias.

At what stage of processing do these semantic errors take place? There are three possibilities, i.e., some kind of disfunction or errors may take place 1) at the level of semantic access; 2) in the transmission of the retrieved semantic code to the output system; or 3) in the output system itself where the phonological specification of the word for the oral production is to be obtained. On the modified Peabody test (Table 3.9), Y.H.'s performance was somewhat below normal, accompanied by some semantic errors, indicating that access to the semantic representation of some of the kanji words (level 1) is incomplete or underspecified and the comprehension of word meaning is attained only within broad semantic spheres. A greater impairment, however, might be suspected at the production stage, i.e. either at level 2 or level 3 above, as reflected in the large gap between her comprehension (72 per cent correct) and her oral reading (12 per cent correct), accompanied by a high incidence of semantic paralexias. Our present data do not tell us, however, which of the two levels of impairment plays a greater role in producing these semantic errors, although it is clear that her deficit at the production stage is not due to a peripheral motor impairment, as is shown by her good performance (80 per cent correct responses) on the oral repetition of single words and non-words of 2–3 syllables. Taken together, these findings indicate that the underlying deficits responsible for the semantic errors in Y.H. are multiple across the different stages of word recoding.

Another observation of note is the general scarcity of visual errors particularly in kanji in Japanese patients. Y.H., for instance, made no visual error at all on kanji and only 3 on kana out of her total 28 paralexic errors (3/28 or 10.7 per cent); while K.K. made only one visual error on kanji and 2 on kana out of his total 74 paralexic errors (1.3 and 2.6 per cent, respectively). The relative incidence of visual errors in the four reported cases, though not given specifically, does not seem to be very high, either. This scarcity of visual errors in Japanese patients may be attributed, at least in part, to the high degree of configurational distinctiveness that kanji characters generally have.

Moreover, a scrutiny of Y.H.'s three errors for kana reveals that all these errors are nominal responses and are more concrete than the stimuli, i.e. a verb and 2 function words (ひ ら く open →

さ く ら cherry blossoms, ぐ ら い about → さ く ら cherry

blossoms, き り only → の り seaweed) and that the first error has

a semantic component as well. In other words, her visual errors do seem to occur in relation to some linguistic variables as was pointed out by Shallice and Warrington (1975), indicating that the locus of these errors would not be earlier than that stage of processing where the direct access is made from the visual code to the lexical/semantic system.

K.K.'s two instances of visual errors on kana, on the other hand, are characterized not only by the visual but also by the phonological similarity existing between the stimuli and his responses (つもり → つまり, mo/ma; ほそい → おそい, o/ho), which can be interpreted as reflecting a phonological component as well as a visual one.

3 Compound-formation among Japanese patients

One of the distinctive tendencies of our deep dyslexic patients is that of producing semantically related nominal compounds when asked to read aloud single kanji. Some of these compound formations change a more or less abstract concept expressed by a single kanji into a more concrete imageable concept as shown in the following example exhibited by Y.H.: 先 priority → 先生 teacher.

We do not know whether this compounding tendency is as pervasive a phenomenon among the users of alphabetical orthography as it is among our patients, but it certainly deserves attention in terms of its possible underlying mechanisms. One explanation can be made in terms somewhat similar to one presented by Saffran, Schwartz and Marin (1976). Since each kanji character has its own meaning, various degrees of semantic constraints can be imposed by combining two or more characters to form a compound. That is to say, the compounding of two or more kanji characters may have the effect of restricting the context in which they are used, which in turn may be effective in narrowing down the 'sphere of meaning' to be activated so that the probability of the correct retrieval of the target word within the semantic field is substantially increased.

Another possible explanation could be made from a linguistic point of view. Our patients who make compound formation errors also exhibit to some extent 1) a tendency for errors to be nouns in response to verbs and adjectives, and 2) a tendency to nominalize verbs and adjectives. Some of the compound formations are in fact nominalizations, such as 水泳 to swim → 泳ぐ swimming. In

Bisazza and Sasanuma (in preparation) it is suggested that there is a connection between the compound formation tendency and the facilitation of noun responses (including nominalizations). Following Bisazza (in preparation), it might be possible to explain both of these tendencies if we assume a hierarchy of lexical items defined by the complexity of the contextual and/or morphological features attached to lexical units which determine the number of frames into which they can enter. This idea is partially similar to ideas presented in Marshall, Newcombe, and Holmes (1975), and Fodor, Garrett, and Bever (1968).

Concluding remarks

The major purpose of this chapter was to present various patterns of acquired dyslexia in Japanese and to look into their underlying mechanisms so as to be able to compare our data with previous findings on dyslexia among users of alphabetical orthographies, as well as to determine the extent to which the dual access hypothesis of reading applies to the symptomatology of Japanese dyslexics.

The findings obtained in the present study would seem to be in accord with a tentative conclusion that the dual access model of reading provides a useful, as well as valid, framework within which symptom patterns exhibited by Japanese dyslexic patients (both language specific symptom patterns and those which find their counterparts in the alphabetical dyslexias) can be analyzed and explained.

Notes

1 The standard 'dual-coding' model of reading assumes two pathways for the processing of written words, one for direct visual coding and the other for phonological coding. According to this model, there are at least two possible ways for a written word to attain a correct reading with comprehension. One is via direct processing and the other is via phonologically mediated processing. The direct processing makes use of visual coding, i.e., the written word form achieves direct access to the internal lexicon so as to be recognized and comprehended and from this internal representation obtain its phonological specification for the output. In other words, the correct oral production of the word is attained post lexically (post-lexical phonology). The phono-

logically mediated processing, on the other hand, makes use of pre-lexical phonological coding in order for a written word form to gain access to the internal lexicon, i.e. the written word form is converted to its phonological representation by means of grapheme-phoneme conversion rules, and then from this phonological code obtains lexical access. In other words, the lexical access is preceded by the phono-logical processing of the graphemic code (pre-lexical phonology).

The formulation of the above model was originally based on experi-mental studies of reading processes in normals. In pathology, however, it has been shown that either one of these two pathways may be selectively impaired, giving rise to specific types of dyslexia with different degrees of dissociations between the two pathways, thus providing strong support for the model.

2 Each mora consists of either consonant plus vowel, vowel alone, mora nasal or mora obstruent, and functions as the unit of length in the language. The notion of mora is traditionally used in describing Japanese utterances, and there are some phonological rules which depend on the number of morae rather than syllables. For the sake of familiarity, however, the word 'syllable' rather than 'mora' will be used hereafter in this chapter, except when the use of the latter becomes absolutely necessary.

3 Two experimental findings relevant to this observation are 1) normal adults read more complex *kanji* more easily than less complex *kanji*, when frequency of usage is controlled (Kawai, 1966); and 2) the optimal stroke number for kanji characters in terms of perception is 11 to 12, ±4 (Leong, 1973). Both of these findings may indicate that there is a certain range of complexity carrying an optimal redundancy of 'stroke' information for recognition.

4 Deep (or phonemic) dyslexia, as described by these authors, is an acquired impairment of reading caused by brain damage of the left (dominant) hemisphere. The cardinal features of this syndrome include the following: 1) an inability to read aloud orthographically regular non-words, which is interpreted as reflecting an impaired knowledge of non-lexical grapheme-phoneme correspondence rules; 2) syntactic word class effects: the word reading performance of these patients is influenced by the syntactic word-class (part of speech) of stimulus words, with nouns being impaired least of all and function words (or grammatical formatives) being most impaired, and adjectives/verbs coming between; 3) a concreteness/imageability effect: words with high concreteness/imageability are usually less impaired than words with low values of these attributes; and 4) the major paralexic error types include semantic errors, derivational errors and visual errors.

5 The author is indebted to Dr Y. Fukusako, Head of the Speech Pathology Service, Tokyo Metropolitan Geriatric Hospital (TMGH), for her generous cooperation in providing all the facilities needed for executing the study of Y.H. and K.K.

6 In constructing the kanji and kana versions of the following tests we

tried to select kanji and kana words in terms of words which are normally written in kanji and kana, respectively.

7 The written form of verbs and adjectives in Japanese orthography consists of kanji (representing the root) plus kana (representing the inflectional ending) in general, as is shown in Table 3.1. Since Y.H. and K.K. demonstrate kana/kanji dissociations in opposing directions, it may be predicted that the presence of kana endings in verbs and adjectives may affect their performance in opposite directions, i.e. disturbing versus facilitatory effects for Y.H. and K.K. respectively. The results obtained, however, do not seem to bear out these predictions in any clear-cut manner, as can be seen in Table 3.5

8 The term 'function' is used here in a very broad sense to include all these 'small' words. Generally, these words are written only in kana.

9 What we are looking at in this test will not be equivalent to what is measured by a lexical decision task in alphabetical languages. Since each kanji character has its inherent meaning(s), what is required of the subject by this test would be a judgment of the 'wordness' in terms of its semantic integrity rather than in terms of its configurational/ (phonological) plausibility. In this respect, we devised another test which, we thought, would be closer to the English version in the sense that it requires a judgment in terms of configurational plausibility. That is to say, we used 40 single characters, 20 of which were real kanji and the remaining 20 of which were computer-generated kanji-like characters not in use in present-day Japanese. We asked the subjects whether these characters were real words. Both Y.H. and K.K. performed perfectly on this test.

References

Allport, D. A. (1977) On knowing the meaning of words we are unable to report: the effects of visual masking. In S. Dornic (ed.) *Attention and Performance*, VI. Hillsdale: Lawrence Erlbaum.

Asayama, T. (1912) Aphasia in Japanese. *Neurologia Japonica, 11*, 473–80 (in Japanese).

Asayama, T. (1914) Uber die Aphasie bei Japanern. *Deutsches Archiv fur die klinische Medizin, 113*, 523–9.

Bisazza, J. (in preparation) *The Structure of Linguistic Competence: Templates for Verbal Behavior.*

Bisazza, J. and Sasanuma, S. (in preparation) Nominalization and compound-formation by brain-damaged Japanese: a possible explanation from lexico-syntactic theory.

Dunn, L. M. (1965) *Expanded Manual for the Peabody Picture Vocabulary Test*, American Guidance Service, Circle Pines.

Fodor, J. A., Garrett, M. and Bever, T. G. (1968) Some syntactic determinants of sentential complexity, II: verb structure. *Perception and Psychophysics*, vol. 3, 6, 453–61.

Fujimura, O. and Kagaya, R. (1969) Structural patterns of Chinese characters. *Annual Bulletin No. 3, Research Institute of Logopedics and Phoniatrics*, University of Tokyo, 131–48.

Goldstein, K. (1917) *Die transcortikalen Aphasien*. Jena: Fischer.

Imura, T. (1943) Aphasia: characteristic symptoms in Japanese. *Psychiatrica et Neurologia Japonica, 47*, 196–218 (in Japanese).

Kawai, Y. (1966) Physical complexity of the Chinese letter and learning to read it. *Japanese Journal of Educational Psychology, 14*, 129–38 and 188 (in Japanese).

Kitao, N., Hatta, T., Ishida, M., Babazono, Y. and Kondo, Y. (1977) Concreteness, hieroglyphicity and familiarity of *kanji* (Japanese form of Chinese characters). *Japanese Journal of Psychology, 48*, 105–11 (in Japanese).

Kotani, S. (1935) A case of alexia with agraphia. *Japanese Journal of Experimental Psychology, 2*, 333–48 (in Japanese).

Leong, H. K. (1973) Hong Kong. In J. Downing (ed.), *Comparative Reading: Cross-National Studies of Behavior and Processes in Reading and Writing*. New York: Macmillan.

Luria, A. R. (1966) *Higher Cortical Functions in Man*. New York: Basic Books.

Marcel, T. and Patterson, K. (1978) Word recognition and production: reciprocity in clinical and normal studies. In J. Requin (ed.), *Attention and Performance*, VII. Hillsdale: Lawrence Erlbaum.

Marshall, J. C. (1976) Neuropsychological aspects of orthographic representation. In R. J. Wales and E. Walker (eds), *New Approaches to Language Mechanisms*. Amsterdam: North Holland.

Marshall, J. C. and Newcombe, F. (1973) Patterns of paralexia. *Journal of Psycholinguistic Research, 2*, 175–99.

Marshall, J. C. and Newcombe, F. (1977) Variability and constraint in acquired dyslexia. In H. A. Whitaker and H. Whitaker (eds), *Studies in Neurolinguistics*, vol. 3. New York: Academic Press.

Marshall, J. C., Newcombe, F. and Holmes, J. M. (1975) Lexical memory: a linguistic approach. In R. A. Kennedy and A. L. Wilkes (eds), *Studies in Long Term Memory*. New York: Academic Press.

Niki, R. and Ueda, S. (1977) A case of 'pure' alexia showing a remarkable recovery more than a year after the onset. *Yoyogi Hospital Medical Report, 14*, 4–16 (in Japanese).

Ohashi, H. (1965) Aphasia. In *Clinical Cerebral Pathology*, chapter 1. Tokyo: Igaku Shorin (in Japanese).

Patterson, K. E. (1978) Phonemic dyslexia: errors of meaning and the meaning of errors. *Quarterly Journal of Experimental Psychology, 30*, 587–607.

Patterson, K. E. (1979) What is right with 'deep' dyslexic patients? *Brain and Language, 8*, 111–29.

Patterson, K. E. and Marcel, A. J. (1977) Aphasia, dyslexia and phonological coding of written words. *Quarterly Journal of Experimental Psychology, 29*, 307–18.

Saffran, E. M. and Marin, O. S. M. (1977) Reading without phonology:

evidence from aphasia. *Quarterly Journal of Experimental Psychology, 29,* 515–25.

Saffran, E. M., Schwartz, M. F. and Marin, O. S. M. (1976) Semantic mechanisms in paralexia. *Brain and Language, 3,* 255–65.

Sakamoto, S. (1940) A contribution to *kanji* and *kana* problems in aphasia. *Medical Journal of Osaka Nisseki, 4,* 185–212 (in Japanese).

Sasanuma, S. (1974) Kanji versus Kana processing in alexia with transient agraphia: a case report. *Cortex, 10,* 89–97.

Sasanuma, S. and Fujimura, O. (1971) Selective impairment of phonetic and non-phonetic transcription of words in Japanese aphasic patients: Kana vs. Kanji in visual recognition and writing. *Cortex, 7,* 1–18.

Sasanuma, S. and Fujimura, O. (1972) An analysis of writing errors in Japanese aphasic patients: kanji versus kana words. *Cortex, 8,* 265–82.

Sasanuma, S. and Monoi, H. (1975) The syndrome of Gogi (word-meaning) aphasia: selective impairment of Kanji processing. *Neurology, 25,* 627–32.

Shallice, T. and Warrington, E. K. (1975) Word recognition in a phonemic dyslexic patient. *Quarterly Journal of Experimental Psychology, 27,* 187–99.

Suzuki, T. (1963) *A Semantic Analysis of Present Day Japanese with Particular Reference to the Role of Chinese Characters,* Keio Institute of Cultural and Linguistic Studies, Tokyo.

Warrington, E. K. and Shallice, T. (1979) Semantic access dyslexia. *Brain, 102,* 43–63.

Yamadori, A. (1975) Ideogram reading in alexia. *Brain, 98,* 231–8.

Yamadori, A. and Ikumura, G. (1975) Central (or conduction) aphasia in a Japanese patient. *Cortex, 11,* 73–82.

4 A new attempt at an interpretation, or, an attempt at a new interpretation

John Morton and Karalyn Patterson

The logogen model has an old and honoured relationship with deep dyslexia. In 1966 it took great succour from the Marshall and Newcombe report, though the account given (Morton, 1968) was not that embraced by Marshall and Newcombe. The basis of the old model was a categorisation system, called the logogen system, which was founded on the premise that the production of a single word response should be mediated by the same element irrespective of the origin of the information which led to the response. For this reason the results of visual analysis and auditory analysis of verbal material were fed into the same system where they interacted with contextual ('semantic') information from higher-order processes (variously called semantic system, cognitive system, etc.).

The logogen system could send information to two other systems. In the first place a phonological code was sent to the response buffer from whence an overt response could emerge. This channel was generally thought of as being limited in its capacity, allowing only one item at a time. The other output from the logogen system was to the cognitive system. This system, in the usual diagrammatic form of the model, included all the higher-order processing not explicitly covered in the other parts of the model. In particular it would produce the appropriate semantic code from the information transmitted to it by the logogen system for, it must most strongly be noted, the logogen system itself *contains* no semantic information and, as such, is widely different from the lexicons proposed by a number of other authors.

We are grateful to M.-C. Goldblum for discussing many of the issues in this paper.

The two relatively independent outputs from the logogen system, illustrated in Figure 4.1, comfortably encompassed the most dramatic feature of the Marshall and Newcombe (1966) report on G.R., namely the presence of semantic paralexias. Thus with *storm* being presented the response was 'thunder'; *uncle* led to the response 'nephew'. This phenomenon posed for most models of perception at the time a grave philosophical problem similar to that posed by perceptual defence phenomena – 'How can something be understood without being recognised?' To the logogen model there was no such problem. Consciousness was associated with a response being available in the response buffer and not with the semantics. Terms like 'recognise' had no meaning independent of the model. The *storm* → 'thunder' sequence required only that the categorisation element or logogen responsible for the morpheme *storm* have a blocked output to the response buffer. Given that the two outputs were independent there would be no need for the one to the cognitive system to be affected. Thus information could still be sent to the cognitive system where a semantic description for *storm* could be found. The semantics would then serve as the basis for a response which would be in the same semantic field as the stimulus word.

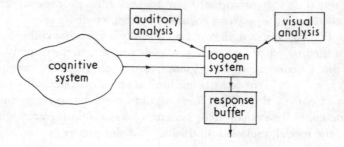

FIGURE 4.1 Elements of the pre-1977 version of the logogen model

In the last two years the form of the logogen model has changed. In addition we have a good deal more detailed information on deep dyslexic patients. It is time to assess whether the relationship is still a comfortable one.

The revised logogen model

The reason for the change in the form of the model is a series of experiments on facilitation. Briefly, the original model required that whenever a single word response was made, for whatever reason, then for some subsequent period of time there should be facilitation of recognition of that word under conditions of stimulus impoverishment (i.e. in a tachistoscope or, with auditory presentation, in noise). This requirement was upset by Winnick and Daniel (1970), who showed that when a subject named a picture of (e.g.) a butterfly there was no subsequent facilitation of recognition of the word *butterfly* presented visually. This result was confirmed by Clarke and Morton[1] who also demonstrated (a) that there was very little transfer from auditory presentation to subsequent visual recognition, and (b) that the amount of facilitation of visual recognition from prior visual presentation was virtually unaffected by the actual response (the word presented or its opposite). To complement these results Jackson and Morton[2] showed that there was very little transfer in a task of auditory recognition, following prior visual experience of the same words.

As a result of these findings the original logogen system has been divided into three components, as illustrated in Figures 4.2a and

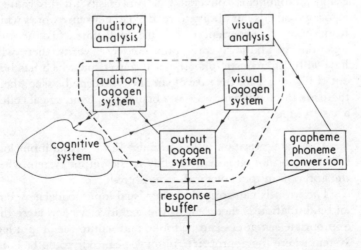

FIGURE 4.2a The 1977 version of the logogen model; the original logogen system has been split into three components

4.2b. Figure 4.2a is presented in roughly the same format as Figure 4.1; the dotted line encompasses the processes now considered necessary to perform the functions of the old unitary logogen system in figure 4.1. Figure 4.2b is topologically equivalent to 4.2a but has been redrawn for clarity and for compatibility with a subsequent picture. Now that input and output logogens (once a single system) have been separated, the question of a direct connection between them must be considered. It is an open question, but we do not wish to devote space here to rehearsing the arguments. Some of these arguments appear in chapters 5 and 12 of this book. For present purposes, the existence of this input-output connection in the normal system will be assumed.

Facilitation in the word-recognition experiments described above is seen as a property of the modality specific input logogen systems, which would not be operative in a task of picture naming. The processes involved in categorising a picture would be located in the cognitive system which sends a semantic code to the output logogen system where the appropriate phonological code is produced. Equally the recognition of a visually presented word would not touch the auditory input logogen nor an auditorily presented word the visual input logogen.

One feature added for Figure 4.2 is the form of analysis known as grapheme-phoneme conversion. The necessity for this route in the logogen model is our ability to read aloud nonsense words which are being visually experienced for the first time. (To account for repetition of auditorily presented nonsense words, there will also have to be an acoustic-phonological conversion which has been left out of Figure 4.2 for the sake of simplicity.) It can be seen, then, that there are three different ways of obtaining a phonological code given a visual input:

1 After categorisation of the stimulus in the visual input logogen system, information is sent directly to the output system where the appropriate phonological code is produced.
2 The word is categorised in the visual input logogen system and information is then sent to the cognitive system. Here the appropriate semantics can be found and sent to the output logogen system where the appropriate phonological code could be obtained.
3 The stimulus is treated as a sequence of graphemes and converted by rule into a phonological code.

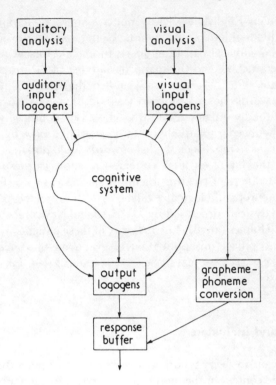

FIGURE 4.2b The 1977 version of the logogen model
re-drawn; this is topologically equivalent to Figure 4.2a

The only one of the three which is in principle error-free even in the
normal system is the first of these processes. The route via the
cognitive system depends first on the precision of the rules which
relate the morphemic element identified by the input system to a
semantic code, and then on the precision with which the semantic
code uniquely identifies a phonological code. There is no theory
which enables us at present to make predictions about the vulner-
ability of this sequence of events; but data from the patients may
provide some clues as to the structure and precision of the semantic
system. Errors in the grapheme-phoneme route are going to arise as
a result of over-generalisation or lack of complete contextualisation.

Pronunciation in English is clearly not a simple one-to-one conversion of individual letters into sounds. Under appropriate circumstances normal subjects can be induced to make errors in reading
which can be attributed to the inappropriate use of the grapheme-
phoneme route. Thus Morton (1964) noted that subjects reading
aloud a list of words chosen randomly from the dictionary (including
a majority of totally unknown and thus effectively nonsense words)
often mispronounced a relatively common word like *ration* by giving
it a long vowel as in *rate*. Since the list of words could not, in general,
be read via the input logogen system, the subjects presumably
adopted the strategy of treating them all as nonsense words. The
best known neuropsychological evidence comes from the patients
with 'surface' dyslexia described by Marshall and Newcombe (1973,
1977) and by Holmes (1978). The majority of these patients' reading
errors seem to reflect misapplication of grapheme-phoneme conversion rules, e.g. *guest* → 'just', *bike* → 'bik' and *listen* → 'Liston . . .
that's the boxer'.

Exclusions and inclusions

Before we go on to describe the symptoms of some deep dyslexic
patients in the context of the model there are two cautionary notes
which we would like to make.

1   We have, at the moment, nothing to say about the anatomical
location of any of the elements in the model. This comes in three
parts:
(a)   We have no opinion as to whether any of the elements are
localised.
(b)   If localised we have no opinion as to whether the localisation
will be the same for all people.
(c)   We wish to remain as neutral as possible with respect to disconnection vs process dysfunction in the description of aphasic
disorders.
In principal, we agree with Oatley's (1978) recent assessment of
lesion studies: we look to such studies for identifying components
of behaviour rather than localising them.

2   We do not believe that there *is* such a thing as a deep dyslexic identifiable by some 'qualifying examination'. We are primarily looking at individual patients and it is only required that our accounts be self-consistent for each individual. Inasmuch as other patients correspond symptomatically to the ones we describe, then the same accounts might but need not hold. There will always be a number of ways of producing a particular symptom. What will decide the appropriate description within a particular model will be the pattern of symptoms.

The pattern of symptoms we shall discuss here is largely that summarised by Shallice and Warrington in Chapter 5 as characteristic of deep dyslexia:

1   The occurrence of semantic, derivational, and visual paralexias in reading single words aloud; also omissions.
2   Severe if not total impairment in any task (such as reading nonsense words) which requires a non-lexical route from graphemic to phonological code.
3   Part-of-speech effects in word reading: nouns > adjectives > verbs > function words.
4   Abstractness effects in word reading: imageable/concrete words > abstract ones.

The patient data presented here come primarily from D.E. and P.W., for whom clinical profiles and psycholinguistic descriptions can be found in Patterson (1978, 1979) and Patterson and Marcel (1977). These two patients also figure prominently in some of the other chapters in this book.

We shall now go through the symptoms in turn, exploring the interpretations offered by the model. For reasons of our own, we choose to deal with reading errors (the various kinds of paralexias and omissions) before grapheme-phoneme impairment. But it will be easier to follow our accounts of reading errors if we make one basic assumption clear at the outset: for the deep dyslexic patients, non-lexical grapheme-phoneme coding is believed to be impossible. By this assumption, if a patient gives a reading response to a word, that word must have been categorised by the visual input logogen system.

Semantic paralexias

Both D.E. and especially P.W. produce semantic paralexias like *paddock* → 'kennel' when reading single words aloud.

Interpretation

All accounts require that the route from the visual input logogen system to the output system is unusable at least in part. The first question to decide is whether this alone would be sufficient to account for the semantic errors. The argument here would be that the semantic code produced in the cognitive system would in some cases be inadequate and could apply to another word (and, thus, phonological code) as well as to the correct response. While accepting that this is a perfectly good account of some of the errors for P.W. and D.E. and may well account for all the semantic errors of other patients, we feel it is not the whole story. The primary reason is that the semantic information available to our patients is frequently sufficient to enable them to distinguish between the stimulus words and their own semantic paralexias. Patterson (1978) has shown (a) that the patients often know when they have made a semantic paralexia (which contrasts with visual errors where it is more often the case that the patients believe their paralexic responses to be correct); (b) that in an auditory-visual matching task (one printed target word, several spoken alternatives), the patients can usually select the correct targets in preference to their own semantic paralexias to those target words. And while it is possible in principle for these judgments and matches to be based on some code other than a semantic one, the patients' difficulty with other codes (in particular non-lexical grapheme-phoneme or phoneme-grapheme) makes semantic information a plausible basis. This assumption receives further support from the fact that under certain circumstances the patients seem unable to discriminate between target word and semantic paralexia: (a) when the two are close synonyms, e.g. *gift* → 'present', *merry* → 'jolly', and (b) when the words are highly abstract, e.g. *earnest* → 'genuine', *oblivion* → 'infinity' (Patterson, 1978). These are the types of relationship where a slightly loose semantic specification might plausibly fail to discriminate, such that with no other source of information the occurrence of semantic paralexias would be likely and undetected. Thus we conclude that some semantic paralexias may arise simply because the deep dyslexics' only reading route to the output logogen system is through the semantic system; but this restriction will not account for the many paralexias which are neither synonymous nor abstract and where the patients know that their responses are wrong.

We have a second reason for feeling that the normal limitations of a semantic specification will not account for all semantic paralexias. If the patients' semantic errors accurately represent the pre-morbid mapping relationships between semantic and phonological codes, then these individuals must have made semantic errors in spontaneous speech with a high frequency. The same, then, should be true for all of us. This is not in fact the shattering *reductio ad absurdum* it might appear to be at first sight. Indeed Morton (1964) long ago suggested that pauses before content words in spontaneous speech allowed the speaker to select a specific lexical item following inadequate specification of the item in the speech plan. But such inadequacy was considered to be the exception rather than the rule.

The preceding discussion has been on whether the normal operation of the semantic route would, in the absence of an input-output connection, be sufficient to account for the semantic paralexias. The alternative means of producing semantic errors include 1) response blocking and 2) problems with the semantic code.

1 Response blocking is the up-to-date version of the explanation proposed under the original version of the model. The account demands that the output logogens for certain items have outputs which are blocked, or at least have greatly raised thresholds. The correct and full semantic code would be sent from the cognitive system to the output logogen system. The appropriate output not forthcoming and a response being called for by the situation, the logogen nearest to threshold activation would be selected. The printed word and the response word would thus be semantically similar; but often there would be enough semantic difference between the two words to enable the patient to identify his paralexia as an error.

A phenomenon which may pose difficulty for the notion of response blocking is that when a patient gives more than one reading response to a word, occasionally the sequence includes the correct response. P.W., trying to read the word *pilot*, said 'air or pilot or navigator . . .'; reading the word *twisted*, he said 'tight or little or twisted or . . .'. He makes no sign on these occasions that the correct response has any special status for him. D.E. does not show this sort of responding (in fact he rarely gives a series of responses), but there is a related phenomenon shown by both patients. When asked to give confidence ratings on their own reading responses, though usually confident about correct responses, they just occasionally judge a correct response to be wrong (Patterson, 1978). It goes without saying that the correct output logogen must be functional when these phenomena occur. Because these are rare events, and because they do not preclude the possibility of response blocking for 'normal' semantic paralexias, we will not discuss them further. But these occurrences should be noted, if not for their implications regarding response blocking, then for the questions they raise about how the patients (or normals!) know when they have produced 'the right word'.

If the output blocking account of some semantic paralexias is correct, we would expect to find difficulties of the same kind with responses produced in situations other than reading, since the same output logogens are required. Unfortunately, the appropriate data are mostly unavailable and in some cases may be unobtainable.

(a) Spontaneous speech: Although expressive dysphasia is apparently not a necessary concomitant of deep dyslexia, both D.E. and P.W. are severe non-fluent Broca's dysphasics. They have very limited expressive vocabularies, and most of the words yielding semantic paralexias would probably not appear in their spontaneous speech anyway. In fact many words which they *can* read correctly never occur in their speech, so the form of the comparison is not clear.

(b) Repetition of spoken words: The patients can repeat words which they cannot read; but as they are also reasonably good at repeating non-words (Patterson and Marcel, 1977), the acoustic-phonological route must be available and word repetition might be based on this non-lexical process. One way of forcing word repetition to mobilise the logogen system might be to present the words in noise such that they could only be recognised given a context. This test has not been attempted.

(c) Picture or object naming: This task does produce semantic errors (D.E., shown a thimble, responded 'needle') and circumlocutions (P.W., shown a picture of a tennis racquet, responded 'Wimbledon . . . uh, tennis'). However, 1) we do not have nearly enough naming data to attempt a comparison with reading. 2) Many words which yield semantic paralexias are not picturable and so cannot be tested; we are preparing tests for the picturable ones. But in any case (and this applies to (a) and (b) as well), 3) semantic paralexias themselves are not especially consistent. A word yielding a semantic paralexia on one occasion might be read correctly on another; and both patients have in fact produced as a semantic paralexia a word which they have been unable to read on another occasion (D.E.: *view* → 'scene'; *scene* → 'tely'; P.W.: *competitor* → 'event'; *event* → 'athletics'). Thus the response block or augmented threshold would have to be a fluctuating one; and any comparison across sessions, much less tasks, will be of uncertain value.

2 Finally, there are various kinds of problem with the semantic code which could give rise to semantic paralexias. Central damage – in the cognitive system itself – is ruled out to the same extent and for the same reasons as the notion that semantic paralexias reflect the normal imprecision of semantic specifications. The primary argument against such notions is that the patients often know that their semantic paralexias are errors. An alternative possibility is that the correct code is produced in the cognitive system but is distorted in transmission to the output logogen system. The consequences of such an impairment are not clearly different from those of response blocking for the processes of reading, spontaneous speech or object naming. Word repetition, on the other hand, might differentiate between the two (provided the repetition response utilises the output logogen, see (b) above) if there is an intact connection from auditory input logogen to output logogen.

Derivational paralexias

Both patients frequently produce a paralexia which appears to share its base morpheme with the word presented but which has a different inflectional or derivational form. Many of these (discussed in more detail by Patterson in Chapter 14) are straightforward suffix deletions (*directing* → 'direct'), substitutions (*edition* → 'editor') or additions (*courage* → 'courageous'). Other paralexias which we have tended to classify as derivational may more properly be considered visual (*bit* → 'bite') or semantic (*buy* → 'bought'); but since most derivationally related words are both visually *and* semantically similar, it is difficult to separate the dimensions.

Interpretation

The visual input logogen system is believed to be morpheme-based rather than word-based, primarily due to Murrell and Morton's (1974) demonstration: recognition of a word like *sees* is facilitated by prior presentation of *seen* but not by a different morpheme of equal visual similarity such as *seed*.[3] The assumption then is that affixes are severed from the base morpheme and dealt with separately. In the normal system, information about affixes must be made available both to the cognitive system (the normal reader understands the difference between *sees* and *seen*) and to the output system. Both types of information appear to be deficient in deep dyslexics: as well as making frequent derivational paralexias, the patients have difficulty discriminating between derivationally related words in comprehension tests (Patterson, 1979) and in auditory-visual word matching (Patterson, 1978). The presence of an affix does not however go unremarked by the patients: although they do sometimes add gratuitous affixes in reading aloud (*coil* → 'coiled'), the likelihood that the reading response will have an affix is greater if the word presented has an affix (Patterson, Chapter 14). Thus it seems that the system produces (albeit unreliably) a 'plus-affix' tag; but the linguistic part of the cognitive system which is sensitive to affixes is impaired in the patients, and the tag often results in production of the wrong affix. Even when the patients produce wrong affixes (i.e., not corresponding to the printed word) they are always appropriate affixes (legitimate for that base morpheme). Thus we find *slavery* → 'slaving' but never 'slavely', *courage* → 'courageous' but never 'couraging'. This suggests that at the level of output logogens, whole words are represented or at least each base morpheme has stored with it a list of legitimate affixes.

Visual paralexias

Both patients make reading errors which have no semantic relationship with the stimulus word but where there is visual/graphemic similarity. Sometimes the degree of similarity is very high (e.g. *tying* → 'typing'; *narrow* → 'marrow'); in other cases it is not (*political* → 'police'; *ceremony* → 'cemetery'). As objective criterion for visual errors we require 50 per cent of the letters in the response word to be present in the stimulus word; more subjectively, we also expect those letters to have *some* semblance of correct order. Thus *own* → 'now' is called a visual paralexia; but P.W.'s *encumbered* → 'broken' (which does satisfy a strict 50 per cent criterion) is classified as '?', not as a visual paralexia.

These 'visual' errors do not show impressive visual regularities. There is something of a tendency for response words to be shorter than their stimuli: in a sample of 74 visual paralexias by D.E., 32 involved a shortening, 19 a lengthening and 23 no change; of 37 visual errors by P.W., 18 were shorter, 10 longer and 9 the same. Stimuli and responses tend to match at the beginning of the word rather than the end: 48 of D.E.'s 74 examples shared the first two letters but only 20 shared the last two; for P.W., 23/37 had the first pair of letters in common while 12/37 shared the final pair. (See also Shallice and Warrington, 1975, for an analysis of position effects in visual paralexias.) These appear to be the only structural regularities. No individual letters seem to be either particularly vulnerable or particularly favoured.

Interpretation
The nature of the errors guarantees that they are to be attributed to a stage in the system within the range of a visual code. Thus, in logogen terms, they cannot arise later than the interface between the logogen system and the cognitive system. The possibilities are the visual analysis system, the visual logogen system, or the entry to the cognitive system.

(a) *Visual analysis system.* One argument against a fault in this system is that it should produce the kind of regularity we failed to find. (Note: there is always the logical possibility of having a fault which consists of random perturbations – an injection of noise, as it were. If we allow this possibility, we cannot rule out the visual analysis system as a source of the visual errors. We will not however consider this further.) In addition, if there were errors in the visual analysis system we would expect words to be changed into non-words and vice versa. The generally high accuracy of the patients' performance in lexical decision tests thus argues against a major fault in analysis. Yet another piece of evidence is the relative indifference of the patients' reading performance to the quality of the visual display. P.W. can sometimes read the handwriting of one of the authors when the other author finds it illegible. Saffran and Marin's (1977) deep dyslexic patient could read words in aLtErNaTiNg case or words with a p+l+u+s sign separating contiguous letters. If the visual analysis system were already impaired, such manipulations might be expected to wreak havoc.

(b) *Visual logogen system*. The account of visual paralexias given by Patterson (1978) was that the input logogens for certain morphemes had abnormally high thresholds. The logogen for another word sharing visual/graphemic features with the presented word was then allowed to exceed threshold to produce a replacement output to the cognitive system. This account does require that some (yet un-specified) control mechanism knows that a particular logogen exists and would have responded if it could have done. Otherwise it would be impossible to distinguish between the state of the input logogen system following presentation of a blocked item and the state following presentation of a similar nonsense word. In other words, if we try to explain the visual paralexia *scandal* → 'sandals' purely on the basis of an inaccessible logogen for *scandal*, we would have to expect the non-word *smandal* to produce a false positive response in a lexical decision task and the oral response 'sandals' in a reading task. Such false positives do occur on occasion, and their frequency rises if the non-words differ by a single letter from reasonably long, low-frequency abstract words (Patterson, 1979). Under these conditions, however, the false positive rate for normal subjects also rises; indeed the patients, while clearly above the mean, were within the range of control false positive rates. We therefore conclude that the patients' responses to non-words probably do not occur with sufficient frequency or generality to allow a simple account of visual paralexias at the input logogen level. The process would have to be the rather complicated one already mentioned above: the correct logogen (e.g. for *scandal*) would categorise the input, and though the results or output from this categorisation would be unavailable, its occurrence would have to be remarked to enable a response from another logogen.

We will not expend more explanatory energy on this notion, because it may have to be rejected on other grounds. There is an indication that, as compared with words which yield semantic paralexias, for example, words yielding visual paralexias are relatively abstract. This is only a strong tendency, not an invariable rule; but the tendency does seem to exist for our patients, for K.F. (Shallice and Warrington, Chapter 5), and for P.D. (Coltheart, Chapter 16). This result has clear implications for the source of visual paralexias. There is no semantic information at the level of the input logogen system. The emergence of a semantic dimension like abstractness in the domain of visual paralexias thus poses serious problems for this account.

(c) *Access to the cognitive system.* Suppose that there are no problems in the input logogen system and that the categorisation of the stimulus word proceeds normally with the appropriate access code being sent to the cognitive system. What could then go wrong to produce a visual error? What we have to suppose is that for some items (plausibly abstract words) the semantic information is not forthcoming. Our reasons for this supposition are that (a) the patients tend to think their visual paralexias are correct and (b) they often choose their visual paralexias rather than the correct target words in an auditory-visual matching task (Patterson, 1978). Neither of these results should occur if a semantic code were available for the presented word. So far so good; but why should the patient then produce a visual paralexia rather than an omission? The answer depends in part upon how the input logogen system is conceived to operate, whether it can produce only one or more than one output at a time.

If only one output is allowed at a time, then we must invoke a control mechanism something like the one discussed under (b) above. This mechanism would sense that a code had been sent from the logogen system to the cognitive system but had failed to yield a semantic representation. The mechanism would then initiate a second analysis of the stimulus. In addition, the procedure would probably require 1) inhibition of the first (correct) logogen, or else it would respond again; 2) absence of any conscious record of the first logogen's response, or else the patient would know that his subsequent reading response was second best (i.e. that *scandal* ≠ 'sandals').

The alternative to this rather tortured process is to allow multiple concurrent logogen outputs, as suggested by Shallice and Warrington (1975); their account of visual paralexias (translated into our terminology) is that the word produced corresponds to the most active logogen which manages to yield a semantic code. It seems to us that this notion encounters difficulty in the low rate of false positives to non-words. We have already introduced this counter-argument in (b) above, but will spell it out again here. According to the multiple-output story of a visual paralexia like *scandal* →

'sandals', the *sandal(s)* logogen responds to presentation of the word *scandal* because the latter contains sufficient visual/graphemic features to exceed the threshold of the former. It is clear, though, that a logogen can know nothing of the formal properties of the stimulus. In particular it cannot know whether the letter-string being analysed is actually a word. (The eventual response of a logogen is in fact the earliest possible basis for a word/non-word decision.) Thus we cannot see any way round the prediction, by this account, that the *sandal(s)* logogen should be just as likely to respond to *smandal* as to *scandal*. As already indicated, the data (such as they are) do not support this prediction. It therefore seems that we are forced to reject the notion of simultaneous production of multiple candidates – and are left, however reluctantly, with the 'tortured process'.

In summary, while we do not see the interpretation of visual paralexias as fully resolved, our interim solution is this. The visual input logogen corresponding to the stimulus word (e.g. *moment*) responds but cannot provoke a semantic code from the cognitive system; the reading response ('monument') is the result of a second attempt by the logogen system to produce an understandable outcome. The absence of the direct input-output connection means that a semantic code is required to produce any response.

Finally, we will mention just briefly other sorts of 'visual error' which may need attention in the complete account to which we eventually aspire. 1) Some visually related erroneous reading responses appear to be deliberate, as when the patient produces a word and indicates that he knows it is wrong (*while* → 'white, but no') or produces part of a word and indicates that he knows something is missing (*manner* → 'man, something'). 2) The same phenomena both occur with non-words. With short non-words which the patients readily reject in lexical decision, they can be persuaded to give 'reading' responses which they know to be wrong. These responses are always visually similar real words (*gat* → 'gate'; *deet* → 'diet'); indeed, in the kind of system we have described, what else could they be? With longer non-words, the part-reading occasionally appears, e.g. *digersity* → 'dig, something'. 3) With long non-words which are minimally different from words, some real (that is non-deliberate) visual errors occur. This is not only true in lexical decision, as described above, but also in reading (e.g. *appead* → 'applaud' and *sovemnity* → 'solemn'), even though the patients were told that many of these items were non-words which they need not try to read. (See Coltheart, Chapter 16 this volume, for a further discussion.)

Omissions

Often the patients can make no reading response to a word, which they indicate by saying 'no', 'don't know', 'sorry' or 'pass'. The main observation in the literature regarding omissions has been their relationship with word class and/or part-of-speech: omissions are much more frequent with abstract words, and their rate could be said to soar with function words.

Interpretation

Omissions might arise from failure at any or all of the input logogen system, cognitive system, and output logogen system.

(a) *Input logogens.* If the input logogen for a word is damaged or has an inaccessibly high threshold (and barring, for the moment, any clever mechanisms which observe that fact and initiate procedures to obtain a substitute response), then presentation of that word for reading should yield an omission and presentation of that word for lexical decision should yield a 'no' response. D.E. performs in precisely this manner on some abstract words, and it is possible that this does reflect a visual logogen failure. Since there are however many words which yield omissions in reading but correct 'yes' responses in lexical decision, malfunctioning input logogens cannot account for all omissions. It has been suggested for example (on the basis of selectively impaired performance in many different contexts) that possibly function words had no or inadequate representation in the logogen system (Saffran and Marin, 1977). But this seems refutable on the basis of 1) near-perfect performance by both of our patients in lexical decision with function words (Patterson, 1979) and 2) impressive performance by P.W. in comprehension of individual function words (Morton and Patterson, Chapter 13). Thus we rule out the input logogen system as a major source of omission errors.

(b) *Cognitive system.* If the input logogen for a word were intact but its semantic representation impaired or absent, an omission in reading would also be predicted.[4] It is not altogether clear how to differentiate the predictions of this account from those of the previous one. Lexical decision performance might seem a potential vehicle, since an impaired input logogen should clearly cause misses in lexical decision, while an intact logogen with impaired semantics might be thought to allow correct lexical decisions. But there is evidence to suggest that in lexical decision, semantic representations may normally be accessed (James, 1975) and may even be required (Warrington, 1975). Such a description would indeed make more sense of the fact that D.E.'s misses in lexical decision seem to be related to abstractness, a clearly semantic dimension. And it must be remembered that for the omissions per se there are strong part-of-speech and abstractness effects. Thus with omissions as with visual errors we may be forced toward the cognitive system as the source of the problem.

Though these first two options may seem to have similar results in these particular circumstances, we might digress for just a moment to say that there are other patients who provide rather clear evidence that input logogens can be intact when the corresponding semantic representations are lost. One such patient, a pre-senile dementia patient described by Schwartz, Saffran and Marin (1979 and Chapter 12 this volume) could correctly read words whose meaning she did not know. This was even true for words like *come* with an irregular spelling-sound correspondence, making it unlikely that the reading responses were produced via non-lexical grapheme-phoneme rules (though see Shallice and Warrington, Chapter 5). This patient, then, seemed to have visual input logogens, output logogens, and the direct connection between them intact, but a severe deficit in the semantic system.

(c) *Output logogens.* If both the input logogen and semantic representation for a word were intact but the output logogen were blocked, then omissions in reading could arise.[5] We would, however, expect adequate performance on such words in lexical decision and comprehension tests. We need more data on comprehension, in particular for P.W. on abstract words which he recognises in lexical decision but omits in reading. But there is at least a suggestion from the available data that the patients comprehend some words to which they make no overt reading response (Morton and Patterson, Chapter 13; Patterson, 1979). Note that effects of imageability and part-of-speech on omissions do not have a ready explanation at the level of output logogens.

In summary, it seems possible that there are at least two classes of omissions, early (semantics) and late (output logogen).

Grapheme-phoneme impairment (or why they have been called phonemic dyslexics . . .)

The patients are completely unable to read aloud visually presented nonsense words which are easy for normals to pronounce. Indeed it appears that the failure is not just in *overt* production of non-lexical phonological codes but in obtaining them in any accessible form. 1) Unlike normals, the patients' lexical decisions are unaffected by the phonological status of non-words (Patterson and Marcel, 1977). That is, neither speed nor accuracy is reduced for the patients when the non-words sound like real words (e.g. *chare*). 2) The patients are very poor at auditory-visual matching of non-words. Their performance is better than chance (how much better depends on how similar the alternatives are); but Patterson (1978) has argued that their strategy is lexically-based. Just as a lexical strategy ('find a visually similar real word') will provide reading responses to non-words which are roughly appropriate (*gat* → 'gate') or even under special circumstances correct (*flore* → 'floor'), the same strategy will support a certain level of matching spoken to written non-words.

Interpretation
We follow other writers (including ourselves) in ascribing these results to a total loss of the grapheme-phoneme route. There are three potential sources of the impairment.
(a) There could be a fault in the transmission of the graphemic information to the system responsible for the application of the rules. In the absence of evidence to the contrary, however, we suppose that the graphemic information used by the non-lexical route is comparable to that used by the visual logogen system. Such information generally appears to reach the logogens in good condition, so there is no obvious reason to suppose otherwise for the grapheme-phoneme system.
(b) There could be a breakdown in the rule system itself. This has probably been the most common assumption, and seems compatible with the fact that the patients cannot even (very well) identify a spoken non-word ('deet') as matching a written non-word (*deet*). However, a careful interpretation of this result reflects only that the patients cannot *access* non-lexical phonological codes and not that the system is incapable of obtaining them. It is thus difficult in

principle to distinguish between a breakdown at this level and the next option.

(c) The fault could be in transmission of phonological information, adequately obtained by application of intact grapheme-phoneme rules, to the response buffer. This would obviously require a demonstration of functioning grapheme-phoneme rules, which is likely to be a difficult order. The only even potentially relevant evidence we know is patient V.S.'s (Saffran and Marin, 1977) good ability to judge which of two printed non-words (e.g. EVAR vs. DVCE) is more word-like. Saffran and Marin interpret this as reflecting pure orthographic knowledge, and we are in sympathy with that conclusion; but we acknowledge (as they did) that regularity of orthography and ease of grapheme-phoneme conversion co-vary, making it difficult to be certain which is the relevant variable. Our motivation for hypothesising that the fault might be in code transmission rather than code production (and it does need to be motivated when there is no evidence that these patients can produce phonological codes non-lexically) is as follows. If there were impaired access to the response buffer for a non-lexical phonological code, it might become plausible to postulate impaired access to the response buffer for any phonological code. In this way we could account for the patients' other problems in reading and manipulating phonological codes without postulating yet another source of trouble. Since we cannot for the present resolve the question of the non-lexical grapheme-phoneme impairment, we shall go on briefly to discuss two tasks involving lexically obtained phonology.

1 *Rhyme judgments.* Deep dyslexic patients (our two plus Saffran and Marin's) understand the concept of rhymes, can accurately judge whether an auditorily presented pair of words rhymes, and can judge whether a visually presented pair rhymes *provided that* visual similarity is correlated with presence/absence of rhyme. Thus they will correctly respond 'yes' to *coast-toast* and 'no' to *land-heel* with visual presentation, but will generally respond 'no' to *come-sum* and 'yes' to *bear-fear*. This result could be viewed as something of a puzzle, as the task requests lexically obtained phonology, not non-lexical grapheme-phoneme conversion. Provided the patient can read the two words in a pair, he ought to be able to judge whether they rhyme. It is not clear, however, what proportion of these words the patients could read: Saffran and Marin report no reading data; we collected reading data on the words used in the

rhyme task but not at the same time, and reading performance by these patients is much less than perfectly consistent. If taken with that caveat, however, our reading data contain at least some cases where both words were read correctly of a pair on which the rhyme judgment was incorrect (e.g. *loose-juice* and *cough-bough*). This suggests either (a) that though the phonological codes for these words were available, the patients did not make use of them in the rhyme decision, preferring perhaps to operate a purely visual strategy; or (b) that they were trying to use a phonological code but have a generalised problem in accessing, storing and/or comparing phonological codes. If we accept the latter sort of account, we must explain how rhyme judgments are correctly made on visually presented pairs like *coast-toast* and on auditorily presented pairs. For the former, we could postulate that the patients attempt a combination of visual and phonological strategies which will usually provide the right answer for *coast-toast*. With auditory presentation, the judgments could be based on an acoustic code, perhaps involving pre-categorical acoustic storage (Morton, 1970). This might be tested by inserting an interval between the two words to be compared, or by asking for rhyme judgments on non-words.

2 *Syllable manipulations.* P.W. can, at least under certain conditions, remove a syllable from a phonological code prior to producing a response. As described by Morton and Patterson, he has over the years been given phonological cues to help him read function words aloud. These include a variety of types, some much more successful than others, but one type of especial interest involves syllable manipulations. Mostly these require him to delete a syllable from a familiar (non-function!) word to obtain the function word, as in *Wendy* → *Wen(dy)* → 'when'. These cues do not always work. Sometimes when the cue is not only several syllables but also several words (as in *evensong* → *even(song)* → 'even') he deletes the wrong one, such that *even* → 'song'. This is even better evidence for phonological manipulation than his successful responses for it demonstrates that he is following a procedure. The procedure involves internal generation of the mediating word (*evensong*) in a phonological form, followed by division at a syllable boundary. One of these syllables/words has then to be selected. If he always produced the correct response it could be argued that he had set up a new 'S-R' connection. The error demonstrates the procedure – which then requires an account.

Part-of-speech and word class effects

Whether a deep dyslexic patient will be able to read any given word is somewhat predictable as a function of the word's part-of-speech and also how abstract it is.[6] These effects are obviously not wholly independent; Shallice and Warrington (1975) attempted to separate them, and concluded that some but not all of the part-of-speech effect was probably attributable to abstractness. In any case, for present purposes we do not require a more refined description than this: the patients can read imageable nouns and adjectives well (giving either correct reading responses or meaning-preserving semantic or derivational paralexias), verbs rather poorly, and function words and abstract content words very poorly indeed. Both of the latter classes yield many omissions but also some paralexias, which for the function words tend to be substitutions of a different function word.

Interpretation
We have already discussed some aspects of these phenomena in previous sections. There is no reason to suppose that linguistic and semantic dimensions should be germane to logogens (either input or output) and these effects are therefore attributed to impairments and/or biases in the cognitive system. In any case, a problem at the level of visual input logogen is ruled out by the fact that in lexical decision both patients are virtually perfect on function words. The impairment cannot be assigned simply to semantics, since we have shown (in our other chapter in this book) that P.W. has a startling degree of comprehension for individual function words. We thus assume that in order to read a function word aloud, the simple route of input logogen → semantic system → output logogen will not suffice, that there must be cooperation from an additional system. We had in the past toyed with the idea that this additional system might be non-lexical grapheme-phoneme conversion, but 1) there is no good reason why that mechanism should be sensitive to linguistic variables, and 2) Coltheart (Chapter 10 this volume) has persuaded us that there is no good evidence for the operation of grapheme-phoneme coding in normal reading. A much better candidate seems to us to be the linguistic processor in the cognitive system. Linguistic processing is severely impaired in our patients, both in production and comprehension. We hypothesise that, without an input-output

logogen connection, and unlike content words for which a purely semantic specification will suffice, function words cannot be produced or acted upon unless there is structural relational information forthcoming from the linguistic processor. This notion seems compatible with our surprising observation that P.W. knows about the meaning of the printed word *on* (he can pair it with *above* rather than *below*) but cannot correctly perform the written instruction *Put the book on the saucer.*

One of the most intriguing phenomena regarding function word reading is the frequency of other function words as responses. The rate is higher when the patients are reading homogeneous lists of function words; but even when mixed with content words, function words selectively and frequently yield other function words as responses (26 per cent of responses in a mixed list of function and content words. The proportion of function word responses to content words is as near to zero as we can determine). The implications of this are that (a) function words as a class are peculiar in some way(s) to which the patients are sensitive, certainly semantic and possibly orthographic as well (at least for th- and wh- words); (b) the problem in producing function words is probably not response blocking. Various function words are by no means equally probable as substitution responses, but words occur as substitutions which cannot be produced when presented as stimuli.

We have less to say on the topic of abstractness. For highly abstract words which D.E. misses in lexical decision, a simple conclusion of impaired (or even absent) semantics will suffice, especially since he misses many of these same words in auditory lexical decision. But P.W. (whose reading of abstract words is scarcely better than D.E.'s) does not miss these words in lexical decision, and even D.E. only misses one-third of them while failing to read almost 90 per cent of them. As already indicated, a satisfactory account will have to wait until we have more data on comprehension of those abstract words which are successfully recognised as legitimate words. For abstract words which are not comprehended, it makes sense that reading should yield a high rate of omissions and some visual paralexias. There are, however, also semantic paralexias on abstract words (e.g. *conscience* → 'honesty', *oblivion* → 'infinity') and in auditory-visual matching on these, the patients tend to choose the paralexic response in preference to the correct word (Patterson, 1978). We interpret this set of words as partially comprehended but producing a semantic specification which, on its own, is inadequate to select the correct output logogen.

A *pro tem* summary

This summary will be far from complete but it is the most that we can agree upon for the moment. The conclusions are primarily germane to reading behaviour but other tasks occasionally creep in.

1   The non-lexical grapheme-phoneme route is non-functional, though we cannot yet pinpoint the exact nature of the breakdown. This accounts for the poor or non-existent performance on any non-lexical phonological manipulations, and for the fact that all reading responses (even to non-words) are real words.
2   The connection from visual input to output logogens is non-functional. This predicts that the patients should never produce as a reading response a word which they do not at least partially understand (barring of course the possibility of totally random perturbation in the addressing from semantic code to output logogen).
3   There is no firm evidence that the visual input logogens are malfunctioning, since all of the behaviours which might have been thought to show this (omissions, visual paralexias, misses in lexical decision) reveal semantic dimensions such as abstractness effects. Thus,
4   Semantics for certain words (particularly abstract ones) are probably impaired, accounting for visual paralexias, some omissions, and misses in lexical decision.
5   It is only for some words that the semantic code uniquely identifies one output logogen; this may even be true for normal readers. For the patients, who have no other code, abstract words and words with close synonyms will yield semantic paralexias which are unidentifiable as errors.
6   Either the output logogens for some words (though what defines the set and how consistently is embarrassingly unclear) have heightened thresholds; or there is a problem in transmission from semantic code to these output logogens. One of these options accounts for some omissions and those semantic paralexias which the patients can identify as errors.

7 The linguistic processor in the cognitive system is impaired, accounting for derivational paralexias and possibly function word errors.

8 Very tentatively, there may be impeded access to the response buffer, which would produce difficulty in all kinds of responding. This would simplify some aspects of the account, though we would still have to explain the unequal degree to which the response buffer seems to accept different sorts and sources of input.

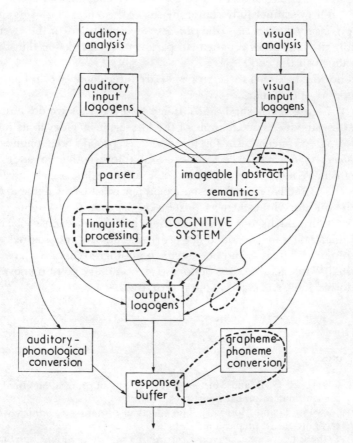

FIGURE 4.3 An expansion of Figure 4.2b; the hypothesised locations of functional impairments in our deep dyslexic patients are indicated by dotted lines

We have attempted a pictorial representation of this summary in Figure 4.3, which no doubt requires some comment.

(a) The cognitive system has been elaborated into several processes, some notions about which can be found in Morton (1968). To give a very minimal idea here, we mean by

1   *semantics* – the processes which allow a patient to pair the word *up* with *top* (rather than *bottom*) and to produce the reading response *oblivion* → 'infinity'.

2   *parser* – the processes which allow a patient to judge that a sentence is ungrammatical (see our other chapter in this book) even if he cannot fully comprehend the sentence.

3   *linguistic processing* – the processes which would (if they were functioning) allow a patient to perform the instruction 'Put the saucer on the cup'.

The way in which these processes are inter-connected in Figure 4.3 is pure speculation.

(b) Figure 4.3 is surely incomplete both in ways we do and don't know about. As an example of the former, it includes in its present format no mechanism for the effects of pseudo-homophones (e.g. *brane*) in normals (see Coltheart, Chapter 10 this volume). Such effects require that the result of grapheme-phoneme conversion, either directly or via the response buffer, must be available to either the auditory input logogen system or the cognitive system.

(c) Our conclusions about the impairments in deep dyslexia are indicated by heavy dotted lines surrounding the impaired system or impaired access from one system to another. Where we have been unable to decide among options (e.g. summary point 6 above), the dotted lines encompass both alternatives.

Notes

1   Clarke, R. G. B. and Morton, J. The effects of priming on visual word recognition. In preparation.

2   Jackson, A. and Morton, J. The effects of priming on auditory word recognition. In preparation.

3   If the time interval between pre-training and recognition were of the order of several seconds, it might be possible to account for the facilitation on the basis of the semantic relationship between *sees* and *seen* (e.g. Meyer, Schvaneveldt and Ruddy, 1975). Since the interval

was as long as 45 minutes, we do not feel this is a plausible alternative.
4 Since this was the description tentatively offered for generation of visual paralexias, we must explain how it can yield omissions as well. We have little to say except that the two events might commence in the same way, terminating in a paralexia if a highly activated alternative candidate is available and in an omission if one is not. Even this notion feels inadequate: the degree of visual/graphemic similarity shown by some visual paralexias suggests a lenient, not a strict criterion, such that some alternative ought almost always to be available. For the present, this remains a problem.
5 In parallel with the previous footnote on omissions vs. visual paralexias as produced by a semantic system fault, we need to explain when response blocking should yield an omission and when a semantic paralexia. Once again we can offer only the obvious: a paralexia if another candidate word fits the semantic specification well enough, an omission if none other will do. And there is the same cause for unease: the relationship between word presented and semantic paralexia is often loose enough to make the omissions seem a puzzle.
6 We prefer to refer simply to the 'abstractness effect', finessing the question of whether it is imageability or concreteness or operativity (or whether, indeed, these are separable dimensions) that is the relevant opposite of abstractness. Where we require a single word for this quality, we shall use 'imageability' on the basis of Richardson's (1975) evidence on patients and Marcel and Patterson's (1978) on normals.

References

Holmes, J. M. (1978) 'Regression' and reading breakdown. In A. Caramazza and E. B. Zurif (eds), *Language Acquisition and Language Breakdown: Parallels and Divergencies*. Baltimore: Johns Hopkins Press.

James, C. T. (1975) The role of semantic information in lexical decisions. *Journal of Experimental Psychology: Human Perception and Performance, 104,* 130–6.

Marcel, A. J. and Patterson, K. E. (1978) Word recognition and production: reciprocity in clinical and normal research. In J. Requin (ed.), *Attention and Performance*, VII. Hillsdale: Lawrence Erlbaum.

Marshall, J. C. and Newcombe, F. (1966) Syntactic and semantic errors in paralexia. *Neuropsychologia, 4,* 169–76.

Marshall, J. C. and Newcombe, F. (1973) Patterns of paralexia: a psycholinguistic approach. *Journal of Psycholinguistic Research, 2,* 175–99.

Marshall, J. C. and Newcombe, F. (1977) Variability and constraint in acquired dyslexia. In H. A. Whitaker and H. Whitaker (eds), *Studies in Neurolinguistics*, vol. III. New York: Academic Press.

Meyer, D. E., Schvaneveldt, R. W. and Ruddy, M. G. (1975) Loci of contextual effects on visual word-recognition. In P. M. A. Rabbitt and S. Dornic (eds), *Attention and Performance*, V. London: Academic Press.

Morton, J. (1964) A model for continuous language behaviour. *Language and Speech*, 7, 40–70.

Morton, J. (1968) Grammar and computation in language behaviour. In J. C. Catford (ed.), *Studies in Language and Language Behaviour.* C.R.L.L.B. Progress Report No. VI, University of Michigan.

Morton, J. (1970) A functional model for memory. In D. A. Norman (ed.), *Models for Human Memory.* New York: Academic Press.

Murrell, G. A. and Morton, J. (1974) Word recognition and morphemic structure. *Journal of Experimental Psychology, 102,* 963–8.

Oatley, K. (1978) *Perceptions and Representations: The Theoretical Bases of Brain Research and Psychology.* London: Methuen.

Patterson, K. E. (1978) Phonemic dyslexia: errors of meaning and the meaning of errors. *Quarterly Journal of Experimental Psychology, 30,* 587–601.

Patterson, K. E. (1979) What is right with 'deep' dyslexic patients? *Brain and Language, 8,* 111–29.

Patterson, K. E. and Marcel, A. J. (1977) Aphasia, dyslexia and the phonological coding of written words. *Quarterly Journal of Experimental Psychology, 29,* 307–18.

Richardson, J. T. E. (1975) The effect of word imageability in acquired dyslexia. *Neuropsychologia, 13,* 281–8.

Saffran, E. M. and Marin, O. S. M. (1977) Reading without phonology: evidence from aphasia. *Quarterly Journal of Experimental Psychology, 29,* 515–25.

Schwartz, M. F., Marin, O. S. M. and Saffran, E. M. (1979) Dissociations of language function in dementia: a case study. *Brain and Language, 7,* 277–306.

Shallice, T. and Warrington, E. K. (1975) Word recognition in a phonemic dyslexic patient. *Quarterly Journal of Experimental Psychology, 27,* 187–99.

Warrington, E. K. (1975) The selective impairment of semantic memory. *Quarterly Journal of Experimental Psychology, 27,* 635–57.

Winnick, W. A. and Daniel, S. A. (1970) Two kinds of response priming in tachistoscopic recognition. *Journal of Experimental Psychology, 84,* 74–81.

5 Single and multiple component central dyslexic syndromes

Tim Shallice and Elizabeth K. Warrington

A variety of acquired dyslexic syndromes have now been described. Certain types of reading difficulties may be grouped together, in that they all result in the patient not attaining a satisfactory visual word-form.[1] These include dyslexia consequent upon neglect (Kinsbourne and Warrington, 1962a), attentional dyslexia (Shallice and Warrington, 1977) and spelling dyslexia (Wolpert, 1924; Kinsbourne and Warrington, 1962b), which we view as damage to the visual word-form system itself (Warrington and Shallice, 1978; 1980). This group we term the peripheral dyslexias.

Another group of acquired dyslexias may be regarded as the central dyslexias. In the central dyslexias the visual word-form system is assumed to be operating normally and the disorder results from damage to one or more of the 'routes' by which words are read (with phonological recoding or by direct access to meaning) and/or from a deficit at the level of semantic processing.

This classification has little in common with that current in neurology where the emphasis is on the pattern of concomitant deficits, but much in common with that proposed by Marshall and Newcombe (1973). We have introduced different terms because it is clear that Marshall and Newcombe's classification – visual, surface and deep – does not exhaust the variety of dyslexic disorders that exist, and therefore a more global terminology seems appropriate.

In this paper we intend to consider deep/phonemic dyslexia (defined as in Appendix 1) in the light of the range of central

We are grateful to Dr P. Rudge, Dr W. Gooddy and Professor P. K. Thomas for permission to study and report our findings on patients under their care. This research was supported by a Project Grant from the Medical Research Council.

119

dyslexic syndromes of which we are aware. We accept the standard view (e.g. Marshall and Newcombe, 1973) that the neuropsychological evidence, like that from experimental psychology, supports the existence of two main reading routes.[2] On our approach they consist of the 'direct' (or 'visual') route from the visual word-form system to the semantic system and the 'phonological route' from the visual word-form system to phonological processing systems. However, as we now consider that deep/phonemic dyslexia, as commonly described, represents a class of multi-component dyslexic syndromes, it becomes relevant to assess them within the framework of cases which we will argue represent single-component central dyslexic syndromes.

Single-component dyslexic syndromes

1 Semantic dyslexia – impairment of direct route reading

Marshall and Newcombe (1973) have argued for the existence of a syndrome 'surface dyslexia', which they view as characterized by the relative preservation of reading by phonological recoding and with a gross impairment of 'direct reading' (resulting in what we will call 'phonological reading'). In fact, one would expect theoretically a number of different syndromes to have in common the phenomenon of phonological reading. For instance, phonological reading would be predicted to occur either if there is an inability to transmit information from the visual word-form system to the semantic system or if the semantic system itself is impaired. In either case, the properties of the reading performance would depend not only on the nature of the information transmitted by the phonological route but how this information is used by the semantic systems. Marshall and Newcombe (1973) characterize the errors made by their surface dyslexics as 'partial failures of grapheme/phoneme correspondence rules'. However, their examples are of two forms. Some, e.g. 'disease'-'decease', may be characterized as misapplications of valid correspondence rules (*s* normally being soft in 'dis' (Wijk, 1966)). Others, e.g. 'resent'-'rissend', where the term 'partial failure' seems appropriate, support their claim that not only was the direct route damaged but so was the phonological route to a lesser extent.

In view of the relative dearth of case reports of such patients, and the possible problem of interpretation, we describe a patient whose reading could be characterized by the failure of the 'direct' route.

Case report 1

R.O.G. (born 1904) a left-handed housewife had a subarachnoid haemorrhage in 1960. She made a good recovery apart from occasional epileptiform fits which have occurred since then. In 1975 after an attack of giddiness and vertigo she observed that her reading and spelling had become impaired. There was evidence of cortical atrophy on the EMI scan. It was thought most probable that a recent vascular accident was responsible for her reading and spelling difficulties.

R.O.G. was tested on a shortened version of the WAIS and obtained a verbal IQ of 93 and a performance IQ of 111. Her expressive speech was fluent and there were only occasional word finding difficulties. Her object naming was satisfactory (14/15 correct), on naming objects from their description her performance was weak (10/15 correct) and on the shortened version of the Token Test her performance was entirely normal (14/15 correct). (For further details of these tests for dysphasia see Coughlan and Warrington, 1978.) Her spelling was very poor (but not formally tested) and her reading was quite impaired: she scored 25/100 correct on the Schonell graded word list and 0/25 correct on the first half of the New Adult Reading Test (NART) (Nelson and O'Connell, 1978). It was observed that she read very slowly and that she had particular difficulty with words which were not regular in their spelling.

R.O.G. was able to point to named letters (26/26 correct). She had some difficulty in naming letters and often produced the letter name after uttering the letter sound. She named 13/26 letters directly and she 'sounded' the remaining 13 letters.

On the Coltheart word list (Coltheart, Davelaar, Jonasson and Besner, 1979) she read 36/39 regular words and 25/39 irregular words. This reading was achieved very slowly; her reading rate was 5.6 seconds and 6.4 seconds per word for the regular and irregular words respectively. Her attempt to read the Schonell words was timed and her reading rate appears to be related to the number of syllables in the word. Considering only those words which she read accurately, her reading rate for 1 syllable words (N = 12) was 4.2 seconds per word, for 2 syllable words (N = 9) was 10.2 seconds and for 2+ syllable words (N = 4) 26.5 seconds. All the reading errors recorded involved the misapplication of a grapheme/phoneme conversion rule (including the application of an inappropriate conversion rule) e.g. *nephew* → 'nepu' and *broad* → 'brōd'. Words correctly pronounced appeared to be comprehended.

In R.O.G. the primary defect appears to be in the transmission of information from the visual word-form system to the semantic system, which is in line with Marshall and Newcombe's (1973) interpretation of their two patients. Another class of patients, however, who it has been claimed, have deficits of the semantic memory system itself – those cases of associative agnosia described by Warrington (1975) – also appear to read using the 'phonological route'. She described three patients who appeared to have special difficulty reading words which did not obey standard grapheme-phoneme rules. Thus one of the three patients, E.M., read 28/39 regular words correctly, but only 5/39 irregular words from the Coltheart list at a time when her dementing illness was very advanced. Moreover, when trying to read the irregular words her errors were nearly always attempts to produce phonologically appropriate renderings.

These three patients were selected for study for reasons entirely independent of their reading and it appeared that their phonological processing was virtually normal. It would therefore be plausible to explain their reading performance as resulting from a deficit in reading by the direct route to the semantic system thus allowing the characteristics of phonological reading to become apparent. These observations would then support the position for which both Green and Shallice (1976) and Coltheart (1978) have argued, namely that the phonological route operates primarily pre-lexically, using word components (misleadingly termed grapheme components by Green and Shallice) or graphemes.

Such a view, however, may be over-simple. Schwartz, Marin and Saffran (1979) have studied the reading of a patient W.L.P. whose deficits of semantic processing are in many respects similar to those of the patients studies by Warrington (1975).[3] She was able to read 20 pairs of high frequency words having similar spellings but dissimilar pronunciations, e.g. home-come. As these words may have been within her vocabulary, given her Peabody picture-vocabulary raw score of 56, this is not compelling evidence that she was able to read irregular words she did not comprehend; but it does indeed raise the possibility. More detailed examination of E.M.'s reading performance during an earlier phase of her dementing illness, provides further evidence for the view that irregular words are not entirely dependent on direct route reading. At a time when she obtained only 69/100 on the Peabody test, she scored 47/60 on the 60 most difficult words of the Schonell, which included 12/16 words judged irregular by Coltheart (personal communication) such as *smoulder, nourished, conscience* and *beguile.*

These results might appear to be most easily explained on a three-route theory in which an additional route is postulated for transmitting information about whole word-forms from the visual to the articulatory system (referred to by Morton and Patterson (in Chapter 4) as the connection between the visual input logogen and the auditory output logogen). Phonological reading then requires that two systems be inoperative, the direct route to the semantic system and this latter route.

In our view a preferable position is to assume that only two routes are required but that phonological recoding does not just operate on graphemes as Coltheart (1978) suggests, but also on larger visual units including syllables and short words. The ease of operation of the route would vary with the frequency in the language with which a particular letter combination occurs with a particular sound and inversely with the frequency with which alternative pronunciations of the letter string occur. For such a process to work, different possible parsings of a letter string may have to be made with the phonological system accepting the most word-like as valid. On this view as the phonological route becomes increasingly impaired so the frequency with which a particular visual-auditory mapping of a letter combination would need to occur in order to be utilized, would increase.

Some support for this position is obtained by examining the errors made by E.M. on the Schonell, on the occasion on which she scored 47/60. Ignoring her attempts to read rows 19 and 20 (the most low frequency words) her errors were on *choir, intercede, siege, colonel, susceptible* and *scintillate. Choir* and *colonel* are probably the most irregular words on the Schonell list, and were pronounced 'chore' and 'col . . on . . el' respectively. *Scintillate,* a regular word, was pronounced 'sk . . .'. Although the regular pronunciation of sci is (s) there are far more examples of an initial sc as (sk) in English. Over four times as many types occur in the Thorndike-Lorge word list. Thus an infrequently applied if correct rule is being dominated by one more frequently applied, even though in this situation it is incorrect because it does not respect a constraint. Even in the case of W.L.P. reading short high frequency words, the one word she failed was *bury* in which the (er) sound is a unique rendering of 'ur' (except for *burial*) (Wijk, 1966). It therefore seems plausible for E.M., and even possibly for W.L.P., that even when many somewhat irregular words can be read, the most irregular words which utilize the least frequent visual to auditory mappings, can still produce difficulty.

On this view, the performance of E.M. at this early stage of her illness represents the phonological recoding mechanisms operating in a relatively normal fashion. The later results with E.M. would reflect a stage in which the disease process had affected these mechanisms such that words which deviated in any way from the most frequently applied rules could virtually never be read. Thus she could read virtually none of the words (5/39) judged as in any way irregular by Coltheart (personal communication).

If this view is correct, then the implications for the interpretation of deep/phonemic dyslexia are important. If a patient cannot utilize grapheme-phoneme correspondences, the phonological recoding mechanisms would be so impaired that all forms of phonological reading would be impossible. Any observed reading abilities must then depend upon the operation of the 'direct' semantic route alone.

A terminological problem is posed by the phonological reading that arises in conjunction with associative agnosia. A dyslexia resulting primarily within the domain of semantic processing should presumably be a 'deep dyslexia'. Yet it manifests itself as a 'surface dyslexia'! Thus these terms seem inappropriate for the syndromes to which they have been applied.

2 Phonological dyslexia – impairment of 'phonological route' reading

The effects of a specific deficit to the phonological route have been a matter of theoretical concern over the last few years. A number of authors have either argued that the phonological route is necessary for certain classes of words to be read (e.g. function words, verbs, abstract nouns) or have held that this was at least a possibility (e.g. Allport, 1977; Marcel and Patterson, 1978; Saffran, Schwartz and Marin, 1976; Shallice and Warrington, 1975). The existence of patients who have an impairment of the phonological route but no deficit for any particular class of words then becomes important theoretically. Beauvois and Dérouesné (1978) have described four patients of this type.

We have recently studied two such patients in whom there appeared to be a highly selective deficit involving grapheme/ phoneme transformations. So selective was this deficit that though their reading skills for English approached very closely to an average adult level, neither nonsense syllables nor nonsense words could be attempted with any degree of success. For clinical reasons our observations on one of these patients are very incomplete but are referred to here as they provide some corroborative support for the phenomenon of a patient being able to read real words but not nonsense words.

Case Report 2

G.R.N. (born 1940) a right-handed school teacher, who had trained at a teacher training college, sustained a closed head injury one year prior to being referred to the psychology department for assessment of her language difficulties.

She was tested on a shortened version of the WAIS and obtained a verbal IQ of 94 and a performance IQ of 104. The only verbal test on which she scored below the average level was Digit Span (5 digits forwards, 3 backwards). Her expressive speech functions appeared to be relatively intact, and only occasional word finding difficulty was noted in her spontaneous speech. On the Oldfield naming test she scored 19/26. She scored 18/50 on the NART (Nelson and O'Connell, 1978) which is equivalent to a reading IQ of 102. She read 16/20 words from the first column of the Schonell graded reading test which prorated gives a Schonell reading IQ of 101 (Nelson and McKenna, 1975). Her performance on this test was essentially unchanged two years later (73/100). At this time she was able to score 84/100 on a written word/picture matching test (adapted from the Peabody picture vocabulary test). In contrast her spelling was markedly impaired. On the Schonell graded spelling test she scored 1/20 on the first column (oral) and 6/20 on the second column (written) which is the level of a 6–7-year-old child. Two years later (1978) she was only able to score 3/40 (oral), 22/60 (written), which reflects quite a marked deficit. Individual letters were named with only very occasional errors but she had much more difficulty in 'sounding' the individual letters. Two years later this was no longer a problem.

She attempted to read 40 high frequency words (AA) and 40 pronounceable non-words (3, 4, 5 letters in both sets) which were presented in blocks of 10 using an ABBA design. She read 39/40 real words correctly but only 3/40 non-words. In 10 of the 32 errors on the non-words, real words were produced as responses e.g. *tix* → 'trick'. Twelve errors involved consonants alone as in *vit* → 'vick'; 7 involved vowels alone as in *clest* → 'calest'; 13 involved both as in *nup* → 'yem'. Twenty monosyllabic (4–5 letters) words, ten of which had frequencies of A or AA and ten of which had frequencies in the range 3–39, were presented in random order with 20 pronounceable non-words (4 and 5 letters). She read correctly 19/20 real words but only 1/20 nonsense words.

Case Report 3

B.T.T. (born 1948) a left-handed 29-year-old systems analyst was admitted to the National Hospital having sustained a subarachnoid haemorrhage. Angiography demonstrated an aneurism arising from the origin of the left posterior communicating artery. She was successfully treated surgically and she made a rapid recovery. She was referred to the psychology department post-operatively for assessment of her residual language difficulties which in fact were resolving very rapidly.

She was seen in the psychology department between 16 and 18 January 1978. She was tested on the shortened version of the WAIS and obtained a verbal IQ of 76 and a performance IQ of 102. Her digit span was particularly poor (4 forwards, 2 backwards). She succeeded in scoring at an average level on the Similarities subtest but her expressive speech was halting and her phrase length was short, and this is reflected in her below average score on the Vocabulary subtest. On the Oldfield naming test she scored 26/26 correct and she scored 13/15 correct in naming words from their description but only 7/15 on a shortened version of the Token test.

At this time she was unable to spell aloud any of the words from the Schonell graded word list. Her reading was relatively unimpaired whereas she had considerable difficulty in reading nonsense syllables.

She read 20 high frequency words (10 high concrete and 10 low concrete) without error. She read 27/30 low frequency high concrete words and 24/30 low frequency, low concrete words, and she read 10/10 function words. In contrast she was only able to read 9/18 nonsense syllables. She showed a tendency to read these nonsense syllables as real words (e.g. *bef* → 'beef'; *fod* → 'food'; *vag* → 'vague').

How closely the deficits of these patients corresponded to those of the patients studied by Beauvois and Dérouesné (1978) is as yet unclear. The crucial point however, is that they, too, were unable to read pronounceable non-words and at the same time had relatively normal word reading.

The obvious interpretation of this syndrome is that if the direct route is operating normally, then even a gross impairment of the phonological route is not by itself sufficient to produce the syndrome observed in G.R. and K.F. It might be argued, however, that the deficit in nonsense syllable reading arises from an output deficit. Yet, as one patient had relatively intact expressive speech functions and could reproduce auditorially presented nonsense syllables easily and the other had virtually no difficulty in word repetition, this possibility seems very implausible. In addition the patients of Beauvois and Dérouesné were described as not aphasic.

The preceding argument that elimination of the phonological route would not be sufficient to produce the deep/phonemic dyslexic syndrome, depends upon the acceptance of a two-route position. On the three-route position damage to the grapheme-phoneme route, as in phonological alexia, would not necessarily reveal the characteristics of the 'direct' route, as a third route would be available for transmission of information about whole word-forms as discussed earlier. A further neuropsychological argument which does not require acceptance of the two-route position can also be advanced to reject the possibility that deep dyslexia reflects the sparing of the 'direct' route with all other reading systems being inoperative. Consider the comparison between deep/phonemic dyslexia and the dyslexic difficulties of a patient A.R., recently reported by us (Warrington and Shallice, 1979). A.R.'s pattern of word reading was very different from that found in previously reported patients but he, too, appeared to be reading by means of the 'direct' route. There was relatively little effect of part-of-speech and much less effect of imageability than that reported previously in deep/phonemic dyslexic patients. Thus even when a large number of errors are produced by a patient who is attempting to read by the 'direct' route the pattern of performance previously reported is not necessarily found. Moreover, A.R.'s pattern of deficit cannot be attributed to the deep/phonemic dyslexic syndrome together with an additional deficit, as on some classes of words (e.g. function words, verbs, abstract nouns) he performs much better than the more typical patients and only on one class of word, namely concrete nouns, worse.[4]

Beauvois and Dérouesné (1978) have suggested that the highly specific syndrome consequent upon the lack of the phonological route should be called 'phonological alexia'. We agree, that the term we previously suggested for the less specific syndrome, namely 'phonemic dyslexia' was inappropriately applied, and we would now wish to use it as a synonym for their 'phonological alexia'.

Multi-component dyslexic syndromes

In our view the deep/phonemic dyslexic cases reported to date (see Appendix 1) represent one, or as we will claim, more than one subclass of the multi-component central dyslexic syndromes. This view has been partially anticipated by Marshall and Newcombe (1973) and Patterson (1978) who have suggested that a deficit additional to that of the phonological route is implicated in deep/phonemic dyslexia. However, there is little agreement as to the locus of this additional deficit. Four possible candidates seem plausible. 1) the visual logogen (Patterson, 1978); 2) access to the semantic system; 3) processing within the semantic system (Weigl and Bierwisch, 1970; Patterson, 1979); 4) phonological retrieval following semantic processing (Marshall and Newcombe, 1966; Marcel and Patterson, 1978; Patterson, 1978).

The last of these alternatives has been the most popular one. Thus Marshall and Newcombe argue that G.R.'s deficit arises after the 'full dictionary entry' has been attained as a result of breakdown 'in encoding this specification into the appropriate phonological form'. Marcel and Patterson (1978) write that 'phonemic dyslexics have impaired access to output phonology from left hemisphere semantics' and Patterson (1978) attributes a major role to a failure of the output logogen in her patients D.E. and P.W. Difficulties in naming are indeed common in aphasics. If we turn to the domain of nominal dysphasia, there is ample evidence that semantic errors occur. Thus Schuell and Jenkins (1961) found that 29 per cent of non-correct responses were semantic errors in naming by aphasics when presented with *both* a picture and the written word corresponding to it. Coughlan (1976) found that of all non-correct responses (i.e. including omissions) 12 per cent of object naming responses and 14 per cent of naming from description responses were semantic errors. Moreover semantic errors have been shown to occur when comprehension has been demonstrated to be intact (e.g. Weisenburg and McBride, 1935, cases 4, 28 and 48); thus in the somewhat special case of optic aphasia reported by Lhermitte and Beauvois (1973) the patient misnamed many objects he could identify as shown by mime, and the misnamings were very frequently semantic errors. In addition, it is known that nominal errors can be category specific (Goodglass *et al.*, 1966; McKenna and Warrington, 1978). Indeed more recently it has been claimed that they can be specific to the written word (Hécaen and Kremin, 1976). Thus a (possibly specific) nominal deficit seems a not implausible candidate for the additional defect in the deep/phonemic dyslexic.

There is indeed considerable support for such a position. Thus patient V.S. of Saffran and Marin (1977) performed at an IQ level of 120 on the Peabody Picture-Vocabulary Test with written words, very little inferior to her auditory performance. She was also able to demonstrate comprehension of over 80 per cent of words with frequencies ranging down to 1 per million by providing a synonym, or an appropriate gesture or mime. It is clear that a considerable proportion of these words could not be read aloud. Thus it seems reasonable to assume that the semantic representation has been adequately accessed and therefore by inference to make the suggestion of a post-lexical phonological ('nominal') deficit plausible. Evidence supporting a 'nominal' interpretation has also been obtained from the use of the lexical decision test. Patterson (1979) has shown that P.W. performs at a normal level on this test for abstract words only a few of which can be read. It remains unclear how specific a semantic representation is required to perform lexical decision satisfactorily, but as will be discussed below, it would seem to require a relatively high degree of specificity (except possibly for function words). However, not all deep/phonemic dyslexics can perform it (see Shallice and Coughlan, 1980).

By contrast, though, there is evidence that deficits other than 'nominal' ones must be involved in deep dyslexia in addition to that of the pre-lexical phonological route. In particular it appears that a specific deficit in achieving the semantic (and syntactic) representation of words from visual input can exist at a level higher than the visual word-form unit. As mentioned earlier we have recently reported the dyslexic difficulties of a patient A.R., which have properties 1 and 4 in common with deep dyslexia but not 2 and 3 (Warrington and Shallice, 1979).

On a variety of tests of written word comprehension which demanded the accessing of a relatively specific semantic representation – the Peabody test and miming tasks – and also lexical decision and upper-lower case matching, which should be done satisfactorily if this facility were available, he performed very poorly and far below his level with auditory input. Taking into account his general level of reading, he performed little above chance for words that cannot be read. By contrast, he was able to assign words which cannot be read to an appropriate category at well above chance levels and in some instances, nearly perfectly (see Table 5.1). It therefore appeared that for many words the precise meaning could not be accessed from visual input but broad categorical information could be. This difficulty is not present with auditory input. We argued that the word reading process involves the accessing of information in the cognitive/semantic system through a process of increasing specification of meaning. It would mean that one tends to know that a canary is a bird, before one knows that it is yellow or that it is a cage bird or that it sings well. A.R., we thought, had a deficit in this process of obtaining the increasingly specific semantic representation. As an explanation of certain dyslexic difficulties it bears some resemblance to theories of an inability to access more than the appropriate 'sphere' or 'field' of word-meaning (Goldstein, 1948 (after Lotmar, 1919); Weigl and Bierwisch (1970); Saffran, Schwartz and Marin (1976)). The existence of a semantic access difficulty in a patient who makes semantic errors does not of course necessitate that semantic errors be caused by difficulties of semantic access. Such errors might result from an additional minor nominal deficit.

TABLE 5.1 *Two-choice categorization performance of A.R. for visually presented words he was unable to read (from Warrington and Shallice, 1979)*

Categories used	Reading performance	Categorization of non-read words
Surnames/forenames	9/60	49/51
Boys/girls names	1/60	55/59
Boys/girls (100msec)	2/40	37/38
Authors/politicians	14/100	69/86
Subject/measurement	12/50	31/38
Five concrete categories	38/125	68/87

Following Coltheart (Chapter 6) one can attempt to specify in more detail the nature of the semantic relation between stimulus and response in semantic errors. On an access theory account one might predict that superordinates, or possibly coordinates, should occur. They do occur, particularly coordinates, but errors with a more distant relation are more frequent. One example, which does show a semantic error being induced as part of the access process is the following protocol obtained in a session where A.R. was trying to verbalize on the nature of his reading difficulties. Presented with the written word *honey* he categorized it as an animal. Then he said it was a 'small animal, flying like a bat, smaller than a bat'. Then he said 'buzz' and 'picture of a bee'. By contrast, when it was presented auditorily he said 'made from bees, very nice, very pleasant eating stuff . . . instead of sugar'. Another example which indicates the potentially non-nominal nature of some semantic errors is his response to *thumb* as 'finger . . . no . . . things . . . no . . . thimble'. Such a deletion of a semantically related response for an unrelated one (things) would not be expected for a nominal error, where the patient *knows* what the word means. (A similar phenomenon occurred with K.F., see Shallice and Warrington, 1975). Overall it appears likely but by no means conclusive that semantic errors can occur from difficulties in semantic access.

A specific deficit in attaining the semantic representation of visually presented words can also occur in deep/phonemic dyslexia. We performed one test with K.F. in 1973, the Coughlan and Warrington (1978) Auditory Choice Vocabulary Test, in which the patient has to decide which of two auditorially presented alternatives is a synonym of the stimulus word. With auditory presentation of the stimulus K.F. scored 47/60 (the mean of Coughlan and Warrington's unselected LH group is 48.2). With visual presentation of the stimulus he scored 32/60, significantly worse (McNemar Test p <.01). It should be noted that about 80 per cent of the stimuli are abstract words, such as *precise, lethal, drastic, adept* and *subside*.

More recently one of us has been engaged with Tony Coughlan in a more detailed investigation of the word comprehension abilities of a deep/phonemic dyslexic patient P.S. (see Shallice and Coughlan, 1980). The series of tests was mainly based on the simple categorization method used with A.R. in which auditory presentation acts as a control for visual presentation. The results are shown in Table 5.2. It can be seen that categorization performance on these tests falls into two main classes. On certain tests, labelled A, performance was far superior on auditory presentation to visual presentation of words. Performance on the written words was near chance and auditory performance at ceiling. By contrast on other tests (labelled B) performance was virtually equally good on the auditory and visual version.

There seem to be two possible reasons for the difference in performance on the two types of test (A and B). It could relate either to the nature of the words or the nature of the test. The words involved in type A test may differ qualitatively from those used in type B test. Alternatively, if one presupposes that the semantic representation of words has an underlying structure (e.g. Katz and Fodor, 1963; Warrington, 1975; Miller and Johnson-Laird, 1976) it could be that the underlying structure is more easily 'tapped' by type B tests, so that the access problems are simpler. Thus on the approach developed by Warrington (1975) and Warrington and Shallice (1979) a pleasantness judgment should be more difficult than, say, a subject/measurement judgment because the broad taxonomic category information most easily and rapidly accessed can be used for the latter but not the former judgment. For the present purposes it is not necessary to distinguish between these alternatives, which, in any case, may be related, as it seems likely that the concept of the relatively abstractness of words will only become understood in terms of their structures. However, by contrast with A.R. the difficulties of P.S. and K.F. have to be specific to the more abstract words given their very good performance on concrete words. These results clearly demonstrate that in two deep/phonemic dyslexics there is a specific inability to attain at least some aspects of the semantic representation of visually presented abstract words.

A simple explanation can be given for this finding, which has some similarity to that given by Shallice and Warrington (1975) and Schwartz, Saffran and Marin (1977) for the deep/phonemic dyslexia syndrome, if one assumes that the organization of the semantic representation of words is categorical (using the term 'categorical' in its broadest sense), and that one major subdivision is related to the abstractness of the words. This assumption will be examined in more detail later. The failure of P.S. and K.F. to comprehend abstract words is then explained by assuming that within one of the subdivisions of the verbal semantic system a semantic representation cannot be adequately attained given visual input, even though the visual word-form system is assumed to be operating normally.

This explanation is compatible with the account of visual errors

TABLE 5.2 *Two-choice categorization performance of P.S. on different types of categorical judgment. I and II refer to testing periods, separated by an interval of one year. The 'reading' column includes semantic errors and paraphasic responses where appropriate. (From Shallice and Coughlan, 1980)*

Task		Reading	VISUAL Categorization performance			AUDITORY Categorization
			Unread stimuli	(Chance)	All stimuli	
Words						
A Pleasant/unpleasant	I				30/60	58/60
	II	14/60	28/46	(23)	42/60	57/60
A Financial/thought	II	4/40	17/36	(18)	21/40	40/40
A Coughlan synonyms	I	–	–		18/30	25/30
A Difficult picture						
vocabulary[a]	I	3/35	11/32	(8)	14/35	56/75
B Surnames/forenames	I	18/40	21/22	(11)	38/40	–
	II	15/30	12/15	(7½)	27/30	29/30
B Boys/girls names	I	25/45	16/20	(10)	41/45	–
B Subjects/measurements	I	8/30	18/22	(11)	26/30	–
	I	15/50	26/35	(17½)	41/50	–
	II	15/50	28/35	(17½)	42/50	47/50

[a] Four-choice.

put forward by Shallice and Warrington (1975) and Saffran and Marin (1977). If, in general, the word-form system can activate (differentially) the semantic representations of more than one word – a possibility discussed theoretically by Shallice and McGill (1978) – and in particular patients semantic representations of abstract words (but not concrete words) cannot be adequately activated, given visual input, visual errors then occur. The semantic unit corresponding to a visually similar concrete word may become the most strongly activated semantic unit and so dominate the semantic unit of the correct abstract word. Thus the visual error is produced 'because' the correct abstract meaning cannot be attained.[5]

An alternative explanation of visual errors, given by Patterson (1978), is that they occur because of a deficit within the word-form system. If it is assumed that the visual word-form system is not organized in terms of semantic (and syntactic) classes of words then on this latter theory visual errors should occur roughly equally frequently for all semantic (and syntactic) classes of words. On the more central theory classes of words which are read well should have a lower rate of visual errors (see also Morton and Patterson, Chapter 4). This, in fact, appears to be the case for the deep/phonemic dyslexics in which it has been studied (see Appendix 2), which provides support for the 'central' theory. A second line of argument that visual errors can arise from a more central locus than the visual word-form system is provided by considering the relative difficulty of tachistoscopic reading compared with reading 'across-the-desk'. Damage to the visual word-form system can be assumed to lead to a special difficulty with tachistoscopic presentation as found in spelling dyslexia (Kinsbourne and Warrington, 1962a; Warrington and Shallice, 1978). However, the reading performance of A.R., who made a high rate of visual errors, was as good with the tachistoscope presentation as when given unlimited time (Warrington and Shallice, 1979).

It therefore seems likely that in certain deep/phonemic dyslexic patients semantic errors, visual errors, the effect of concreteness on reading and failures in the comprehension of the written word can all have a common explanation; namely that with written input an adequate semantic representation cannot be achieved for certain classes of words (e.g. abstract nouns), but it can be for other classes (i.e. concrete nouns).

Different forms of deep/phonemic dyslexia

Comparison of deep/phonemic dyslexic patients is hindered by the rarity with which the same tests have been administered to different patients. It remains, for instance, possible that these patients have a similar pattern of multiple deficits, a rather uninteresting conclusion except, perhaps, to adherents of the right hemisphere theory. However, there appear to be at least three known empirical differences between the patients. V.S. performs nearly as well on the written version of the Peabody test as she does on the spoken version (Saffran and Marin, 1977), but P.S. (Shallice and Coughlan, 1980) performs much worse on the written than the spoken version. Secondly, P.W. (Patterson, 1979) performs normally on lexical decisions for abstract words, but P.S. by contrast was quite impaired (only 19/34 correct for abstract words that could not be read). Thirdly, in deep/phonemic dyslexics there are striking differences in the relative frequency of different error types (see Table 5.3).

TABLE 5.3 *The proportion of different types of error made by certain deep/phonemic dyslexic patients (in percentages). The final column gives the percentage of all non-correct responses that were explicit errors (i.e. not omissions). It should be noted that these results were collected on different word pools. However, variation between word pools is very unlikely to account for the variability in the Semantic/Visual differences (e.g. maximum Semantic for A.R. of 6 pools is 8 per cent) or the E/NC effect (ranges: K.F. (5 pools) 15–31 per cent; A.R. (6 pools) 22–45 per cent).*

Patient	Semantic	Visual and/or Semantic	Visual	Derivational	Other	E/NC
P.W.	54	4	13	22	6	82
G.R.	56	?	22	11(?)	11	47
D.E.	23	6	35	32	4	47
W.S.	21	17	35	4	23	59
V.S.	19	16	48	10	7	99
P.S.	10	7	51	9	23	76
K.F.	4	10	61	19	6	25
(A.R.	5	12	57	6	20	34)

Data from Marshall and Newcombe (1966); Patterson (1978); Schwartz, Saffran and Marin (1977); Saffran (personal communication); Shallice and Coughlan (1980); Shallice and Warrington (1975); Warrington and Shallice (1979).

We will consider then the possibility of there being different forms of deep/phonemic dyslexia arising from damage to different functional systems, always in conjunction with an impairment of the phonological route. In particular we would suggest that three types can theoretically be distinguished, one resulting from output difficulties from the verbal semantic system, another from input/ access difficulties (with the visual word-form system operating normally) and another – which will not be discussed further – from damage to verbal semantic memory itself (i.e. associative agnosia together with phonological route damage).

If there are a number of possible causes, why should deep/ phonemic dyslexia have been interpreted as a coherent syndrome? In particular, why should the semantic/syntactic pattern of word reading failures be so similar and why should the same type of errors occur?

The pattern of word-reading errors can be simply explained by the commonly held assumption that neurological differentiations, such as that between the representations of concrete and abstract words, exist within the semantic system (see Shallice and Warrington, 1975; Schwartz, Saffran and Marin, 1977; Marcel and Patterson, 1978). If any part of the system is damaged at either input or output then reading performance will reflect the functioning of the other part. Why this semantic dissociation should exist is unclear, but a frequent suggestion relates to the way children acquire the meaning of words (Goodglass, Hyde and Blumstein, 1969; Shallice and Warrington, 1975; Marcel and Patterson, 1978).[6]

Good independent evidence for the existence of dissociations of this nature derives from that of nouns with verbs and function words in spontaneous speech (see Goodglass and Geschwind, 1976). More directly relevant is the remarkable preservation of the comprehension of abstract words in a patient whose comprehension of concrete words was very bad (Warrington, 1975). For instance, this patient who had no idea of the meanings of *hay*, *poster*, *needle* and *acorn* defined *supplication* as 'making a serious request for help' and *arbiter* 'he is a man who tries to arbitrate. Produce a peaceful solution'. This very strongly supports the existence of a dissociation between abstract and concrete semantic systems.

Such a dissociation does not, however, provide a common explanation for the presence of seemingly similar types of errors. In particular semantic errors need to be explained in different ways. As 'nominal' errors, they would reflect a failure in the process of retrieving an appropriate label. Other types of aphasic nominal errors can show only a loose semantic connection between stimulus and response. Thus Lhermitte and Beauvois (1973) give the examples of *cap* → 'jockey', *helmet* → 'cassock', *comb* → 'toothbrush' in picture naming.

As 'input' errors they would reflect a failure of semantic access. In our earlier paper on deep/phonemic dyslexia, we differentiated semantic errors from what we termed 'paraphasic responses' i.e. responses of a circumlocutory nature using an implicit input/ nominal split. We argued that (input) semantic errors should be either (a) highly semantically similar (e.g. *pencil* → 'Biro'), or (b) lack precision unless abstractly defined (e.g. *fiction* → 'acting') such that the stimulus and response require the operation of the abstract comprehension system in order to be differentiated. Depending upon one's theory of semantic access it is probably necessary to widen these criteria to include, for instance, superordinate and, possibly, coordinate relations as we discussed earlier. However, as Patterson (personal communication) has pointed out, if one assumes that no information can be conveyed by the phonological route, errors occurring prior to the complete semantic representation being attained can only be known to be errors if re-use of the same process produces a different result. In particular, it should be difficult for deep/phonemic dyslexic patients to know that they have made an (input) semantic error. Using our rather narrow criteria Patterson (1978) has shown for both of her deep/phonemic dyslexic patients that if a semantic error satisfies the above criteria, it is significantly more likely to be accepted as the stimulus in a recognition test. This fits well with the assumption that semantic errors can arise from two different causes.

Finally the assumption that semantic errors can arise in two different ways helps to explain why they occur with different rates in different deep/phonemic dyslexic patients (see Table 5.3). The alternative explanation that a highly damaged phonological route can be used by some as a checking process seems unlikely to be the total answer, if only because of the low rate of semantic errors made by K.F. as he appeared to make no use of the phonological route, not being able to sound even single letters.[7] In our view those deep/ phonemic dyslexics whose additional deficit is of the 'input' variety, e.g. K.F. and P.S., would make fewer such errors (by comparison with visual ones) than would patients, e.g. P.W. and V.S., of the 'output' variety. Any unitary theory of deep/phonemic dyslexia seems to have difficulty in accounting for this great variability in error patterns.[8]

In conclusion, we have argued that there are a variety of central acquired dyslexia syndromes and that it is convenient to subdivide these not only in terms of the major route affected but also according to whether it is primarily a single-component dyslexia or a multi-component dyslexia. After presenting evidence for the existence of single-component dyslexic syndromes we have given our argument for regarding deep/phonemic dyslexia as a multi-component syndrome. Further we have attempted to differentiate two distinct types of deep/phonemic dyslexia, each having as their common feature an inoperative phonological route but a different locus for the additional component. For one type an adequate semantic representation of certain classes of visually presented words cannot be achieved; in the other type subsequent to adequate semantic processing, the appropriate verbal label cannot be obtained (a nominal deficit for the written word). If this last differentiation is valid, then it follows that the same anatomical lesion site would not be responsible for all the deep/phonemic dyslexic syndromes. In particular, the view that deep/phonemic dyslexia is the product of right-hemisphere reading systems (Coltheart, Chapter 16, this volume; Saffran, Bogyo, Schwartz and Marin, Chapter 17, this volume) becomes less likely.[9]

We would argue then that the common features of the deep/ phonemic dyslexic syndrome arise from a mosaic of the relative impairment/sparing of the more central systems involved in reading. Among the central dyslexic syndromes, such complexity is not solely a characteristic of deep/phonemic dyslexia. Thus 'surface' dyslexia or 'semantic' dyslexia, as originally described by Marshall and Newcombe (1973) involves *either* or *both* the inability to attain the semantic systems (from visual input) *and* damage to the semantic systems themselves, *together with* a relatively less severe impairment to the phonological route.

The necessity for multi-component explanations of the reading difficulties observed in individual patients might seem to reduce their explanatory power. However, we have attempted to show that the variety of central dyslexic syndromes (when considered as a group) each studied as an individual syndrome, can be explained by assuming the existence of a number of subsystems underlying reading which are differentially impaired. In addition, it has been shown that single component syndromes do exist, e.g. phonological alexia. Moreover our approach allows for predictions to be made about the existence of syndromes that have not yet been recorded. For instance, patients should exist that read irregular words correctly only if they are imageable nouns (i.e. phonological route intact but the direct route only available for concrete nouns), to give an example of a syndrome yet to be observed, or that have a disproportionate difficulty with concrete words by comparison with abstract nouns (see Warrington, in preparation) to give an example of one that has.

Appendix 1

For reasons given in the section on single-component dyslexic syndromes we do not consider either 'deep dyslexia' or 'phonemic dyslexia' satisfactory terms for the syndrome which is the primary topic of this symposium and which we view as one of the mixed central dyslexias. For convenience we will use the term 'deep/phonemic dyslexia' to refer specifically to certain patients such as those described by Marshall and Newcombe (1966, 1973, cases 5 and 6); Shallice and Warrington (1975), Patterson and Marcel (1977), Saffran and Marin (1977), Schwartz, Saffran and Marin (1977) and Kapur and Perl (1978), whose difficulties appear to have certain characteristics in common. Given the variety of symptoms that have been described in such patients – Coltheart (Chapter 2) lists twenty which have been thought relevant – it becomes very difficult to determine which should be considered core symptoms and which merely associated deficits due to an anatomical relation between the relevant lesion sites. Somewhat arbitrarily we assume that the syndrome can be defined by four key features:

1   The patient has a very great difficulty in using the phonological route in reading, as shown, for instance, by a very poor performance in reading nonsense syllables.
2   Word reading performance is influenced by part-of-speech, in the order: nouns (best), adjectives, verbs, function words (worst).
3   There is a large effect of imageability/concreteness on word reading performance. (Even though imageability is operationally the more effective criterion (e.g. Richardson, 1975; Shallice and Warrington, 1975) we use the terms concrete and abstract so as to emphasize that in our view imagery is not a relevant process.)
4   Errors of visual, semantic and derivational types are all made.

Two individual case studies, in addition to those mentioned above, are known to us in which sufficient quantitative data is available to make it worth considering whether the patient should or should not be placed in this category. The patient of Low (1931) must be considered at best borderline as there appeared to be no effect of abstraction: monosyllabic concrete nouns 84 per cent correct, monosyllabic abstract nouns 90 per cent correct. The patient, P.S., of Shallice and Coughlan (1980) performed relatively rather better on function words. However, this can be ascribed to her ability to use the phonological route not being totally abolished for short words. Her improved ability to read function words can therefore be attributed to their short length rather than to their syntactic and/or semantic properties. She will therefore be provisionally included. Otherwise her overall level and pattern of reading performance was very similar to that of K.F.

It should be noted that to define deep/phonemic dyslexia just in terms of the presence of semantic errors is unsatisfactory given the presence of a clearly differentiated syndrome, namely that of A.R. (Warrington and Shallice, 1979).

Appendix 2

Information on the pattern of words on which visual errors are made is available to us on three patients, G.R., K.F. and P.S. Marshall and Newcome (1966) found that for G.R. visual errors occurred on only 3.5 per cent of nouns stimuli compared with 13.3 per cent of adjectives and 10.2 per cent of verbs. Correct responses occurred on 45, 16 and 6 per cent of these words respectively. Therefore for G.R. the stimuli which produce most correct responses, also produce least visual errors.

Shallice and Coughlan (1980) found that in a set of 200 words, half of which were below the median concreteness and half above, 27 visual errors were made by P.S. on the former words and 7 on the latter; only one error was made in the highest concreteness quartile (i.e. $C>6$).

For K.F. the situation is more complex. The four samples used in our 1975 study did not give completely similar results. For the AA words 11/99 (11 per cent) of the visual errors occurred on words representing concrete objects (i.e. the sort of words that can be read) by comparison with 23 per cent of the total. Thus visual errors are significantly less likely to occur on such words than would be expected by chance ($\chi^2 = 7.71$, $p<.01$). For A words there was an insignificant trend in the same direction. 18/91 (20 per cent) of the visual errors occurred on words representing concrete objects by comparison with 27 per cent of the total pool ($\chi^2 = 2.29$, $.1<p<.2$).

A comparable criterion for the Brown and Ure (1969) and Paivio, Yuille and Madigan (1968) words is to use $C\geq6$ for concreteness and $C\geq6$ for imageability respectively. For the Brown and Ure list one obtains 7/52 (13 per cent) of the visual errors with $C\geq6$ by comparison with 26 per cent of the total pool, just significantly less than chance expectations ($\chi^2 = 3.98$, $p<.05$). (However, there is no trend over the other quartiles: 16, 17, 12). By contrast for the Paivio words, 15/32 (47 per cent) of the visual errors were on stimuli with $C\geq6$ by comparison with 35 per cent of the total pool. There is an insignificant trend in the opposite direction ($\chi^2 = 2.1$, $.1<p<.2$).

Overall if one considers classes of words defined by either syntactic or semantic criteria, it appears that deep/phonemic dyslexics have a relatively low rate of visual errors on classes of words for which there is a high reading rate. Visual errors are therefore unlikely to result entirely from a dysfunction prior to the stage at which semantic and syntactic variables are relevant.[10]

Notes

1 For the purposes of this classification it will be assumed that an essential stage in both reading direct to semantics and by phonological recoding is the attainment of a visual word-form. A unit which performs this level of analysis may be characterized as parsing (multiply) a letter string into familiar components and attaining a visual specification of the components. The components can range in size from graphemes through syllables to the letter string as a whole (if a morpheme). It is performing a related but not identical function to that undertaken by the visual logogen in Morton's (1979) approach. In this paper we have used the concept in a somewhat different fashion from our previous usage (sometimes under the term 'grapheme') (e.g. Shallice and Warrington, 1975; Shallice and McGill, 1978; Warrington and Shallice, 1979), and made it functionally rather different from a 'visual logogen'. We now assume that one set of outputs of the unit is to the phonological system and that such outputs need not represent morphemes.

2 We will ignore letter-by-letter reading, which involves the use of letter names and a spelling check, as although neurologically important (see Warrington and Shallice, 1978; 1980) it is relevant specifically to the peripheral dyslexias and is presumably not used in normal reading.

3 The reading of this patient is discussed in more detail in Chapter 12.

4 A.R.'s ability to use the phonological route was, although greatly impaired, somewhat better than that typically reported in deep/phonemic dyslexia (nonsense syllable reading 20 per cent and 28 per cent correct, on two separate tests). This cannot account for the different reading pattern. Use of the phonological route would be expected to be most beneficial for short words. Yet he was inferior to deep/phonemic dyslexic patients on concrete nouns and better on abstract nouns, which are on average longer. It might be argued that the lack of effect of word class on reading in A.R. reflects his using, in isolation, the hypothetical 'third' route (visual logogen to auditory output logogen), which was, however, impaired. Such an explanation would not, though, account for his making semantic errors, for the level of comprehension of words that could not be read or for the variability in his word reading responses.

5 The objection has been raised that the deep/phonemic dyslexic patient should on this theory make visual errors to non-words as frequently

as to abstract words, which they do not (see Morton and Patterson, Chapter 4). This argument depends critically on how well matched words and non-words are in their overall similarity to words and on the subjects' conception of their task. We believe the argument to be not-proven. For instance P.S. in attempting to read 375 words made 7 word responses to the 15 non-word stimuli which were included without prior warning (Shallice and Coughlan, 1980). This value is somewhat lower than her substantive errors/all non-correct error rate (E/NC) for real words (76 per cent) (but overall visual similarity to potential error responses was not controlled).

6 Whether the difference in performance of deep/phonemic dyslexic patients on different classes of words can be interpreted in terms of some dimension related to the abstract/concrete one remains in our view an open question. In either case the same type of argument could be advanced for the word class effects as for the abstract/concrete effects.

It should be noted that contrary to the interpretation of our 1975 paper made by Marshall and Newcombe (1977), we have never held that there was any necessary connection between deep/phonemic dyslexics' good performance on imageable words and the process of imagery itself.

7 The idea has been floated by Ellis and Marshall (1978) that K.F.'s semantic errors are a chance phenomenon because only 4 per cent of his responses had a semantic similarity to the stimulus word but no visual similarity (e.g. *little* → 'small'). This suggestion can be simply disproved. As 90 per cent of his error responses are either derivational, visual or visual and/or semantic errors, only 45 (10 per cent of all errors) have no visual similarity to the stimulus word. It is within this restricted set that it is appropriate to contrast a theoretical 'chance' rate of occurrence of semantic errors with the observed rate of non-visually similar semantic errors. In fact 19 (42 per cent) of this restricted set of errors are semantically related, much higher than the chance rate estimated by Ellis and Marshall to be 6–9 per cent. One wonders what Ellis and Marshall think of Marshall and Newcombe's (1973) claim that their patient K.U., who made only two semantic errors, be considered deep dyslexic!

8 The rate of derivational errors does not show any obvious correlation with either visual or semantic errors. This suggests that this category has a cause distinct from either of the above or can arise for multiple reasons (see Morton and Patterson, Chapter 4).

9 The standard argument for the right hemisphere theory is the similarity between the properties of deep/phonemic dyslexia and those of the intact right hemisphere in split-brain patients. This argument is gravely weakened by the strong suggestion of abnormal language lateralization in the split-brain patients, prior to the sectioning of the corpus callosum (Gazzaniga, Le Doux and Wilson, 1977). According to these authors, the one exception is a patient, W.J. who 'apparently developed normally until age 30' and 'shows

no sign of right hemisphere language under standard testing conditions'.

10 It should be noted that the prediction that visual error responses are more concrete than the stimuli, as found in both K.F. and P.S. (Shallice and Warrington, 1975; Shallice and Coughlan, 1980), is made by both of the theories of visual errors being considered.

References

Allport, D. A. (1977) On knowing the meaning of words we are unable to report: the effects of visual masking. In S. Dornic (ed.), *Attention and Performance*, VI. Hillsdale, N.J.: Lawrence Erlbaum.

Beauvois, M.-F. and Dérouesné, J. (1978) Phonological alexia: a study of a case of alexia without aphasia or agraphia. *Experimental Brain Research, 32,* R5.

Brown, W. P. and Ure, D. M. N. (1969) Five rated characteristics of 650 word association stimuli. *British Journal of Psychology, 60,* 223–50.

Coltheart, M. (1978) Lexical access in simple reading tasks. In G. Underwood (ed.), *Strategies of Information Processing.* London: Academic Press.

Coltheart, M., Besner, D., Jonasson, J. T. and Davelaar, E. (1979) Phonological encoding in the lexical decision task. *Quarterly Journal of Experimental Psychology, 31,* 489–508.

Coughlan, A. D. (1976) An investigation of selected verbal skills and verbal memory following left-hemisphere lesions. Ph.D. Thesis. University of London.

Coughlan, A. D. and Warrington, E. K. (1978) Word-comprehension and word-retrieval in patients with localized cerebral lesions. *Brain, 101,* 163–85.

Ellis, A. W. and Marshall, J. C. (1978) Semantic errors or statistical flukes? A note on Allport's 'On knowing the meaning of words we are unable to report'. *Quarterly Journal of Experimental Psychology, 30,* 569–75.

Gazzaniga, M. S., Le Doux, J. E. and Wilson, D. H. (1977) Language, praxis and the right hemisphere: clues to some mechanisms of consciousness. *Neurology, 27,* 1144–7.

Goldstein, K. (1948) *Language and Language Disturbances.* New York: Grune & Stratton.

Goodglass, H. and Geschwind, N. (1976) Language disorders (aphasia). In E. Carterette and M. Friedman (eds), *Handbook of Perception*, vol. 7. New York: Academic Press.

Goodglass, H., Klein, B., Carey, P. and Jones, K. J. (1966) Specific semantic word categories in aphasia. *Cortex, 2,* 74–89.

Goodglass, H., Hyde, M. R. and Blumstein, J. (1969) Frequency, picturability and availability of nouns in aphasia. *Cortex, 5,* 104–19.

Green, D. W. and Shallice, T. (1976) Direct visual access in reading for meaning. *Memory and Cognition, 4,* 753–8.

Hécaen, H. and Kremin, H. (1976) Neurolinguistic research on reading disorders resulting from left hemisphere lesions: aphasic and 'pure' alexia. In H. Whitaker and H. A. Whitaker (eds), *Studies in Neurolinguistics*, vol. 2. New York: Academic Press.

Kapur, N. and Perl, N. T. (1978) Recognition reading in paralexia. *Cortex, 14,* 439–43.

Katz, J. J. and Fodor, J. A. (1963) The structure of a semantic theory. *Language, 39,* 170–210.

Kinsbourne, M. and Warrington, E. K. (1962a) A variety of reading disabilities associated with right hemisphere lesions. *Journal of Neurology, Neurosurgery and Psychiatry, 25,* 339–44.

Kinsbourne, M. and Warrington, E. K. (1962b) A disorder of simultaneous form perception. *Brain, 85,* 461–86.

Lhermitte, F. and Beauvois, M.-F. (1973) A visual-speech disconnection syndrome: report of a case with optic aphasia, agnosic alexia and colour agnosia. *Brain, 96,* 695–714.

Lotmar, F. (1919) Zur Kenntnis der erschwekten Wortkindung und ihre Bedeutung fur das Denken der Aphasischen. *Schweizer Archiv fur Neurologie und Psychiatrie, 5,* 206.

Low, A. A. (1931) A case of agrammatism in the English language. *Archives of Neurology and Psychiatry, 25,* 556–97.

McKenna, P. and Warrington, E. K. (1978) Category specific naming preservation: a single case study. *Journal of Neurology, Neurosurgery and Psychiatry, 41,* 571–4.

Marcel, A. J. and Patterson, E. K. (1978) Word recognition and production: reciprocity in clinical and normal studies. In J. Requin (ed.), *Attention and Performance*, vol. 7. Hillsdale, N.J.: Lawrence Erlbaum.

Marshall, J. C. and Newcombe, F. (1966) Syntactic and semantic errors in paralexia. *Neuropsychologia, 4,* 169–76.

Marshall, J. C. and Newcombe, F. (1973) Patterns of paralexia: a psycholinguistic approach. *Journal of Psycholinguistic Research, 2,* 175–99.

Marshall, J. C. and Newcombe, F. (1977) Variability and constraint in acquired dyslexia. In H. A. Whitaker and H. Whitaker (eds), *Studies in Neurolinguistics*, vol. 3. New York: Academic Press.

Miller, G. A. and Johnson-Laird, P. N. (1976) *Language and Perception.* Cambridge, Mass.: Harvard University Press.

Morton, J. (1979) Word recognition. In J. Morton and J. C. Marshall (eds), *Psycholinguistics* Series, vol. 2. London: Elek.

Nelson, H. E. and McKenna, P. (1975) The use of current reading ability in the assessment of dementia. *British Journal of Social and Clinical Psychology, 14,* 259–67.

Nelson, H. E. and O'Connell, A. (1978) Dementia: the estimation of premorbid intelligence levels using the new adult reading test. *Cortex, 14,* 234–44.

Paivio, A., Yuille, J. C. and Madigan, J. A. (1968) Concreteness, imagery and meaningfulness values for 925 nouns. *Journal of Experimental Psychology Monograph Supplements, 76* (1).

Patterson, K. E. (1978) Phonemic dyslexia: errors of meaning and the meaning of errors. *Quarterly Journal of Experimental Psychology, 30,* 587–608.

Patterson, K. E. (1979) What is right with 'deep' dyslexic patients? *Brain and Language, 8,* 111–29.

Patterson, K. E. and Marcel, A. J. (1977) Aphasia, dyslexia and the phonological coding of written words. *Quarterly Journal of Experimental Psychology, 29,* 307–18.

Richardson, J. T. E. (1975) The effect of word imageability in acquired dyslexia. *Neuropsychologia, 13,* 281–8.

Saffran, E. M. and Marin, O. S. M. (1977) Reading without phonology: evidence from aphasia. *Quarterly Journal of Experimental Psychology, 29,* 515–25.

Saffran, E. M., Schwartz, M. F. and Marin, O. S. M. (1976) Semantic mechanisms in paralexia. *Brain and Language, 3,* 255–65.

Schuell, H. and Jenkins, J. J. (1961) Reduction of vocabulary in aphasia. *Brain, 84,* 243–61.

Schwartz, M. F., Marin, O. S. M. and Saffran, E. K. (1979) Dissociations of language function in dementia: a case study. *Brain and Language, 7,* 277–306.

Schwartz, M. F., Saffran, E. M. and Marin, O. S. M. (1977) An analysis of agrammatic reading in aphasia. Paper presented at the International Neuropsychology Society meeting, Santa Fe.

Shallice, T. and Coughlan, A. K. (1980) Modality specific word comprehension deficits in deep dyslexia (submitted).

Shallice, T. and McGill, J. (1978) The origins of mixed errors. In J. Requin (ed.), *Attention and Performance,* vol. 7. Hillsdale, N.J.: Lawrence Erlbaum.

Shallice, T. and Warrington, E. K. (1975) Word recognition in a phonemic dyslexic patient. *Quarterly Journal of Experimental Psychology, 27,* 187–99.

Shallice, T. and Warrington, E. K. (1977) The possible role of selective attention in acquired dyslexia. *Neuropsychologia, 15,* 31–41.

Warrington, E. K. (1975) The selective impairment of semantic memory. *Quarterly Journal of Experimental Psychology, 27,* 635–58.

Warrington, E. K. and Shallice, T. (1978) Spelling dyslexia: impairment of the visual word-form. *Experimental Brain Research, 32,* R50.

Warrington, E. K. and Shallice, T. (1979) Semantic access dyslexia. *Brain, 102,* 43–63.

Warrington, E. K. and Shallice, T. (1980) Word-form dyslexia. *Brain* (in press).

Weigl, E. and Bierwisch, M. (1970) Neuropsychology and linguistics. *Foundations of Language, 6,* 1–18.

Weisenburg, T. and McBride, K. (1935) *Aphasia: A Clinical and Psychological Study.* New York: Commonwealth Fund.

Wijk, A. (1966) *Rules of Pronunciation for the English Language.* Oxford University Press.

Wolpert, I. (1924) Die Sinultanagnosie Storung der Gesantauffasung. *Neurologie und Psychiatrie, 93,* 397–415.

6 The semantic error: types and theories

Max Coltheart

This chapter has two aims. The first is to examine the *nature* of the semantic relationships which exist between stimulus and response when a deep dyslexic produces a semantic error in attempting to read aloud a single printed word. The second aim is to review and to assess theories which have attempted to explain how semantic errors in reading aloud come about.

Detailed inspection of a sufficiently large number of instances of semantic error suggests, at least to me, that there are two rather different types of semantic error. Consider the word *merry*. When patient 13* was asked to read this word aloud, he responded 'happy'. When patient 7 was asked to read this word aloud, she responded 'Christmas'. The semantic relationship of response to stimulus is surely very different in these two examples. In the first case, the response is a synonym of the stimulus: the two words belong to the same syntactic category and have the same semantic features. In the second case, the stimulus and response differ in syntactic category and have very different semantic features. What links them is not that they share semantic features, but that they are *associatively* related. There are other examples of the same kind: to the word *short*, patient 3 responded 'small', whilst patient 15 responded 'walk'.

Many semantic errors, of course, are related to their stimuli in both ways: *savage* → 'cannibals' is an example. However, it is possible to select a set of examples of semantic error which seem to be clearly associative in character, and another set which seems

* The numerical references to patients follow the tabulation of cases given in Chapter 2.

146

equally clearly to represent a sharing of semantic features between stimulus and response. Table 6.1 gives examples of associative semantic errors; note that the existence of errors such as *cone* → 'ice cream' or *dial* → 'sun' indicates that the associative relationship may sometimes be from response to stimulus. Table 6.2 gives examples of shared-feature semantic errors, divided up into two sub-categories. The first sub-category is the superordinate error: the response is a semantic superordinate of the stimulus. The second sub-category is the co-ordinate error: the stimulus and response are both exemplars of a single semantic category (this includes synonyms). A third sub-category, the subordinate error, is logically possible, but turns out to be very rare. One example is *child* → 'girl' (patient 1); but such examples have only very rarely been reported, and hence Table 6.2 has no subordinate-error sub-category.

TABLE 6.1 *Examples of associative semantic errors*

wrist → 'watch'	(3)	*motor* → 'car'	(15)
brass → 'band'	(3,13)	*free* → 'enterprise'	(14)
antique → 'vase'	(3)	*drove* → 'car'	(13)
next → 'exit'	(3)	*bring* → 'towards'	(13)
pale → 'ale'	(5)	*postage* → 'stamps'	(13)
merry → 'Christmas'	(7)	*wear* → 'clothes'	(8)
comfort → 'blanket'	(8)	*dial* → 'sun'	(13)
ideal → 'milk'	(12)	*sty* → 'pig'	(13)
thermos → 'flask'	(12,13)	*blowing* → 'wind'	(12)
stage → 'coach'	(13)	*shining* → 'sun'	(12)
income → 'tax'	(15)	*cone* → 'ice cream'	(12)
short → 'walk'	(15)		

The term 'superordinate' is used rather loosely in Table 6.2. Semantic errors have been classified as superordinates when it is plausible to argue that any characterization of the stimulus as a list of semantic features would include all the semantic features of the response plus some others. This is clear enough for cases such as *cattle* → 'animals', *minute* → 'time', *robin* → 'bird', and *bride* → 'girl'. It is arguable for cases such as *product* → 'work' (a product is defined as that which results from work), *phase* → 'moon' (a phase, in this sense, is defined as one of the stages through which the moon passes) or *oxygen* → 'air' (oxygen is defined as one of the constituents of air). Some of the examples of Table 6.2 may be arguable, but a comparison of Tables 6.1 and 6.2, it seems to me, provides good reason for believing in the reality of the distinction between associative semantic errors and shared-feature semantic errors, and hence for accepting the view that at least two different types of semantic error exist.

TABLE 6.2 *Examples of shared-feature (superordinate and co-ordinate) semantic errors*

Superordinates		Co-ordinates	
bush → 'tree'	(3,13)	dad → 'father'	(1)
cattle → 'animals'	(3)	wed → 'marry'	(2)
cousin → 'relations'	(3)	niece → 'aunty'	(3)
minute → 'time'	(5)	hurt → 'injure'	(5)
robin → 'bird'	(8)	little → 'small'	(5)
hours → 'time'	(8)	or → 'diamant'	(6)
dream → 'sleep'	(12)	est → 'nord'	(6)
product → 'work'	(12)	May → 'January'	(7)
competitor → 'event'	(12,13)	tulip → 'crocus'	(8)
phase → 'moon'	(13)	cane → 'crutch'	(9)
oxygen → 'air'	(13)	big → 'tall'	(10)
inhabitant → 'people'	(13)	cow → 'donkey'	(11)
mutton → 'meat'	(13)	nephew → 'auntie'	(12)
classes → 'school'	(13)	girl → 'boy'	(12)
pilot → 'air'	(13)	merry → 'happy'	(13)
tandem → 'cycle'	(13)	carnation → 'narcissus'	(13)
bride → 'girl'	(15)	nephew → 'cousin'	(13)
cushion → 'seat'	(15)	elk → 'yak'	(13)
seed → 'plant'	(15)	movies → 'pictures'	(15)
		city → 'town'	(15)

It will probably be clear already to the reader that this distinction, though it emerges here from thinking about a large corpus of semantic errors, turns out to be a familiar one in psychology. Wundt (1907), for example, discussed the distinction between associations based on contiguity ('outer associations') and associations based on similarity ('inner associations'), which corresponds to the distinction between associative semantic errors and shared-feature semantic errors. More recently investigators of word association have distinguished between two types of response produced by subjects in a word-association task: paradigmatic and syntagmatic responses:

Paradigmatic associations are those in which the stimulus and response fit a common grammatical paradigm and syntagmatic associations are, in general, sequential elements or at least elements which usually occupy different positions within phrases or sentences. Syntagmatic associations are, more often than not, like the transitional frequencies between words in the language itself and are, therefore, in general contiguous. A paradigmatic association, however, need not be contiguous and usually is not. 'It is hard to think of the word *hot* as providing the principal or even a moderately frequent linguistic environment for *cold*' (Deese, 1965, pp. 103–4).

On this definition, there is clearly some similarity between Table 6.1 responses and syntagmatic responses, and also some similarity between Table 6.2 responses and paradigmatic responses.

Yet another similar dichotomy has been proposed, this one specifically in connection with aphasic speech: the distinction between similarity and contiguity elaborated by Jakobson (1971), who considered that aphasic patients could be classified into two categories: those patients whose speech showed a similarity disorder, and those whose speech showed a contiguity disorder.

Words which are related by *contiguity* are those which exemplify the figure of speech known as metonymy: use of the name of an attribute of a thing instead of the thing itself, such as 'crown' for *king*. Patients with a similarity disorder fall back on contiguity as a principle for selecting a word when word-finding difficulties occur. Examples given by Jakobson of such contiguity relationships are:

knife → 'fork'
lamp → 'table'
pipe → 'smoke'
toaster → 'eat'
black → 'what you do for the dead. Dead.'
hut → 'thatch, litter, poverty'
house → 'stands, burns, broken, old, little'

Jakobson's view of the nature of these errors is evident in the following quotation:

metonymies may be characterized as projections from the line of a habitual context into the line of substitution and selection:

a sign (e.g. *fork*) which usually occurs together with another sign (e.g. *knife*) may be used instead of this sign. Phrases like 'knife and fork', 'table lamp', 'to smoke a pipe' induce the metonymies *fork*, *table*, *smoke*; the relation between the use of an object (toast) and the means of its production underlies the metonymy *eat* for toaster. (Jakobson, 1971, p. 62)

Words which are related by *similarity* exemplify a different figure of speech: not metonymy but metaphor. Patients with contiguity disorder rely on similarity when selecting a word during word-finding difficulty:

the patient . . . deals with similarities, and his approximate identifications are of a metaphoric nature, contrary to the metonymic ones familiar to the opposite type of aphasics. *Spyglass* for *microscope*, or *fire* for *gaslight* are typical examples of such quasi-metaphoric expressions as Jakobson termed them, since, in contradiction to rhetoric or poetic metaphors, they present no deliberate transfer of meaning. (Jakobson, 1971, p. 64)

Examples given by Jakobson of word pairs related by similarity are:

house → 'cabin'
hut → 'cabin, hovel, palace, den, burrow'
microscope → 'spyglass'
gaslight → 'fire'

Jakobson used the terms 'external' and 'internal' in connection with the distinction between contiguity and similarity: 'the two opposite tropes, metaphor and metonymy, present the most con-densed expression of two basic modes of relation: the internal relation of similarity (and contrast) underlies the metaphor; the external relation of contiguity (and remoteness) determines the metonymy'. His use of 'external' and 'internal' here corresponds exactly to Wundt's use of 'outer association' and 'inner association'. We also know that Jakobson's distinction corresponds to the distinction between syntagmatic and paradigmatic word associa-tions, because Osgood asked Jakobson point blank whether this was so (see Jakobson, 1971, pp. 118–19):

Osgood: 'word-association shows a very clear split, with two types relating to your distinction between similarity and contiguity. They are the paradigmatic type, in which the association is in the same substitution class, versus the sequential type of association. An example of the first type would be table versus chair; of the second type, man versus walks.'

Jakobson: 'In connection with Dr Osgood's question . . . the stimulus "house" responded to by "cabin" or some other word for a certain kind of house, or perhaps by a mere synonym for "house" . . . these are paradigmatic responses, whereas syntagmatic responses add to the word "house" some predicate or attribute: "stands", "burns", "broken", "old", "little". This duality corresponds to our observations on similarity versus contiguity.'

It is evident, then, that in Wundtian psychology, in relatively recent work on word association, in Jakobson's linguistic aphasiology, and in the analysis of the semantic errors of deep dyslexics, the same dichotomy of response types arises. Various pairs of terms have been used to describe this dichotomy: for clarification these are listed in Table 6.3, together with Osgood's example of each response type.

TABLE 6.3 *An example of the two basic types of stimulus-response relationship, and a list of the terms which have been used to describe each*

table → 'chair'	man → 'walks'
similarity	contiguity
inner association	outer association
metaphor	metonymy
internal relation	external relation
paradigmatic association	syntagmatic association
shared-feature semantic error	associative semantic error

Jakobson considered that the two error types did not coexist in individual aphasic patients: 'of the two modes of relation, similarity and contiguity, the aphasic suffers impairment or at least greatest deterioration of only one mode in his verbal behaviour'. This does not seem to apply in the case of deep dyslexia; as far as can be discovered at present, individual patients produce both shared-feature and associative semantic errors, with shared-feature errors being by far the more frequent of the two error types.

In word-association tasks, children produce predominantly syntagmatic responses whilst adults produce predominantly paradigmatic responses (Ervin, 1961; Entwistle, Forsyth and Muuss, 1964). Amongst adults, the tendency towards syntagmatic response depends upon the syntactic class of the stimulus; Deese (1962) found that the percentage of syntagmatic responses was 21.4 for nouns, 48.1 for verbs, 49.9 for adjectives and 72.8 for adverbs. Comparison of Tables 6.1 and 6.2 suggests that something comparable may be true for the deep dyslexic: nouns tend mainly to evoke shared-feature semantic errors, whilst adjectives and verbs produce a larger proportion of associative semantic errors. This result, and indeed Deese's result, may however be a consequence of output bias towards nouns.

Having provided some evidence for the view that at least two different kinds of semantic error occur, I turn now to the question of how the occurrence of semantic errors is to be explained.

The Marshall-Newcombe account of semantic errors

Marshall and Newcombe (1966) proposed that reading aloud of single words is sometimes achieved by retrieving a word's semantic representation from its lexical entry and using this representation to gain access to the word's phonological form. They adopted the theory of Katz and Fodor (1963) concerning the nature of the lexical representation of semantic information. The Katz-Fodor view is that semantic representations are hierarchically organized; a proposed entry for *bush*, for example, would be noun/plant/ with branches/ arising from or near the ground. The top of the hierarchy is a syntactic-class specification: the bottom is a *distinguisher* which indicates whatever is idiosyncratic about the particular word.

If a patient does not proceed fully to the deepest aspect of the semantic hierarchy, he will produce a semantic error: in the example given above, if the distinguisher is neglected, what results is the semantic representation of the word 'tree': hence the response *bush* → 'tree'.

This theory gives a precise explanation for the type of semantic error referred to earlier, in connection with Table 6.2, as a super-ordinate error, since the relationship of response to stimulus is exactly that the response is the stimulus minus its distinguisher. The theory does not explain how co-ordinate errors arise, but a trivial modification to the theory allows this. Firstly, co-ordinate errors which are synonyms are obviously predicted by the theory anyway: if two words have *identical* semantic representations, a reading mechanism in which the only link from stimulus to response was via semantics could not avoid synonymic errors such as *dad* → 'father', *little* → 'small', or *hurt* → 'injure'. To explain non-synonymous co-ordinate errors such as *niece* → 'aunty', *May* → 'January', or *carnation* → 'narcissus', one needs to suppose that, when a determiner is lost, sometimes its loss leaves some trace: the patient knows that a determiner is lost, so supplies one, without having any way of selecting the correct determiner.

On this theory, subordinate semantic errors should not occur if the patient does not introduce semantic features at levels of the hierarchy which are not represented in the stimulus: for example, the response *meat* → 'mutton' should not occur since *mutton* contains semantic features which are more specific (lower in the hierarchy) than any of the semantic features of *meat*. As noted above, although subordinate errors have been observed, they are extremely rare; co-ordinate and superordinate errors are common.

The function-word substitution – responding to a function word by another, unrelated, function-word – is common (see Chapter 2) and on this theory would arise if all but the most general of semantic features are lost, the feature at the apex of the semantic hierarchy being the word's syntactic class. Here all the patient would know is that his response ought to be a function word; he would have no way of deciding *which* function word.

The analysis proposed by Marshall and Newcombe (1966) thus gives a good account of the kinds of errors represented in Table 6.2, namely, shared-feature semantic errors. However, it does not seem applicable to the other type of semantic error, the associative semantic error, because for this kind of error it simply is not the case that the stimulus and the response are located at different levels of a single semantic hierarchy: the stimulus is often syntactically and semantically quite different from the response.

Semantic errors as associative responses

The possibility that the relationship of stimulus to response when a semantic error is made might be the same as it is when subjects are free associating was in fact discussed by Marshall and Newcombe (1966, and see Chapter 7) in relation to the idea that deep dyslexics simply misunderstand the reading-aloud task, treating it as a free-association task. They are clearly correct in rejecting this idea; but to reject it is not to dismiss the view that interword association is the mechanism linking stimulus to response in the semantic error. They argued against *this* view on the ground that antonymic responses are common in free-association tasks but do not occur in the oral reading of deep dyslexics. However, since then antonymic semantic errors have been observed (Marshall and Newcombe, 1973; Weigl and Bierwisch, 1970; Ohashi, 1965, cited in Yamadori, 1975; Shallice and Warrington, 1975).

It can be suggested, then, that semantic errors arise because the internal lexicon incorporates an associative network. When the lexical entry for a word is accessed, the entries for other words linked to this entry by the associative network are also accessed. If the procedure by which a correct choice is made from this set of associatively-related words is disabled in deep dyslexia, the response produced would often be an associate of the stimulus. This idea was proposed by Weigl and Bierwisch (1970, p. 13):

> preliminary analysis subsequently leads to an internal
> generation of the item to be understood by means of
> information stored in the lexjcon. Here an irradiation within
> a particular class or field of lexical items takes place in
> disturbed cases such as the one discussed here. Finally an
> erroneous matching of the stored result of the preliminary
> analysis and the internally generated item leads to the
> significant misreading.

Weigl and Bierwisch considered that lexical irradiation is itself an abnormal phenomenon, but this concept, under the name 'spreading excitation' is currently used to explain a number of aspects of the performance of normal readers (see, e.g., Meyer and Schvaneveldt, 1971; Warren, 1972; Collins and Loftus, 1975) as was pointed out by Saffran, Schwartz and Marin (1976). Consequently the latter authors, whilst agreeing with the basic idea proposed by Weigl and Bierwisch, suggested that the deep dyslexic's problem 'may lie not in the spread of excitation, but in the failure to restrict verbal output to the appropriate element within the activated field'.

On this view, semantic errors reflect the structure of the lexicon's associative network, not, as Marshall and Newcombe (1966) proposed, the internal structure of individual lexical entries. Clearly, the associative view gives an appropriate account of the kinds of associative semantic errors illustrated in Table 6.1. Since at least some of the shared-feature semantic errors illustrated in Table 6.2 are also associatively related in the sense that the stimulus-response pairs occur in word association norms, it is worth considering whether an associative theory may explain all, not merely some, semantic errors.

It seems that this is unlikely. Firstly, many semantic errors are not found in word association norms. The responses *canary* → 'parrot' (Marshall and Newcombe, 1966) and *tulip* → 'crocus' (Saffran and Marin, 1977) were made by none of the one hundred subjects in the word-association study of Marshall and Cofer (1970). Marshall and Newcombe's patient produced the response 'and' to each of the five function words *for, me, before, up* and *other*; 'and' seems an implausible associative response to any of these words, an impression confirmed by consultation of associative norms. In the norms of Keppel and Strand (1970), only one of 186 subjects produced the response 'and' to *me*. In the norms of Ervin-Tripp (1970) only one of 379 subjects responded 'and' to *for*.

A second objection to the associative view is that, if the stimulus is the name of a month, a common response in free-association tasks would be the *following* month. However, a patient described by Saffran, Schwartz and Marin (1976) responded 'August' to *March* and 'January' to *May*. These are co-ordinate errors and hence well described by the theory of Marshall and Newcombe.

A third objection to the associative view is that the deep dyslexic sometimes offers a kind of definition of the word he is attempting to read aloud: for example, *college* → 'school . . . not ordinary' or *canal* → 'not river . . . small river' (Marshall and Newcombe, 1966); or, from patients who were presumably deep dyslexics, *dimanche* → 'c'est un jour de la semaine . . . vendredi' (Dubois-Charlier, 1971) or *Holland* → 'it's a country, not Europe . . . no . . . not Germany . . . it's small . . . it was captured . . . Belgium? That's it, Belgium'

(Luria, 1970). I submit that what one is hearing here is a slow progression down a Katz-Fodor semantic hierarchy, in each case not reaching as far as the determiner. Thus the Marshall-Newcombe view provides a natural interpretation of this kind of response; an associative view does not.

For these three reasons, it seems to me that the associative view gives a good account of some semantic errors – the associative semantic errors – but fails to explain shared-feature semantic errors. Marshall and Newcombe's view explains shared-feature errors but not associative errors. Very few errors fail to be explained by one or the other view. The conclusion I would like to suggest, therefore, is that not only are there two distinct types of semantic error, but also that the two error types require different explanations. Associative semantic errors arise via an associative link between stimulus and response. Shared-featured semantic errors arise because some of the semantic features of the stimulus are lost or not used during the process of deriving response from stimulus via semantic representation; moreover, the lower a semantic feature is in the Katz-Fodor hierarchy, the greater the likelihood of its loss. Neither mechanism in isolation can explain all semantic errors; but if both are postulated, then as far as I can determine a reasonable account can be given of virtually all semantic errors.

Imagery and semantic errors

These two accounts of semantic errors are not the only ones which have been proposed; a third account also exists. This account proposes that stimulus and response are linked, not by an associative network, nor by an incomplete set of semantic features, but by an *image*. For example, Benson and Geschwind (1969, p. 412) suggest that, in their patient, 'it appears possible that certain written words aroused visual images which were then named paraphasically'. This view has also been proposed by Richardson (1975).

As an attempt to explain all semantic errors, this account can be refuted, because many such errors simply could not occur in this way: examples are *niece* → 'nephew', *his* → 'she' (Marshall and Newcombe, 1966); *gray* → 'red', *March* → 'August', *May* →

'January' (Saffran, Schwartz and Marin, 1976); *zebra* → 'giraffe' (Brown, 1972); *me* → 'him' (Marin, Saffran and Schwartz, 1975); *Petersilie* (parsley) → 'Radieschen' (radish), *Ananas* (pineapple) → 'Bananen' (bananas), *Socken* (socks) → 'Sandalen' (sandals), *Manschette* (cuff) → 'Krawatte' (tie), *Bluse* (blouse) → 'Hose' (trousers) (Weigl and Bierwisch, 1970). In every one of these instances, the response could not possibly have been made as an attempt to name an image evoked by the stimulus.

Nevertheless, even if not *all* semantic errors arise in this way, *some* might:

> the responses of our patients to abstract targets frequently suggested mediation by imagery. For example, in reading the word 'success', patient V.S. said 'son . . . college . . . doctor . . .', raising her hand to indicate successive levels of achievement. (Marin, Saffran and Schwartz, 1975)

Other favourable examples for an imagery account are *Dalmatian* → 'spots' (Saffran, Schwartz and Marin, 1976), *child* → 'girl' (Low, 1931), *Kyoto* → 'kansai' (Sasanuma, 1974; Kyoto is a city in the Kansai region of Japan) and *livingroom* → 'Oh I know what that place is, it is the place we go to after dinner to watch TV' (Benson and Geschwind, 1969).

It is, however, hard work finding examples of semantic error which are much more naturally interpretable in terms of imagery than in terms of either of the two other theories I have described earlier. Furthermore, the *success*, *dalmatian* and *child* examples can perhaps be explained as word-association effects, and the *Kyoto* as a semantic-feature effect. Thus it seems fair to conclude that, although imaginal mediation may be occurring in some cases, the evidence is not strong enough to compel us to accept this view; whereas the evidence *does* compel us to accept that both word-association effects of the kind postulated by Weigl and Bierwisch (1970) and Saffran, Schwartz and Marin (1976), and semantic-feature effects of the kind postulated by Marshall and Newcombe (1966), contribute to the occurrence of semantic errors. Thus, the existence of just these two different forms of semantic error must be taken into account by theories of deep dyslexia.

References

Benson, D. F. and Geschwind, N. (1969) In P. J. Vinken and G. W.
Bruyn, (eds), *Handbook of Clinical Neurology*, vol. 4. Amsterdam: North
Holland.

Brown, J. A. (1972) *Aphasia, Apraxia, Agnosia.* Springfield, Ohio: C. C.
Thomas.

Collins, A. M. and Loftus, E. F. (1975) A spreading-activation theory of
semantic processing. *Psychological Review, 82,* 407–28.

Deese, J. (1962) Form class and the determinants of association. *Journal
of Verbal Learning and Verbal Behaviour, 1,* 79–84.

Deese, J. (1965) *The Structure of Associations in Language and Thought.*
Baltimore: Johns Hopkins Press.

Dubois-Charlier, F. (1971) Approche neurolinguistique du probleme de
l'alexie pur. *Journale de Psychologie, 68,* 39–67.

Entwistle, D. R., Forsyth, D. F. and Muuss, R. (1964) The syntagmatic-
paradigmatic shift in children's word-association. *Journal of Verbal
Learning and Verbal Behaviour, 3,* 19–29.

Ervin, S. (1961) Changes with age in the verbal determinants of word
association. *American Journal of Psychology, 74,* pp. 361–72.

Ervin-Tripp, S. M. (1970) Substitution, context and association. In
L. Postman and G. Keppel (eds), *Norms of Word Association.* London:
Academic Press.

Jakobson, R. (1971) *Studies on Child Language and Aphasia.* The Hague:
Mouton.

Katz, J. J. and Fodor, J. A. (1963) The structure of a semantic theory.
Language, 39, 170–210.

Keppel, G. and Strand, B. Z. (1970) Free-association responses to the
primary responses and other responses selected from the Palermo-
Jenkins norms. In L. Postman and G. Keppel (eds), *Norms of Word
Association.* London: Academic Press.

Low, A. A. (1931) A case of agrammatism in the English language.
Archives of Neurology and Psychiatry, 25, 555–97.

Luria, A. R. (1970) *Traumatic Aphasia.* The Hague: Mouton.

Marin, O. S. M., Saffran, E. M. and Schwartz, M. F. (1975) Dissociations of language in aphasia: implications for normal function.
Annals of the New York Academy of Science, 280, 868–84.

Marshall, G. R. and Cofer, C. N. (1970) Single-word free-association
norms for 328 responses from the Connecticut cultural norms for
verbal items in categories. In L. Postman and G. Keppel (eds), *Norms
of Word Association.* London: Academic Press.

Marshall, J. C. and Newcombe, F. (1966) Syntactic and semantic errors
in paralexia. *Neuropsychologia, 4,* 169–76.

Marshall, J. C. and Newcombe, F. (1973) Patterns of paralexia: a
psycholinguistic approach. *Journal of Psycholinguistic Research, 2,* 175–99.

Meyer, D. E. and Schvaneveldt, R. W. (1971) Facilitation in recognizing
pairs of words: evidence of a dependence between retrieval operations.
Journal of Experimental Psychology, 90, 227–34.

Richardson, J. T. E. (1975) The effect of word imageability in acquired dyslexia. *Neuropsychologia, 13,* 281–8.

Saffran, E. M. and Marin, O. S. M. (1977) Reading without phonology: evidence from aphasia. *Quarterly Journal of Experimental Psychology, 29,* 515–25.

Saffran, E. M., Schwartz, M. F. and Marin, O. S. M. (1976) Semantic mechanisms in paralexia. *Brain and Language, 3,* 255–65.

Sasanuma, S. (1974) Kanji vs. kana processing in alexia with transient agraphia: a case report. *Cortex, 10,* 89–97.

Shallice, T. and Warrington, E. K. (1975) Word recognition in a phonemic dyslexic patient. *Quarterly Journal of Experimental Psychology, 27,* 187–99.

Warren, R. E. (1972) Stimulus encoding and memory. *Journal of Experimental Psychology, 94,* 90–100.

Weigl, E. and Bierwisch, M. (1970) Neuropsychology and linguistics; topics of common research. *Foundations of Language, 6,* 1–18.

Wundt, W. (1907) *Outlines of Psychology.* London: Williams and Norgate. (Third English edition, translated by C. H. Judd.)

Yamadori, A. (1975) Ideogram reading in alexia. *Brain, 98,* 231–8.

7 Response monitoring and response blocking in deep dyslexia

Freda Newcombe and John C. Marshall

Introduction

In patients with deep dyslexia, semantic errors in single-word reading may account for as many as 50 per cent of the overt mistakes (Marshall and Newcombe, 1966). These errors occur when the material consists of unrelated words, individually presented, and without the imposition of either time pressure or stimulus degradation.

We report here on the psychological status of semantic errors in one subject, G.R. (Marshall and Newcombe, 1966) with deep dyslexia. We consider and reject three 'artefactual' explanations for such errors. The first two hypotheses are to the effect that the subject misunderstands the nature of the task. The third account explains semantic 'errors' as elliptical circumlocutions which spring from an underlying deficit in word-production. Rejection of these putative explanations strengthens the claim that deep dyslexia is indeed a specific impairment of the *reading* system (Marshall and Newcombe, 1973).

Our subject (G.R.) was injured in 1944 at the age of 19, when a bullet penetrated the brain in the region of the left Sylvian fissure and emerged in the superior parietal lobe of the left hemisphere. The neurological signs, that have persisted, include a right homonymous hemianopia, a right spastic hemiparesis and right-sided sensory loss. Full neurological and clinical details of the case can be found in Marshall and Newcombe (1966) and Newcombe and Marshall (1975) and will not be repeated here. For present purposes it suffices to say that he is an appropriate subject with whom to investigate the 'tip-of-the-tongue plus elliptical circumlocutions' hypothesis. G.R.

has a non-fluent dysphasia: his spontaneous speech is telegrammatic, phrase length is short, and he produces occasional articulatory errors. Word-finding difficulty is apparent in spontaneous speech; he is impaired in object-naming tests both with respect to latency of response and error-rate (Newcombe, Oldfield, Ratcliff and Wingfield, 1971).

Misunderstanding the task?

Presented with a subject who reads *abroad* as 'overseas', *message* as 'telegram', and *nephew* as 'cousin', one's first reaction is to explain away the errors by claiming that the patient is not 'really' reading. Such interpretations typically take one of two forms. In the first case, it is claimed that the subject has failed to understand the instructions. The subject is under the erroneous impression that his task is, for example, 'free-association' rather than reading. This 'explanation' can be speedily rejected. On a number of trials, the subject will produce a circumlocution or a commentary upon what he is doing. Examples of such responses, produced by G.R., are shown in Table 7.1. We suggest that this is not the behaviour of a subject who imagines that he has been asked to free-associate. One does not give spontaneous confidence ratings for the 'correctness' of free-associations. Additional evidence against the hypothesis is found in the relative rarity of antonym responses (*arrival* → 'departure') compared with the frequency of partially or fully synonymous responses (*ill* → 'sick'; *large* → 'long'; *little* → 'short'; *short* → 'small').[1] Moreover, when G.R. is given a free-association test (with an auditorily-presented stimulus), his responses are typically normal (e.g. *dark* → 'light'; *man* → 'beast'; *fruit* → 'vegetable'; *boy* → 'girl'; *good* → 'bad'). He thus appears to know when we have asked him to read and when we have asked him to 'associate'.

One might at this point essay the notion that the patient believes he had been asked to define the words presented to him. Even shorter shrift may be given this idea. Presented with lists of fairly common concrete nouns, G.R. reads at least half of them correctly, producing one response (the correct one) per stimulus. It is unlikely that a man who presented with, e.g. *brush, chicken, helicopter, submarine* etc., and who says, quickly and confidently, 'brush', 'chicken', 'helicopter', 'submarine' is under the delusion that he should define or explain the meaning of the stimulus words.

There seems little doubt, then, that G.R. knows what he is trying to do, namely to read words. However, there is a second form of 'explaining away' that raises issues of a much more serious nature.

TABLE 7.1

enemy	→ 'I know it . . . something . . . different countries fighting together . . . spy'
needle	→ 'I'm not sure . . . thimble'
caution	→ 'danger . . . I'm not quite sure . . . might be'
pneumonia	→ 'something to do with treatment'
guilty	→ 'scaffold . . . something like that'
pink	→ 'I know it . . . a colour . . . not blue'
applaud	→ 'laugh . . . not quite sure'
bake	→ 'cake . . . not quite right'
flour	→ 'wheat . . . not wheat . . . flour'
cheap	→ 'cheap . . . no! . . . not quite'
rubbish	→ 'rubber . . . no! . . . It can't be'

Elliptical circumlocutions?

While there is no doubt that G.R. understands what we want him to do, it does remain the case that a proportion of his responses are unequivocal circumlocutions. We can accordingly construct an argument of the following nature:

When, presented with *tiger*, G.R. simply says 'tiger' we may be sure that he indeed read the word *tiger*.

When, presented with *tomato*, G.R. says 'Can't pronounce it[2] . . . don't like 'em myself . . . they're red', we may be sure that he is *not* reading the stimulus word *tomato* but is giving us a running commentary on his failure to so do. He is also, of course, showing us that he understands the meaning of the printed word *tomato*. (Note, however, that failure cannot be ascribed to a purely peripheral problem of articulation. G.R. may produce and reject a correct response. For example, presented with *office*, G.R. responded 'Yes, the firm, management, office . . . um, I can't say the name now – I know it, manager.') Unless one intends to become a sceptic of truly Berkeleyan proportions, the interpretation of responses at these two extremes is unambiguous.

But what of the examples that most concern us? Could it be that responses of the type *arsenic* → 'poison' are really disguised commentaries? Consider how the argument might proceed: we know that most (if not all) subjects with deep dyslexia show word-finding difficulties in their spontaneous speech; we also know that several of them are 'non-fluent' in the sense of Goodglass and Kaplan (1972). Given this pattern of deficit it would not be unreasonable to suggest that the underlying structure of the overt response 'poison' is something like 'It's on the tip-of-my-tongue but I can't quite say it. However, I know what the word means. It's a poison'. On this account, then, failure to retrieve and articulate 'arsenic' is a symptom of the underlying word-finding difficulty, and failure to produce an explicitly marked circumlocution follows from the patient's generally effortful and elliptical manner of speech.

We shall now test the adequacy of the above hypothesis as an explanation of the semantic errors produced by G.R. We report first the 'confidence' that he has in the correctness of his responses. Confidence ratings on reading by deep dyslexic patients have also been used by Kapur and Perl (1978) and Patterson (1978).

On 26 June 1964, during the first of a series of follow-up examinations of ex-servicemen from World War II (Newcombe, 1969), G.R. was asked to read the hundred words composing Schonell's graded word reading test, R1. The standard form and instructions were used (Schonell and Schonell, 1950) and responses were recorded verbatim. An unusual tendency to semantic substitution was noted. The test was therefore repeated on two subsequent occasions (July 17 and August 4), to check the reliability of the phenomenon. On the third occasion, the subject was asked to rate his confidence in the accuracy of all his responses, using a four point scale ('sure' 3; 'likely' 2; 'not sure' 1; 'don't know' 0).

In August 1965, during a more intensive investigation of G.R.'s dyslexia, he was asked to read some 2000 words drawn from West's (1953) general service list, presented in short sessions over a period of two weeks (see Marshall and Newcombe, 1966 for a report of the general pattern of response). One month later, he was asked to read a sample of one hundred words (from that list) to which he had made semantic errors and/or circumlocutions which indicated that he was at least aware of the semantic field to which the stimulus belonged. Each word was displayed separately, typed on a plain white card. No time pressure was imposed. Immediately after each response, the subject was asked to indicate his degree of confidence in the accuracy of his response. On this occasion, G.R. himself devised the form of rating that he preferred to use: when sure that his response was correct, he would say 'hundred per cent'; lesser degrees of certainty would be rated as 'fifty per cent', 'twenty per cent', 'ten per cent', and so on.

Erroneous responses were scored as follows:

semantic: a single-word response, bearing a semantic relationship to the stimulus word but without an obvious visual resemblance, e.g. *antique* → 'ornament'.

visual: a single-word response bearing a visual resemblance to the stimulus but without an obvious semantic connection, e.g. *saucer* → 'sausage'.

circumlocution (C): a response involving more than one word. Responses that were exclusively semantic were scored C (semantic), e.g. *ceiling* → 'paint . . . painter . . . plaster'. Those in which a visual distortion was also involved were scored C (visual), e.g. *pivot* → 'fly . . . flee . . . aeroplane'.

other: those few errors that could not be assigned to a specific category (e.g. *think* → 'and'), that were ambiguous (e.g. *bucket* → 'basket'), or that might be regarded as derivational (e.g. *refresh* → 'refreshment'; *sandwich* → 'sandwiches'.

TABLE 7.2

| | *Probability ratings* | | | | |
	3	2	1	0	Total
Correct	22	1	0	0	(23)
Semantic	2	1	3	0	(6)
C (semantic)	1	0	3	2	(6)
C (+ visual)	0	0	2	2	(4)
Visual	4	3	3	1	(11)
Other	4	1	0	1	(6)
Total	(33)	(6)	(11)	(6)	56

The results were as follows. G.R. attempted to read 56 of the one hundred words in the Schonell list, and 23 of his responses were correct. Of the 33 erroneous responses, twelve (6 single-word responses and 6 circumlocutory responses) were drawn from the same semantic field as the stimulus word; and an additional 4 responses were semantic errors that also involved a visual error in decoding the stimulus-word. The subject's confidence ratings for his responses are shown on Table 7.2. Individual responses, grouped according to confidence levels are shown on Table 7.3a, b, c, d.

The pattern of G.R.'s responses to the 100 word-stimuli from the West sample (to which he had previously produced paralexic errors) is shown on Table 7.4. Responses are classified according to whether the word-stimuli had initially evoked a semantic or a circumlocutory

TABLE 7.3a *Single-word responses, rated '3' ('sure')*

Correct	Incorrect	
tree	*bun*	→ 'cake'
milk	*crowd*	→ 'crown'
egg	*sandwich*	→ 'sandwiches'
book	*saucer*	→ 'sausage'
school	*canary*	→ 'parrot'
frog	*forfeit*	→ 'forge'
flower	*genuine*	→ 'guinea'
road	*heroic*	→ 'hero'
clock	*think*	→ 'and'
train	*playing*	→ 'play'
light		
picture		
summer		
people		
dream		
biscuit		
shepherd		
island		
orchestra		
colonel		
little		
thirsty		

TABLE 7.3b *Single-word responses, rated '2'*

Correct	Incorrect	
angel	*postage*	→ 'post office'
	university	→ 'versity'
	campaign	→ 'camping'
	sabre	→ 'sword'
	diseased	→ 'disease'

TABLE 7.3c *Single-word responses, rated 'I'*

Correct	Incorrect
	nephew → 'relations'
	audience → 'clap'
	antique → 'ornament'
	sit → 'short'
	intercede → 'interval'
	fascinate → 'fantasy'

TABLE 7.3d *Single-word responses, rated 'o'*

Correct	Incorrect
	slovenly → 'gas-stove'
	applaud → 'applause'

error. On the second trial, he attempted to read 90 words and 18 of these responses were correct. Erroneous responses included 52 semantic errors, 12 circumlocutory errors, and 7 miscellaneous errors. The pattern illustrates both the consistent tendency to produce semantic errors and the variability of response to individual items between trials. Confidence ratings for these second-trial responses are shown on Tables 7.5a and b. The two derivational errors given on the first trial were repeated on the second trial and accorded a 100 per cent confidence rating. Individual responses, grouped according to confidence levels, are shown on Tables 7.6a, b and c.

It is clear that G.R. uses his ratings in a rational fashion; he gives a consistently high rating to correct responses and is correspondingly

TABLE 7.4

Response-errors on first trial	Correct	Identical error	New semantic error	New C (semantic)	Other	Failure	(Total)
Semantic	12	25	16	7	4	3	(67)
C (semantic)	6	1	11	4	2	7	(31)
Other (lexical)	0	1	0	0	1	0	(2)
Total	(18)	(27)	(27)	(11)	(7)	(10)	100

Response on second trial spans columns Correct through Other.

tentative about his circumlocutions. Of the responses rated as 'sure' or '100 per cent' in the 1964 and the 1965 sample, 67 per cent and 37 per cent respectively are in fact correct. (The 1965 reading material – drawn from the subject's previous errors – was more difficult for him.) The corresponding figures for responses rated as 'likely' or '50–80' were 17 per cent and 21 per cent; and none of the responses rated as 'not sure' or '10 to 25 per cent' were correct. He understands, then, the notion of confidence levels and can deploy that knowledge in a manner that corresponds with objective correctness on an ordinal scale.

Regarding error-responses, the data samples are too small for precise interpretation. It can be seen, however, that both (single-word) semantic and (single-word) visual errors receive confidence-ratings that vary across the range of the scales. In this respect, G.R.

TABLE 7.5a *Second-trial responses with ratings to words that evoked a semantic error on the first trial*

Response	Rating			
	100%	*50–80%*	*10–25%*	*Total*
Correct	9	3	0	(12)
Identical semantic error	10	13	2	(25)
New semantic error	6	5	5	(16)
C (semantic)	0	3	4	(7)
Other	2	1	1	(4)
Total	(27)	(25)	(12)	64

TABLE 7.5b *Second-trial responses with ratings to words that evoked a circumlocutory response on the first trial*

Response	Rating				
	100%	*50–80%*	*10–25%*	*No rating given*	*Total*
Correct	3	3	0	0	(6)
Semantic	3	3	5	0	(11)
Identical C (semantic)	0	1	0	0	(1)
Other C (semantic)	0	1	2	1	(4)
Other	0	1	1	0	(2)
Total	(6)	(9)	(8)	(1)	24

appears to be somewhat different from other deep dyslexic patients for whom confidence rating data have been reported. Both Kapur and Perl's (1978) and Patterson's (1978) patients rated their visual errors correct more frequently than their semantic errors.

The second set of material, derived from the subject's own prior paralexic errors, is consistent with the Schonell data in that correct responses are again given with confidence. It is also the case that single-word semantic errors – whilst spread across the three confidence-categories – do tend to cluster in the higher confidence range whereas responses involving circumlocution are given with less certainty.

The fact remains that at least a third of the responses to which G.R. gives a rating of 'sure' in the original Schonell data are, by our standards, wrong. This percentage is increased to two thirds when he is asked to read words that elicited paralexic responses on

TABLE 7.6a *Single-word responses, rated 100 per cent*

Correct	Incorrect	
enemy	*birth*	→ 'born'
mill	*city*	→ 'town'
mouth	*cream*	→ 'ice'
needle	*daughter*	→ 'sister'
race	*dinner*	→ 'food'
reward	*game*	→ 'games'
sport	*joy*	→ 'jolly'
tobacco	*log*	→ 'cabin'
tower	*lunch*	→ 'parcel'
wife	*pay*	→ 'money'
bad	*price*	→ 'money'
flat	*system*	→ 'perm'
	talk	→ 'speech'
	voyage	→ 'ships'
	wage	→ 'money'
	wrist	→ 'watch'
	abroad	→ 'overseas'
	brave	→ 'hero'
	merry	→ 'jolly'
	short	→ 'small'
	south	→ 'east'
	kill	→ 'murder'
	refresh	→ 'refreshment'

TABLE 7.6b *Single-word responses, rated 50–80 per cent*

Correct	Incorrect	
common	*act*	→ 'play'
field	*bucket*	→ 'basket'
flour	*bowl*	→ 'bowling'
polish	*cost*	→ 'money'
throat	*example*	→ 'sums'
uncle	*fair*	→ 'poor'
	harm	→ 'burn'
	hut	→ 'house'
	mail	→ 'post'
	mercy	→ 'angel'
	ruin	→ 'rubble'
	sheet	→ 'paper'
	value	→ 'cheap'
	close	→ 'shut'
	false	→ 'cheat'
	guilty	→ 'scaffold'
	heavy	→ 'hard'
	ill	→ 'sick'
	attack	→ 'fight'
	develop	→ 'camera'
	enjoy	→ 'jolly'
	punish	→ 'prison'
	rob	→ 'crook'

TABLE 7.6c *Single-word responses, rated 10–25 per cent*

Correct	Incorrect	
	caution	→ 'danger'
	fever	→ 'flu'
	fit	→ 'gymnastics'
	industry	→ 'factory'
	jewel	→ 'jews'
	limb	→ 'leg'
	season	→ 'pass'
	start	→ 'first'
	stock	→ 'shock'
	early	→ 'small'
	applaud	→ 'cheerio'
	educate	→ 'school'
	heal	→ 'medicine'
	his	→ 'she'

previous testing. Taken in conjunction with the underlying rationality of his judgments, we interpret this to mean that when he reads, e.g. *canary* as 'parrot', *city* as 'town' and *craft* as 'sculpture', he does indeed believe that he has given a correct 'reading-response'.

A second source of evidence that refutes the output-blocking hypothesis is to be found in word-selection tasks, when no verbal response is required. In May 1978, such a test was carried out during an experiment in which G.R. was asked to sort, read, and select word-names. The stimulus material consisted of 50 words printed on individual cards and drawn from five categories: kinship, animals, tools, vehicles, qualities (e.g. truth, beauty, freedom, justice); and there were ten exemplars in each category. Initially, five cards with the printed category-names were read by the examiner and left on the table. G.R. was asked to sort the 50 word-stimuli appropriately. Then a category-name was exposed on the table with the ten exemplars placed beneath it in two columns of five cards each. G.R. was asked to point in turn to each of the exemplars named by the examiner. He was later asked to read the 50 words presented at first in categories and then in random order. Results are shown on Table 7.7. Predictably, sorting was the easiest condition. The dramatic effects of categorization on reading performance, reported by Beringer and Stein (1930) and Albert, Yamadori, Gardner and Howes (1973) were not found. More germane to our argument is the fact that elimination of the *verbal* response did not eliminate semantic confusions.

TABLE 7.7 *Errors in sorting, selecting, and reading 50 word stimuli*

	Kinship	Animals	Tools	Vehicles	Qualities	Total
Sorting	0	0	3	3	6	(12)
Pointing to exemplar within a category	4	3	4	3	6	(20)
Reading exemplars within categories	4	6	7	2	9	(28)
Reading (shuffled order)	6	5	6	4	10	(31)

We have also hinted earlier at yet another source of difficulty that an 'output-blocking' explanation will run into. The circumlocutions include a number of instances where G.R. has rejected or 'continued past' a response that is in fact correct. Some examples of this phenomenon are shown in Table 7.8.[3]

In fact, we see no way in which the overall pattern of our results is consistent with the notion that semantic errors are really disguised, elliptical circumlocutions. A final rejection of the above hypothesis as the full and entire explanation of semantic errors rests upon evidence that we have recently collected from a word-comprehension test,[4] requiring no overt verbal response.

TABLE 7.8

captain	→	'in charge . . . captain . . . not captain . . . captain'
carriage	→	'I know roughly . . . carriage . . . similar to carriage'
female	→	'female . . . woman'
office	→	'yes . . . the firm . . . management . . . office . . . um . . . I can't say the name now . . . I know it! manager'
remember	→	'it might be remember . . . I'm not quite sure of that'
slow	→	'danger . . . road . . . zig-zag crossings – go slow . . . danger . . . something like that'
stone	→	'inside . . . gall . . . stone . . . bladder inside . . .'
throat	→	'roughly something to do with sore throat . . . gargle . . . I don't know'
pretty	→	'somebody that is sweet . . . pretty, sweet . . . I'm not quite sure of that'
empty	→	'bottles, empty, similar to that word'
thirst	→	'thirsty . . . um . . . dry'
shower	→	'water . . . you know . . . shower . . . I can't say the name'

A 'central' comprehension deficit?

In this task, G.R. was given successively 80 concrete nouns that had to be matched with a picture from an array of 4 or 8 items. Twenty of the arrays contained one *semantic* distractor and a set of filler items. The semantic distractors in this subset bore no visual similarity to the target items (e.g. key/lock). Twenty of the arrays contained a *visual* distractor and irrelevant fillers. The visual distractor bore no semantic similarity to the correct response (e.g. flag/axe). Twenty of the arrays contained a distractor that bore both a *semantic and a visual* similarity to the correct response (e.g. strawberry/raspberry). A final twenty arrays contained distractors that bore no obvious semantic or visual resemblance to the target item. For each of these four subsets there were 10 arrays with four pictures and 10 arrays with eight pictures. Word frequency and position of target were balanced across distractor types.

The pictures for each array were arranged in oval fashion on a sheet of paper (42 cm × 30 cm). The procedure was as follows. There were two conditions: the 80 target words were presented *visually* (typed on a blank white card and placed in the centre of the page) and auditorily (spoken by the examiner), in balanced order. The 80 items were divided into two sets of 40 items (sets A and B) that were equivalent in relation to the pattern of distractor items. The order of presentation was as follows: Set A (auditory version); Set B (visual version); Set A (visual version); Set B (auditory version). An auditory version of the task was presented first on the assumption that he was less likely to make semantic errors in this condition. In addition, there were four practice items for which the target word was presented auditorily to ensure that the subject understood the task. Later, G.R. was asked to read the 80 stimulus-words.

The results of the experiment are shown in Table 7.9.

TABLE 7.9

| Errors | Stimulus presentation | |
	Visual	Auditory
Semantic	7	2
Semantic/visual	6	2
Visual	0	0
Random	2	0

It can be seen that semantic errors are a striking feature of G.R.'s performance even when no overt verbal response is required. Although these unambiguous semantic errors are more frequent with written stimulus presentation (7/20) they do occur with acoustic presentation (2/20). The fact that *no* errors are found when the distractor items bear a purely visual relationship to the target, leads us to suppose that the errors made with semantic + visual distractors are in fact semantic errors. In the latter condition the errors are again more frequent with written (6/20) than with spoken (2/20) stimuli.

Nonetheless, the fact that semantic errors *do* occur with acoustic presentation would appear to indicate that there is an aphasic (multi- or supra-modal) aspect to G.R.'s impairment. It is not the case that semantic errors are restricted to performance with visual language. An instability or loss of modality-free semantic information is accordingly postulated. The table of errors (Table 7.10) does, however, show that the errors made with acoustic presentation are a proper sub-set of those made with written presentation.

TABLE 7.10 *Errors in word-picture matching task*

Auditory presentation		Visual presentation	
lamp	→ bulb	*lamp*	→ bulb
needle	→ cotton reel	*needle*	→ cotton reel
raspberry	→ strawberry	*raspberry*	→ strawberry
swan	→ duck	*swan*	→ duck
		magnet	→ xylophone
		brush	→ comb
		grave	→ coffin
		stool	→ chair
		stethoscope	→ syringe
		violin	→ trumpet
		cigar	→ cigarette
		jug	→ cup
		pen	→ pencil
		nail	→ ear
		bell	→ bat

Thus, he may be considered to have made 13 semantic errors on the visual version and 4 semantic errors on auditory presentation of the relevant 40 test items. The proportion of semantically-related errors produced subsequently by G.R. when asked to read the 80 words used for all conditions of the task was similar to that observed in the *visual* version of the pointing task. The reading errors were as follows: semantic 16; semantic circumlocutions 9; visual 4; other 5.

We are therefore forced yet again to discard the hypothesis that overt (output) response blocking is the sole determinant of semantic error. The evidence thus far points in the direction of a more central disturbance of lexical access, although for this patient the overt expression of this disorder is far more probable when semantic information has to be retrieved in reading or writing than in the comprehension or expression of speech. We must accordingly modify our original claim: it would now seem that in the case of G.R. 'deep dyslexia' both is and is not a specific impairment of the *reading* system.

Notes

1 We have previously reported some relevant data on this topic (Marshall, Newcombe and Marshall, 1970).
2 G.R. often uses this phrase in a stereotyped fashion to express word-finding difficulties.
3 Similar evidence was reported by Simmel and Goldschmidt (1953): '*napkin* → napkin, towel, no! . . . not towels, rags, napkin, tablets.'
4 We are indebted to Dr D. V. M. Bishop for the use of her experimental task.

References

Albert, M. L., Yamadori, A., Gardner, H. and Howes, D. (1973) Comprehension in alexia. *Brain, 96,* 317–28.
Beringer, K. and Stein, J. (1930) Analyse eines Falles von 'reiner' Alexie. *Zeitschrift für die Gesamte Neurologie und Psychiatrie, 123,* 472–8.
Goodglass, H. and Kaplan, E. (1972) *The Assessment of Aphasia and Related Disorders.* Philadelphia: Lea & Febinger.
Kapur, N. and Perl, N. T. (1978) Recognition reading in paralexia. *Cortex, 14,* 439–43.
Marshall, J. C. and Newcombe, F. (1966) Syntactic and semantic errors in paralexia. *Neuropsychologia, 4,* 169–76.
Marshall, J. C. and Newcombe, F. (1973) Patterns of paralexia: a psycholinguistic approach. *Journal of Psycholinguistic Research, 2,* 175–99.
Marshall, M., Newcombe, F. and Marshall, J. C. (1970) The microstructure of word-finding difficulties in a dysphasic subject. In G. B. Flores D'Arcais and W. J. M. Levelt (eds), *Advances in Psycholinguistics,* 416–26. Amsterdam: North Holland.
Newcombe, F. (1969) *Missile Wounds of the Brain: A Study of Psychological Deficits.* Oxford: Oxford University Press.
Newcombe, F. and Marshall, J. C. (1975) Traumatic dyslexia: localization and linguistics. In K. J. Zulch, O. Creutzfeldt and G. S.

Galbraith (eds), *Cerebral Localization: An Otfrid Foerster Symposium.* Berlin: Springer-Verlag.

Newcombe, F., Oldfield, R. C., Ratcliff, G. G. and Wingfield, A. (1971) Recognition and naming of object-drawings by men with focal brain wounds. *Journal of Neurology, Neurosurgery and Psychiatry, 34,* 329–40.

Patterson, K. E. (1978) Phonemic dyslexia: errors of meaning and the meaning of errors. *Quarterly Journal of Experimental Psychology, 30,* 587–607.

Schonell, F. J. and Schonell, F. E. (1950) *Diagnostic and Attainment Testing.* Edinburgh: Oliver and Boyd.

Simmel, M. L. and Goldschmidt, K. H. (1953) Prolonged posteclamptic aphasia. *A.M.A. Archives of Neurology and Psychology, 69,* 80–3.

West, M. (1953) *A General Service List of English Words.* London: Longmans, Green.

8 Transcoding and lexical stabilization in deep dyslexia

Freda Newcombe and John C. Marshall

Our purpose in this note is twofold: we wish to draw attention to one somewhat neglected aspect of the behaviour of some patients with *deep dyslexia*; and we then want to propose a simple diagram that seems to capture the essential characteristics of one subject who manifests the syndrome.

The behaviour in question is the occurrence of 'semantic paragraphias' in a writing-to-dictation task. In our original report on deep dyslexia (Marshall and Newcombe, 1966) we noted that G.R. made paraphasic errors on a task where individual words were dictated for the patient to write down. Some of his responses were also mis-spelt (e.g. 'cousin' → *nephil* (= nephew), and 'parrot' → *canisty* (= canary)). A few more examples were mentioned in the discussion of Newcombe and Marshall (1975). The same phenomenon is reported by Saffran, Schwartz and Marin (1976). Their two patients made such errors as writing *time* for 'hours' and *orchid* for 'lilac'. More recently, Peuser (1978) has described the condition in a German aphasic patient (Hans F.). This man made such semantic or 'associative' paragraphias (with individual words again) as 'Himmel' → *Nacht*, 'Onkel' → *Grossvater*, 'schmecken' → *prüft*, 'gestern' → *morgen*, 'schon' → *niemals*, 'Leben' → *Alles und sein* (!) and 'Liebe' → *Alte (!)*. Morphological and derivational errors were also in evidence ('Arbeiter' → *Arbeit*; 'baden' → *Badschwimme*, 'freundlich' → *freudig*), as were 'visual' (or 'spelling' or 'perceptual') errors ('lieben' → *liegen*). The effects of syntactic class upon the writing-to-dictation of this patient are in excellent quantitative agreement with the effects reported for the reading performance of G.R.

When describing oral reading or dictation we shall adopt the useful terminology of Weigl (1975) and refer to both tasks as involving the process of 'transcoding' (in the one case from the visual to the acoustic modality, in the other from acoustic to visual). We will contrast G.R.'s performance on transcoding tasks with his performance on two analogous but 'within-modality' tasks. Before turning to consider dictation errors in more detail we shall outline a provisional model of lexical organization that will, we hope, clarify the interpretation of transcoding procedures.

The architecture of lexical access and retrieval

Figure 8.1 represents the minimal number of components and interconnections that we currently consider to be required for understanding the process of word-recognition in both normal and aphasic subjects.

The heads of arrows denote the direction of information-flow; arrows with double lines denote a fast ('automatic'), with single a slow or variable, rate of information-flow.

Boxes and arrows are to be interpreted traditionally, that is as 'computational or storage centres' and 'transmission lines' respectively. Any box designated as a 'logogen' is to be interpreted as an 'evidence-collecting' device in the sense of Morton (1979a). Each such device takes input from between 1 and n sources until sufficient evidence has accumulated to exceed the threshold of the 'unit' that corresponds to 'recognition' of a particular stimulus. It is possible that these devices may have to be replaced by the more complex mechanisms postulated in 'cohort theory' (Marslen-Wilson and Welsh, 1978). Although this is an issue of considerable importance, it concerns the internal structure of our postulated boxes and will thus not affect (yet) the validity of our general argument. (An interesting possibility would be that cohort theory is appropriate to auditory perception and logogen-theory to visual perception; the initial plausibility of this suggestion derives, of course, from a comparison of the strictly sequential nature of an acoustic signal versus the wider, and more variable, window-size that characterizes the visual system.)

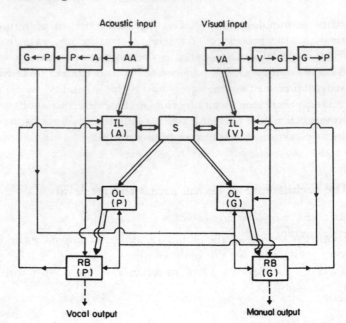

AA   = Acoustic Analysis
VA   = Visual Analysis
A → P = Acoustic to Phonologic
         Conversion
V → G = Visual to Graphemic
         Conversion
P → G = Phonologic to
         Graphemic Conversion
G → P = Graphemic to Phono-
         logical Conversion
IL(A) = Input Logogens
         (Auditory)

IL(V) = Input Logogens (Visual)
S   = Semantic System
OL(P) = Output Logogens
         (Phonologic)
OL(G) = Output Logogens
         (Graphemic)
RB(P) = Response Buffer
         (Phonologic)
RB(G) = Response Buffer
         (Graphemic)

FIGURE 8.1

The above diagram is not, of course, entirely new or indeed original. The idea of a post-semantic 'threshold device' is to be found in our first schema (Marshall and Newcombe, 1973); some of the 'peripheral' devices are discussed in Baron (1977); the diagram as a whole bears a striking similarity to current versions of the 'logogen model' (Morton, 1979 a and b; Morton and Patterson, Chapter 4 this volume). None the less, we do consider Figure 8.1 to be a small advance on all previously published schemata if for no other reason than that it allows for the existence of paragraphic errors.

Much of the diagram is self-explanatory, but its somewhat Byzantine appearance suggests that we should give a brief explanation.

We assume that AA, VA, IL(A), IL(V) and S (and their inter-connections) are all fast-acting, 'automatic' systems, and that in addition the semantic system (S) is subject to 'spread of activation' in the (approximate) sense of Fischler (1977a and b) and Neely (1977). When we say that *acoustic* analysis provides an input to auditory logogens and *visual* analysis an input to visual logogens (via the double-lined arrows) we mean precisely that. We do not believe that the auditory input has to be recoded into a phonologic representation before it can access the (auditory) input logogens (Klatt, 1977; 1979); neither do we believe that the visual input must be recoded into a graphemic (explicit letter) code before gaining access to (visual) input logogens. Anyone who does subscribe to this latter claim has never looked at handwriting. We are nevertheless fully prepared to countenance the existence of both *acoustic-to-phonologic* and *visual-to-graphemic* recoding. But one primary function of such re-coding is, in our view, the 'stabilization' of other components and processes. More specifically, we postulate that the output of *acoustic-to-phonologic* and *visual-to-graphemic* systems feed back into their respective logogen systems, thereby sharpening the definition of the input and ruling out a subset of putative candidates for 'recognition' within the input (logogen) system. This, however, will only be possible if the (physical) signal is sufficiently clear to allow (pre-lexical) *acoustic-to-phonologic* or *visual-to-graphemic* conver-sion. (When listening to spontaneous speech or reading 'normal' handwriting this pre-condition will often fail to obtain.) We postulate, in addition, that the outputs of *acoustic-to-phonologic* and *visual-to-graphemic* re-coding also flow into their respective output logogen systems. In this respect the model differs from that of Morton and Patterson (Chapter 4), where such codes only have access to the appropriate response buffers. The crucial function here is again that of stabilization or selection. We have conjectured that the semantic system is characterized by 'spread of activation' among semantically-related entries once one entry has been addressed via its input logogen. If we grant a certain level of 'random noise' within the semantic system (serving to elevate the resting level of activation of some entries whilst depressing others), it will follow that, occasionally, a wrong (but semantically-related) entry (or series thereof) will be transmitted from the semantic system to the output logogen system. Feeding phonological or graphemic codes into their respective output logogen systems will serve to 'catch' and block such errors before they emerge as overt (external) responses. We have previously noted (Marshall, 1976) that in order for this mechanism to be effective languages must be such that the dimension of physical similarity between words is uncorrelated with the dimension of semantic similarity. (A number of obvious consequences follow when this constraint is relaxed, as to some extent obtains within Chinese and Japanese orthography.) Finally, we hypothesize that the 'true' transcoding peripherals feed into their respective output logogen systems (as suggested by Marcel and Patterson, 1978) and also feed 'directly' into their respective response buffers (which is their only destination in Morton and Patterson, Chapter 4).

Preliminary empirical predictions

Let us now turn to the explication (within the above framework) of the pattern of impaired and preserved performance that is displayed by G.R.

We conjecture that G.R. has two 'lesions'; one 'lesion' that 'disconnects' *acoustic-to-phonological* conversion from *phonological-to-graphemic* conversion, and one 'lesion' that 'disconnects' *visual-to-graphemic* conversion from *graphemic-to-phonological* conversion. Within the traditional interpretation of diagrams such as our Figure 8.1 (Lichtheim, 1885), one cannot distinguish empirically between the preceding hypothesis and the two alternatives that either the *phonologic-to-graphemic* box and the *graphemic-to-phonologic* box have been 'destroyed', or that the outputs of *phonologic-to-graphemic* and *graphemic-to-phonologic* conversion have been 'cut'. For the moment, then, we shall accordingly regard the above three hypotheses as no more than 'notational variants' of each other. We have placed the term 'lesion' in scare quotes in order to emphasize that the notion is being used here solely in conjunction with theoretical schemata rather than in its customary anatomical or physiological sense. Our use of the term 'lesion' is thus equivalent to the idea of 'functional disconnection'.

In its current form, our 'two-lesion' model predicts:

1   Qualitatively, the pattern of performance (including error-analysis) on both transcoding tasks (oral reading and writing to dictation) should be (at least grossly) similar. *Ex hypothesi*, the stabilizing functions of *phonologic-to-graphemic* and *graphemic-to-phonologic* conversion are impaired.
2   Qualitatively, the pattern of performance (including error-analysis) on within-modality tasks (auditory repetition and delayed transcription of visually-presented words) should be (at least grossly) similar. Performance on these tasks should be greatly superior to that on the transcoding tasks. *Ex hypothesi*, the stabilizing functions of *acoustic-to-phonologic* and *visual-to-graphemic* conversion are not impaired.

We turn now to the evidence.

Evidence for the schema

During the course of July 1964 a list of 60 stimuli was prepared; these stimuli – concrete nouns for the most part – were then given to G.R. in four different task-settings: 1) oral reading; 2) writing-to-dictation; 3) immediate oral repetition; 4) immediate written recall to visual presentation. In other studies, line drawings of objects drawn from a wide frequency range were also presented to G.R. for naming. We shall not discuss this task further other than to note that G.R.'s performance was slightly impaired relative to an appropriate control group in terms of both latency to respond and error-rate. In one series of 41 trials, G.R. made one uncorrected semantic error (*anvil* → 'forge'), four corrected semantic errors (e.g. *moon* → 'sky . . . moon'), one semantic circumlocution (*metronome* → 'don't know . . . the time . . . music') and two phonological or articulatory errors.
   The other four tasks were conducted in the following fashion:

1   *Oral reading:* One word was presented at a time and was left in plain view of the subject until he made a response.
2   *Writing-to-dictation:* One word was spoken at a time. G.R. responded (in writing) at his own rate.
3   *Immediate oral repetition:* One word was spoken at a time. G.R. responded (orally) at his own rate.

4   *Immediate written recall:* One written word at a time was
presented for approximately 3 to 5 seconds. The stimulus card
was then removed from view, at which point G.R. attempted to
write down the word.

The results are shown in the following tables. Table 8.1 (a and b)
compares the overall level of performance for the first two ('transcoding') tasks:

TABLE 8.1 (a and b)

	(a) Oral reading	(b) Writing-to-dictation
Correct	39	17
No response ('Don't know')	2	9
Errors	19	34

G.R.'s impairment is clearly greater in the dictation task. Table 8.2
(a and b) compares the nature of the errors elicited in the two tasks:

TABLE 8.2 (a and b)

Errors	Oral reading (a)	Writing-to-dictation (b)
Single word semantic	4	11
Multi-word semantic	13	0
Derivational	0	2
Visual (a) or 'spelling' (b)	2	21
Totals	19	34

It will be seen that semantic errors occur in both tasks, although
sequences of such errors, including frank circumlocutions, only
occur when reading. 'Spelling' errors in the dictation task are far
more frequent than 'visual confusions' in the reading task. Although
the overall error patterns are rather different, we wish to focus on a
significant similarity: semantic errors constitute comparable pro-

portions of the total responses in the two transcoding tasks (28 per cent for reading, 18 per cent for writing).

Some examples of the different error types follow:

Representative examples from reading include:
Single-word semantic: *gnome* → 'pixie'
Multi-word semantic: *port* → 'ship' . . . 'harbour'
        page → 'something in a book'
Visual: *anvil* → 'angel'
Representative examples from dictation include:
Single-word semantic: 'star' → *moon*
Some semantic errors are also mis-spelt: 'parrot' → *canisty*
Derivational: 'tap' → *taps*

The category 'spelling errors' is highly heterogenous. It ranges from responses that have only one letter in common with the stimulus (e.g. 'screw' → *tr*), through complex patterns of addition and deletion (e.g. 'fence' → *freners*) to 'simple' transpositions (e.g. 'shoe' → *sheo*).

We now present the data from the two non-transcoding tasks, oral repetition and written recall. Table 8.3 (a and b) shows the overall level of performance.

TABLE 8.3 (a and b)

	Oral repetition (a)	Written recall (b)
Correct	57	41
No response ('Don't know')	0	0
Errors	3	19

It can be seen that performance here is dramatically better than in the transcoding tasks, although again the task requiring a written output fares worse than that requiring a spoken output. Table 8.4 (a and b) is a classification of the error responses.

TABLE 8.4 (a and b)

Errors	Oral repetition (a)	Written recall (b)
Semantic	0	0
Articulatory (a) or 'spelling' (b)	3	19

Semantic errors do not occur in either task. The articulatory errors in the repetition task are relatively minor and are provoked by such words as 'stethoscope'. The errors in written recall again range from responses having only one letter in common with the stimulus ('parrot' → *pe*), through complex additions and deletions ('toothbrush' → *tooblebresse*) to 'simple' transpositions ('nephew' → *newhep*).

We consider, then, that the simple schema of Figure 8.1 has been reasonably successful in capturing the broad outlines of G.R.'s pattern of impaired and preserved abilities.

Discussion

Our conjecture, then (as previously proposed by Morton, 1968; Patterson, 1978; Morton and Patterson, Chapter 4) is that when G.R. reads *sick* as 'ill' or writes 'bun' as *cake*, he has entered the semantic system via the *correct* node in the input logogen system. It will accordingly be obvious that any success our model may have in accounting for errors rests upon two crucial assumptions.

The first of these is that in the normal case (that is, in subjects who have not suffered brain-damage) the box we have labelled *semantic system* is intrinsically unstable unless it is 'corrected' or 'checked' by its various peripheral devices. By unstable we mean that the product of the input logogen system following categorization of e.g. *sick* is the availability of the semantic codes not only for *sick* but also for *ill*, *unwell*, etc. We take this assumption to be an empirical question. A number of scholars (Marcel, 1974; Marcel and Patterson, 1978; Allport, 1977) have recently reported on data that can be interpreted as giving a positive answer to this question. Specifically, it is claimed that when visually-presented words are pattern-masked (a procedure that may be interpreted as blocking the effective operation of the peripherals) normal subjects produce semantic errors when reporting the stimulus-words. Although some doubt has been cast upon the statistical validity of the phenomenon (Ellis and Marshall, 1978), the status of the claim is still open. It receives partial support from demonstrations that semantic 'priming' may be achieved when the prime itself has been so severely pattern masked as to be totally unavailable to conscious report (Marcel, 1974; Allport, 1977).

Note that Morton and Patterson (Chapter 4) have considered the notion of semantic instability or imprecision and more-or-less reject it as a full account of semantic paralexias. Their primary reason is that Patterson's (1978) two deep dyslexic patients can usually judge that their semantic paralexias are incorrect responses. However this does not hold, or at least not as generally, for G.R. (see Newcombe and Marshall, Chapter 7, this volume).

The postulate of normal instability in the 'core' system is important in that it provides for a principled distinction between central and peripheral devices. There would be little point in conjecturing the existence of peripheral stabilizing systems if the central mechanism were not unstable to begin with; once invoked, however, we see that the same peripheral machinery càn play an important role in decoding unfamiliar material.

We consider, then, that the instability-postulate is quite reasonable in the light of both psychological and physiological evidence (Winograd and Cowan, 1963). And we assume, with Freud (1891), that 'the safeguards of our speech against breakdown' are 'overdetermined, and . . . can easily stand the loss of one or the other element.' We accordingly interpret the data on 'phonological alexia' brought forward by Beauvois and Dérouesné (1978) as indicating that very minimal phonological re-coding can block the overt expression of semantic errors in reading. One notes that their patient did manage to read correctly some 10 per cent of the pseudo-words that he was presented with. But contrasting with the lack of semantic errors in reading, the patient displayed a bilateral tactile aphasia with substantial numbers of naming errors that were semantically-related to the stimulus items. In the case of G.R., however, severe and extensive brain-damage would appear (a) to have destroyed totally one set of stabilizing mechanisms, and (b) to have raised drastically the level of 'noise' within the semantic system (Weigl and Bierwisch, 1970) which would serve to accentuate the normal instability of the semantic system. Further arguments and evidence related to this point can be found in Saffran, Schwartz and Marin (1976). They too give qualified support to the 'normal' instability hypothesis and suggest that, in deep dyslexia, 'the problem may lie not in the spread of excitation, but in the failure to restrict verbal output to the appropriate element within the activated semantic field.' They show that (semantic) contextual constraints (a variable that we have not considered in our pared-down diagram) can 'aid in this restriction process and thus alter the probability of semantic error'.

The second assumption of our model is, of course, the existence of two 'lesions'. One 'lesion' is of the lateral output line of *acoustic-to-phonologic* conversion, and one is of the lateral output line of *visual-to-graphemic* conversion (or their respective notational variants). We have not so far found a satisfactory (that is, descriptively adequate) version of our model in which only a single 'lesion' is postulated. That is, all our attempts to interpret the data by conjecturing a 'lesion' of some kind of 'two-way' *phonologic-to-graphemic* and *graphemic-to-phonologic* device have been either logically incoherent or have failed to cover the full range of data that we have presented. Our failure to construct an adequate 'one-lesion' diagram does not, of course, imply that it is logically impossible to do so. We shall be more than happy if the reader attempts this exercise for him- or herself, and succeeds.

What, then, is the position we have now arrived at? It is clear that, in the case of G.R., we cannot interpret deep dyslexia as a disorder solely of reading. At very least, G.R. has a 'transcoding' deficit that extends across both oral reading and writing-to-dictation. If we extend the notion of transcoding to include tasks in which *pictorial* and linguistic objects must be 'associated' with each other, then the transcoding deficit is even more widespread. We have previously remarked upon the occurrence of semantic errors in an object-naming task (pictorial stimulus → vocal response); we have also noted (Chapter 7) semantic errors in an analogous 'comprehension' task (vocal or graphemic stimulus → manual response to a pictorial array). It would seem that we must complicate our diagram by at least the addition of a pictorial input system, the semantic interpretation of which may again require stabilization, albeit of a nature quite distinct from the 'rule-governed' stabilization that we have postulated for reading and writing tasks. There is, of course, mounting evidence for the independence of pictorial and verbal processing (Morton, 1979a; Scarborough, Gerard and Cortese, 1979).

To achieve a truly plausible model, however, would require far more than the addition of a few more boxes and lines. It would necessitate that we specify in some detail the nature of the computations that our boxes are capable of and the nature of the codes that are 'passed' from one box to another. Even more critically, it would require us to justify a new interpretation of diagrams, an interpretation that does not commit one to the postulation of yet greater numbers of *ad hoc* 'lesions'. We believe we can do this, but that is the topic of another paper.

References

Allport, D. A. (1977) On knowing the meaning of words we are unable to report: the effects of visual masking. In S. Dornic (ed.), *Attention and Performance*, VI. Hillsdale: Lawrence Erlbaum.

Baron, J. (1977) Mechanisms for pronouncing printed words: use and acquisition. In D. Laberge and S. J. Samuels (eds), *Basic processes in reading: perception and comprehension*. Hillsdale: Lawrence Erlbaum.

Beauvois, M.-F. and Dérouesné, J. (1978) Phonological alexia – a study of alexia without aphasia or agraphia. *Experimental Brain Research, 32,* R5.

Ellis, A. W. and Marshall, J. C. (1978) Semantic errors or statistical flukes? A note on Allport's 'On knowing the meaning of words we are unable to report.' *Quarterly Journal of Experimental Psychology, 30,* 569–75.

Fischler, I. (1977a) Semantic facilitation without association in a lexical decision task. *Memory and Cognition, 5,* 335–9.

Fischler, I. (1977b) Associative facilitation without expectancy in a lexical decision task. *Journal of Experimental Psychology: Human Perception and Performance, 3,* 18–26.

Freud, S. (1891) *Zur Auffassung der Aphasien*. Vienna: Deuticke.

Klatt, D. H. (1977) Review of the ARPA Speech Understanding Project. *Journal of the Acoustical Society of America, 62,* 1345–66.

Klatt, D. H. (1979) Speech perception: A model of acoustic-phonetic analysis and lexical access. In R. Cole (ed.), *Perception and Production of Fluent Speech*. Hillsdale: Lawrence Erlbaum.

Lichtheim, L. (1885) On aphasia. *Brain, 7,* 433–84.

Marcel, A. J. (1974) Perception with and without awareness. Paper presented at the Experimental Psychology Society, Stirling, July 1974.

Marcel, A. J. and Patterson, K. E. (1978) Word recognition and production: reciprocity in clinical and normal studies. In J. Requin (ed.), *Attention and Performance, VII*. Hillsdale: Lawrence Erlbaum.

Marslen-Wilson, W. D. and Welsh, A. (1978) Processing interactions and lexical access during word-recognition in continuous speech. *Cognitive Psychology, 10,* 29–63.

Marshall, J. C. (1976) Neuropsychological aspects of orthographic representation. In R. J. Wales and E. Walker (eds), *New Approaches to Language Mechanisms*. Amsterdam: North Holland.

Marshall, J. C. and Newcombe, F. (1966) Syntactic and semantic errors in paralexia. *Neuropsychologia, 4,* 169–76.

Marshall, J. C. and Newcombe, F. (1973) Patterns of paralexia. A psycholinguistic approach. *Journal of Psycholinguistic Research, 2,* 175–99.

Morton, J. (1968) Grammar and computation. In J. C. Catford (ed.), *Studies in Language and Language Behaviour*, C.R.L.L.B. Progress Report No. VI, University of Michigan.

Morton, J. (1979a) Word recognition. In J. Morton and J. C. Marshall (eds), *Psycholinguistics Series*, vol. 2. London: Paul Elek.

Morton, J. (1979b) Some experiments on facilitation in word and picture recognition and their relevance for the evolution of a theoretical position. In P. Kolers, M. Wrolstad and H. Bouma (eds), *Processing of Visible Language*. New York: Plenum.

Neely, J. H. (1977) Semantic priming and retrieval from lexical memory: roles of inhibitionless spreading activation and limited-capacity attention. *Journal of Experimental Psychology: General, 106*, 226–54.

Newcombe, F. and Marshall, J. C. (1975) Traumatic dyslexia: localization and linguistics. In K. J. Zulch, O. Creutzfeldt and G. C. Galbraith (eds), *Cerebral Localization: An Otfrid Foerster Symposium.* Berlin: Springer Verlag.

Newcombe, F. and Marshall, J. C. (1979) Response monitoring and response blocking in deep dyslexia. Chapter 7, this volume.

Patterson, K. E. (1978) Phonemic dyslexia: errors of meaning and the meaning of errors. *Quarterly Journal of Experimental Psychology, 30*, 587–607.

Peuser, G. (1978) *Aphasie.* Munchen: Wilhelm Fink Verlag.

Saffran, E. M., Schwartz, M. F. and Marin, O. S. M. (1976) Semantic mechanisms in paralexia. *Brain and Language, 3*, 255–65.

Scarborough, D. L., Gerard, L. and Cortese, C. (1979) Accessing lexical memory: the transfer of word repetition effects across task and modality. *Memory and Cognition, 7*, 3–12.

Weigl, E. (1975) Neuropsychological approach to the problem of transcoding. *Linguistics, 154/155*, 105–35.

Weigl, E. and Bierwisch, M. (1970) Neuropsychology and linguistics: topics of common research. *Foundations of Language, 6*, 1–18.

Winograd, S. and Cowan, J. D. (1963) *Reliable Computation in the Presence of Noise.* Cambridge, Massachusetts: MIT.

9 Two auditory parallels to deep dyslexia

John Morton

In spite of their trouble with reading, their agrammatism and non-fluency the deep dyslexic patients in Cambridge do not, in general, have any problem with the repetition of words. Their repetition of nonsense words is slightly impaired – about 75 per cent correct with monosyllabic nonsense words (Patterson and Marcel, 1977) – but contrasted with their total inability to read nonsense words this is approaching normality. For these reasons Morton and Patterson (Chapter 4, this volume), in their description of the functional problems of the deep dyslexics, regard the auditory half of the system as untouched. This is clearly shown in their Figure 4.3, which is reproduced here. No attempt is made here to explain the model: it is assumed that the reader will have read Chapter 4.

The symmetry of the underlying model with respect to modality of input leads one naturally to speculate as to whether patients can be found with, roughly speaking, the mirror syndrome to the deep dyslexics. This would constitute:

1 No semantic paralexias.
2 No problem with reading nonsense words.
3 Semantic errors in repetition of words.
4 Inability to repeat nonsense words.

This pattern of problem would correspond to a disruption of the path involving the auditory-phonological conversion together with a

My thanks are due to Dr D. A. Cruse and Dr F. Michel for allowing me to report work in press and allowing me to use some unpublished data. I am grateful to Marie-Claire Goldblum for discussing some of the issues raised.

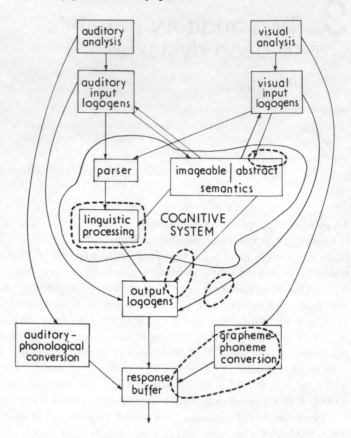

disconnection of the direct route between the auditory logogen system and the output logogen system. A case as pure as this would be too much to hope for and we would expect to find other problems present for anatomical reasons rather than functional ones, as with most of the deep dyslexics.

It is possible that qualifying cases could be found in the literature under the headings of word deafness or conduction aphasia. To attempt to include such patients would involve a lengthy discussion of taxonomy and so I prefer to describe briefly two recent cases who contain the elements of the syndrome I wish to illustrate.

1 Cruse (in press)

This patient has a 'left-sided posterior lesion . . . confirmed by EMI scan', caused by a cerebro-vascular accident 'presumed to be embolic in nature'. This occurred at age 46. A history of his early treatment can be found by Byers Brown and Ives (1969). The patient showed severe problems in auditory recognition and comprehension together with a severe word finding difficulty. Speech was fluent with severe paraphasia.

Cruse did two experiments with this patient. In the first experiment he spoke individual words, all concrete nouns, one at a time to the patient 'whose task was first to attempt to repeat the word, then to give a gloss of its meaning sufficiently detailed to confirm that it was not being confused with any other word'. If the patient failed to repeat the word he was presented with it in written form and was asked first to read it and then to paraphrase its meaning. In all cases but one the patient succeeded in reading the words at hand and supplying a satisfactory definition. The interest lies in his response to spoken words.

The patient's attempts at repetition were classified in three groups:

+S – unambiguously identifiable;
½S – an attempt at the word;
−S – no attempt (usually) or an attempt with no relation to the target word.

A score was also given to the patient's attempt at the definition of each word. Again there were three categories used:

+M – a full account of the meaning, e.g.
      E: 'herring'
      S: 'sea fish . . . very nice grilled . . . the best . . . used for
          kippers . . . North Sea . . . trawlers'
½M – the subject gave a partial account of the meaning or made some reaction indicating that the meaning had been accessed. There were three main kinds of response:
(a) a verbal indication of the correct semantic field, e.g.
    (i) E: 'pheasant'
        S:'some kind of large bird'
    (ii) E: 'fertiliser'

      S: 'Is it something you put on the garden?'
      E: 'What for?'
      S: 'I don't know . . . to kill insects?'

(b) the subject described a visual image evoked by the stimulus
word, e.g.

      E: 'brass'
      S: 'I suddenly got a picture . . . an old-fashioned bedstead
      . . . you know the kind . . . with knobs. Is it something to
      do with sleeping?'

(c) the stimulus word evoked a bodily reaction, e.g.

   (i) E: 'sergeant'
      S: 'I can feel my legs going . . . as if I was marching. Is it
      something to do with the army?'

 (ii) E: 'trombone'
      S: (went through the motions of playing the trombone)
      E: 'What are you doing?'
      S: 'I've got it . . . gymnastics . . . I'm on the tromboline.'

This last response is more complex, involving a nonsense word
which is a blend of 'trombone' and 'trampoline'. We will not
attempt to trace its possible aetiology.

Cruse reports that with the words giving rise to this class of
responses the patient did not behave as if he had recognised the
stimuli. Nor, when given the written form of the word immediately
afterwards, did he recognise it as what he had just heard. However,
he was always able to give a satisfactory definition of the written
form of the word. He described his own state of mind in the (½M)
condition by saying that he was making 'an educated guess'.

(−M) the patient made no attempt at a definition or, very rarely,
suggested an unrelated meaning.

The patient's performance to the spoken stimuli is shown in Table
9.1.

We can describe this matrix in the following way:

1 If he knew the meaning completely then he could nearly always
repeat it adequately.

2 If he could only make an attempt at repeating the word without
getting it unambiguously right (½S) then the odds were that he did
not know its meaning (−M).

3 If he only knew something of the meaning (½M) then the odds were that he had not attempted to repeat it (−S). This is the category of interest, which corresponds most nearly to the semantic errors in deep dyslexia. Since all the stimulus words were mono-morphemic, the subject must have analysed the sound more or less completely in order to get any aspect of the meaning. Cruse rightly points out that this is something of a problem for the published versions of the logogen system. Within that framework one might be tempted to suggest that a 'response block' has developed − similar to the account given of deep dyslexia in Morton (1968). However the subject was able to read out all except one of the stimulus words correctly. In the framework of the old model this would not have been possible if the output from the logogen had been blocked. Indeed, on one occasion the patient actually used the stimulus word as an example of the general category he was trying to illustrate without being aware that it was in fact the stimulus word.

TABLE 9.1

| | | Accuracy of the repetition | | |
		(+S)	*(½S)*	*(−S)*
Accuracy of	(+M)	122	11	0
the	(½M)	6	9	29
definition	(−M)	34	54	13

However, once the visual and auditory input logogens are separated the notion of a response block becomes possible again. Thus, in the new form of the logogen system, I would account for this patient's performance in the following way.

1 The patient has no system for converting directly from an acoustic code to a phonological code. In normal people, this system, equivalent to the grapheme-phoneme system, allows nonsense words to be repeated. With other patients one could imagine that this system provides an alternative way of repeating words when other routes are damaged.

2 There is an exit block in the auditory logogen system such that information cannot pass from the auditory logogen system to the output system. This may apply to all words or only to those in the (½S) and (−S) classes.

3 For the (½M, −S) words, the route from the auditory logogen

system to the output logogen system would be blocked but that to the cognitive system left intact. This meaning could be accessed even though no phonemic code was available. Note that this code does not account for the patient's inability to produce a full semantic description. By analogy with the deep dyslexics we might expect better – that is more complete as well as more accurate – semantic readings. Cruse's account of this is that with the critical words ($-S$, $\frac{1}{2}M$) the phonological representation is lost very quickly, and the semantic processing is interrupted prior to completion. He could not find convincing evidence to support his account but it remains highly plausible. Certainly we need to account for the patient's inability or unwillingness to attempt to respond on the basis of the semantic information he had. This is most comfortably considered in terms of loss of the phenomenal aspect of the stimulus – being aware only of meaning without stimulus (c.f. Marcel, in press).

2 Michel (1979)

This patient suffered a left temporal lesion in 1973 at the age of 45 as the result of a fall. He did not have any particular problems apart from linguistic ones, preserving, for example, good arithmetic ability from the beginning, and no visual or motor problems. His audiogram was almost normal and he had a performance I.Q. of 107. The main contrast in this patient's language function is in the mode of output, his writing being relatively good but his speech being highly aphasic. The outstanding feature of his performance from our current viewpoint is his repetition behaviour. First of all he was completely incapable of repeating nonsense words. He could only repeat concrete nouns and adjectives, with any degree of success, had a lot of difficulty with abstract nouns, verbs and adverbs and would rarely attempt pronouns, prepositions, conjunctions, or articles. With concrete nouns his repetition attempts were typified by semantic paraphasias. In one session where he attempted 50 concrete nouns, he managed to repeat only 24 per cent correctly and made 58 per cent semantic errors. These errors included:

'buffet'   → 'divan'
'jumeau'   → 'bébé'
'ballon'   → 'cerf-volant'
'mendiant'   → 'clochard'

'noyau'　　→ 'pêche'
'chaussons'　→ 'pantoufle'
'sommeil'　　→ 'paupière'

Of a set of 23 adjectives 10 were correct and of 21 verbs only three were repeated correctly. All three were in the infinitive form of the verb, though not all the infinitives were repeated correctly. There were a couple of derivational errors

'mangerais'　→ 'manger'
'lu'　　　　→ 'lire'

where the responses were in the infinitive. The semantic errors included

'coucher'　　→ 'dormir'.

In one of the earlier examinations this feature of the patient's behaviour surprised his examiners and they explained the task again to him, emphasising that he should repeat the stimulus word and not give free associations. Michel reports that the patient was perplexed at this and almost annoyed that they should suspect him of not following instructions. At a later stage he was asked to free associate to the stimulus words and, not unexpectedly, he took longer to produce responses under these conditions than when producing equivalent kinds of responses under the instructions to repeat the words. This confirmed that the semantic errors under the repetition conditions were not strategic but involuntary.

　In contrast to the patient's performance in the repetition task, Michel reports that he could read any word or nonsense syllable. In these respects, then, the patient conforms precisely to the requirements set out at the beginning of the chapter.

　Not unexpectedly, the patient presented a number of other symptoms. His speech was paraphasic; object-naming was very difficult, and the patient preferred to spell the word out loud rather than grope around trying to find phonological form. Performance in a dichotic task was quite dramatic. Four years after his accident he showed a total suppression of the right ear with monosyllabic words or disyllabic words. In addition his responses to the left ear, whether spoken or written, included a number of semantic errors. These included *crabe* being reproduced as *homard*, *auto* as *voiture*, *biche* as *gazelle*. With a task involving pairs of easily identifiable everyday sounds to be labelled, with a written response, the patient scored 90 per cent of the stimuli from the left ear and 70 per cent from the right ear. As Michel remarks, this could be due to the temporal properties of the sounds which did permit a switch of attention from ear to ear.

Finally it is clear that the patient is agrammatic in all modalities. Thus, in a written answer to the written question *Où est la Tour Eiffel?* he wrote *315 mètres*. All French children know the height of the Eiffel Tower and the imagined question is a likely one. In answer to the spoken question 'Who is the president of the U.S.A.?' he began to write a list of all the presidents he could remember.

From the point of view of trying to model deep dyslexia, this patient is very significant. His pattern of performance helps to answer a problem which existed when only the deep dyslexic pattern had been described, namely that the reading functions might be considered more complex or more-vulnerable (since more recently learned) than repetition skills. If this were so, then the functional separation of reading skills and repetition skills need not be asserted. One could simply say that the more complex skills are more liable to disturbance. The existence of these two patients amounts to evidence for a double dissociation and as such is more convincing evidence for a modality separation.

References

Byers Brown, D. B. and Ives, L. (1969) The re-education of a dysphasic adult. *British Journal of Disorder of Communication, 4,* 176–96.

Cruse, D. A. (in press) Aspects of word recognition in an adult aphasic. *Brain and Language.*

Marcel, A. J. (in press) Conscious and unconscious reading: the effects of visual masking on word perception. *Cognitive Psychology.*

Michel, F. (1979) Preservation du langage ecrit malgré un deficit majeur du langage oral. *Le Lyon Medical, 241,* 141–9.

Morton, J. (1968) Grammar and computation. In J. C. Catford (ed.), *Studies in Language and Language Behaviour,* C.R.L.L.B. Progress Report no. VI, University of Michigan.

Patterson, K. E. and Marcel, A. J. (1977) Aphasia, dyslexia and the phonological coding of written words. *Quarterly Journal of Experimental Psychology, 29,* 307–18.

10 Reading, phonological recoding, and deep dyslexia

Max Coltheart

A major characteristic of deep dyslexia is the patient's inability to gain access to, or to create, phonological representations of printed letter-strings. This inability has been demonstrated in a variety of ways. Some examples are:

(a) Deep dyslexic patients have great difficulty in pronouncing aloud even the simplest of pronounceable non-words.

(b) When the non-words are pseudo-homophones (i.e. have the same pronunciations as genuine words – examples are *brane* and *burd*), patients will sometimes pronounce them correctly, but it is clear that they do not do this by deriving a phonological code directly from the letter-string. Instead they use what might be termed 'approximate visual access'; they seek that English word which is *visually* the most similar to the pseudohomophonic non-word, and give this as the response (Saffran and Marin, 1977). This may even be done with non-words which are not pseudo-homophones (Patterson, 1978).

(c) Even in tasks which do not require overt articulation this phonological disability can be observed. For example, one patient chose *cough* rather than *cuff* as a rhyme for *rough*, and *choke* rather than *soap* as a rhyme for *hope*; clearly her rhyme decisions are made on the basis of *visual* similarity (Saffran and Marin, 1977).

(d) Furthermore, when patients are asked to perform the lexical decision task (classifying letter-strings as words or non-words), their 'No' responses are not impeded when non-word strings are pseudo-homophones (Patterson and Marcel, 1977), whereas

I thank Derek Besner and Estelle Doctor for useful discussions.

normal subjects respond more slowly and make more errors to non-words which are pseudo-homophones than to those which are not (Rubenstein, Lewis and Rubenstein, 1971; Coltheart, Davelaar, Jonasson and Besner, 1977; Patterson and Marcel, 1977).

It can be argued with considerable plausibility that this phono-logical disability is an absolutely central component of the syndrome of deep dyslexia, and that other symptoms are secondary ones, caused by the phonological disability. For example, Patterson (1977) has suggested the possibility that derivational errors, rather than representing an independent symptom, could be a consequence of the phonological disability. She has proposed that words which have the same free morpheme but different bound morphemes, i.e. words that are derivationally related to each other, may have a single lexical entry corresponding to this free morpheme. For example, *run*, *runs*, *running* and *runner* may possess only the single lexical entry *run*. If this were so, access to this entry would not be sufficient to enable the reader to know which of these four words he was looking at. In order to pronounce an inflected word aloud, it would be necessary to have a non-lexical representation of the word's bound morphemes. If the non-lexical representation is phonological in form, it would not be available to the deep dyslexic. Hence, when he is asked to pronounce inflected words aloud, he should produce the correct free morpheme but make frequent errors on the bound-morpheme components, i.e. he should make derivational errors; and these patients do so.

It has also been suggested that the semantic error itself is a secondary symptom which arises as a consequence of the patient's phonological disability. The general idea here is that lexical access will not produce a single unambiguous lexical entry; instead, because of the existence of an associative network in the internal lexicon, a set of semantically related lexical entries will be activated when a single word is being read (e.g. the printed word *tree* may activate the lexical entries for tree, leaf, bush, green, oak and so on). Selection amongst these candidates is performed by matching each to a non-lexically derived stimulus record. This record could be visual, or phonological, or both. If it is sometimes (or always) phonological, then correct selection from the set of semantically-related lexical entries will sometimes or always be denied to the patient; thus he will produce semantic errors in reading aloud. An idea of this sort is put forward in Chapter 8.

Allport (personal communication) has taken this line of reasoning still further by pointing out that one might even argue that the deep dyslexics' difficulties with function words are secondary to their phonological disability. It might be argued that function words do not possess lexical entries in quite the same sense that content words do; the role of function words is not to 'convey meaning' but to indicate how to assemble the meanings of individual content words into a phrase unit. If so, when someone is asked to pronounce aloud a single printed function word, he might need to use some non-lexical procedure for converting print to phonology. A patient lacking this procedure would then be unable to pronounce function words aloud.

It has sometimes been suggested (e.g. Pickering, personal communication) that low-frequency words rely for lexical access on a preliminary phonological recoding; and also that abstract words rely more on phonological recoding than concrete words (Shallice and Warrington, 1975). If these suggestions are correct, then a patient who has lost the ability to carry out phonological recoding would, *ipso facto*, be selectively impaired with low-frequency words, and abstract words. These two selective disabilities are in fact demonstrated by deep dyslexic patients.

Some neurologists have made considerably more sweeping suggestions along these lines. Hécaen and Kremin (1976, p. 281) summarize an account of alexia popular amongst neurologists as follows:

> The visual images /of letters/ cannot be evoked in the left
> hemisphere, because of the interruption of the optic radiations.
> They can, however, be evoked on the right side through the
> right optic radiation, *but they cannot be used in reading, since they no
> longer evoke the verbal acoustic components of the letters.* (My italics.)

One who holds this kind of view is Geschwind (1965); his views concerning the reason that reading is impaired by angular gyrus damage were summarized by Benson and Geschwind (1969) as follows:

> The suggestion has been made recently by Geschwind (1965)

that the angular gyrus plays a major role in the formation of associations between vision, somesthesis and audition and thus is basic to the visual-auditory associations involved in reading.

The view expressed here is a simple one: reading occurs by proceeding from print through phonology to meaning, and therefore a lesion which abolishes the ability to proceed from print to phonology must have catastrophic consequences for reading.

What the various views I have discussed so far have in common is the contention that phonological encoding of print is an essential component of the normal reading process, and that therefore an inability to perform such recoding will be sufficient to produce some kind of abnormality of reading. The expected abnormality might take the form of making derivational errors, making semantic errors, being unable to read function words, being unable to read low-frequency words, or being unable to read abstract words; this depends upon the particular theoretical role assigned to phonological encoding. According to some theorists, loss of the ability to derive phonology from print would even abolish reading entirely.

Whilst neurologists and neuropsychologists have been proposing explanations of alexic symptomatology in terms of disruption of phonological recoding, experimental psychologists have been attempting to investigate directly what role or roles phonological recoding actually plays in normal reading. Until very recently, there has been little cross-communication between those who work on the pathology of reading and those who work on normal reading; but, obviously, such communication is essential. For example, if experimental psychologists were to provide convincing evidence that phonological recoding were *not* used in normal reading, it would follow that abolition of the ability to perform phonological recoding would have no consequences whatsoever for reading; reading would remain normal. In this case, all suggestions to the effect that some alexic symptoms occur because of disruption of the ability to perform phonological recoding would have to be abandoned forthwith. On the other hand, if neuropsychological studies were to demonstrate conclusively that some of the symptoms of deep dyslexia were a direct consequence of lack of phonological recoding, then this would be convincing evidence that phonological recoding *does* play a role in normal reading, since normal readers do not display deep-dyslexic symptoms; it would follow that any suggestions by experimental psychologists that phonological recoding plays no part in normal reading would have to be rejected.

What I aim to do in this chapter is to review what experimental psychology currently has to say about the role or roles of phonological recoding in reading, and then, by deducing from this work what the consequences of impaired or abolished phonological recoding would be, to discuss to what extent the deep dyslexic's constellation of symptoms might spring from his undoubted inability to derive phonology from print.

Until quite recently there was no experimental work which provided convincing elucidations of the importance of phonological recoding for adult reading. Despite this, many people were willing to make pronouncements on this issue:

> Adults reading silently to themselves bypass subvocalisation and go directly to the abstract meaning for which the text is only a notation. The articulatory and acoustic representation intervening is unnecessary. (Gibson and Levin, 1975)

> In order to read alphabetic languages one must have an ingrained habit of producing the sounds of one's language when one sees the written words which conventionally represent the phonemes. (Bloomfield, 1942)

> Reading does not need to proceed by the reader's forming auditory representations of printed words. (Kolers, 1970)

> The heart of (reading skill) is surely the process of decoding the written symbols to speech. (Gibson, 1970)

> Reading can be, and for skilled readers often is, a visual process. (Bower, 1970)

> A word to be recognised is recoded phonemically even when it is presented visually. (Rubenstein, Lewis and Rubenstein, 1971)

> Phonemic stage not necessary for reading. (Baron, 1973)

> To read, in effect, is to translate the writing into silent speech. (Egger, 1881, cited by Kleiman, 1975)

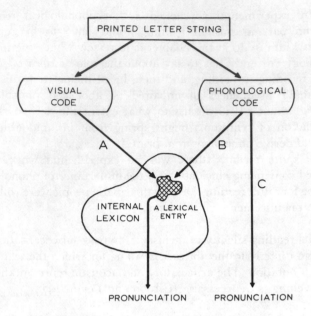

FIGURE 10.1 Ins and outs of the internal lexicon

> Purely visual reading is quite possible, theoretically. (Huey, 1908)

> The printed word is mapped onto a phonemic representation by the reader. (Gough, 1972)

None of these statements was accompanied by any satisfactory supporting evidence. Relevant evidence has been emerging from recent experimental work however, and I will now turn to a discussion of this. My discussion will be organized within the framework set out in Figure 10.1. This framework assumes the existence of an internal lexicon which embodies all the knowledge a person has concerning the words in his vocabulary. Each word he knows is represented in this lexicon as a lexical entry, containing information about how the word is spelled, how it is pronounced, and what it means: orthographic, phonological and semantic information.

A human being can do many things with printed letter-strings:

pronounce them, write them down, spell them aloud, and understand them (if they are words). The scheme shown in Figure 10.1 is limited to the two processes of comprehension and pronunciation; it is assumed that a word is comprehended when access is gained to its lexical entry. Many fairly recent theoretical treatments of reading comprehension have been concerned with questions about the *existence* of some of the pathways shown in Figure 10.1. For example, theories which claimed that access to a lexical entry *requires* phonological recoding (e.g. Rubenstein, Lewis and Rubenstein, 1971; Gough, 1972) amounted to claims that pathway A does not exist; theories which claimed that reading is purely 'visual' (Smith, 1971) were assertions that pathway B does not exist; and 'dual-access' models (e.g. Meyer, Schvaneveldt and Ruddy, 1974) asserted that both of these pathways exist.

It seems to me now that questions concerning the existence of these pathways do not require experimental investigation; such questions can be answered adequately by simple demonstrations. My argument here will rest upon an assumption concerning the nature of phonological recoding. According to Figure 10.1, phonological recoding is a process which can be carried out whether or not a letter-string is a word, and hence is a non-lexical process. It is also non-lexical in the sense that it is pre-lexical, because it is carried out so as to produce a phonological representation which is *subsequently* used to access the internal lexicon. Various possible ways of performing such non-lexical phonological recoding can be proposed:

(a) letters are converted to sounds by grapheme-phoneme conversion rules operating at the level of letters and phonemes;
(b) an internal syllabary may be used, by means of which syllabic letter groups are translated into syllables;
(c) there may exist a phonological lexicon, so that a whole word accesses this lexicon and the phonological representation of the word thereby is obtained.

I have argued elsewhere (Coltheart, 1978) that only the first of these three proposed methods is workable and is consistent with experimental results; thus these issues will be considered only briefly here. A central point is that a system of grapheme-phoneme conversion rules can be formulated which produces the correct pronunciation of *most* English words when applied to their spellings (Wijk, 1966;

Venezky, 1970). However, for a not insubstantial proportion of words, these rules produce the wrong pronunciation. Thus there exist two classes of word: regular words (those which conform to the rules) and exceptions (those which do not). This linguistic distinction has psychological reality, since naming latencies are faster for regular words than for exceptions (Baron and Strawson, 1976; Gough and Cosky, 1977). Theories of non-lexical phonological recoding based on the syllable or the whole word as a unit provide no obvious explanation for this result. Furthermore, they do not provide any obvious explanation for the kinds of reading error characteristic of 'surface dyslexia' (Marshall and Newcombe, 1973); here the patient appears to be neglecting to apply specific grapheme-phoneme correspondences (GPCs), so that this syndrome provides further support for the view that non-lexical phonological recoding operates via GPCs. Finally, there is the fact that we can pronounce non-words. If pronunciation depended upon a whole-word-based phonological lexicon, the latter would need to contain all possible pronounceable non-words; if pronunciation depended upon a procedure which used the syllable as a unit, there would have to be an internal syllabary which contained all the possible syllables of English, even though the number of different syllables which actually occur in English words is far fewer than the number of possible different English syllables (Fudge, 1970). Why should such prodigality occur?

For these reasons, I will assume that non-lexical phonological recoding depends upon the use of GPCs. But if this is so, one can demonstrate that pathway, A, B and C must all exist.

Pathway A must exist because we can pronounce exception words correctly. Incorrect pronunciations would result if pathways B or C were used; thus the correct pronunciation must be achieved via non-phonological access to a lexical entry followed by retrieval of the word's phonological representation from that entry. How else could, for example, *bread* be pronounced correctly? In nearly all English words the vowel digraph *ea* is pronounced as in *steam*. Application of this GPC to the word *bread* would produce the phonological form of the word 'breed' and hence the reader would pronounce *bread* as if it were *breed*. There is a second reason for the existence of a non-phonological route to the lexicon, namely, that many words in printed English are ideographs (examples include Arabic and Roman numerals, mathematical signs, and many abbreviations such as &, lb, and cwt) to which GPCs cannot be applied; yet we can pronounce these correctly. Whether the pathway used for pronouncing ideographs is identical to the pathway used for pronouncing exception words is not yet known, but my guess is that we will need to postulate different visual pathways for ideographs and alphabetically printed words. For one thing, the gross overall visual distortion produced by alternating case (tReE) has surprisingly little effect on readability, whereas one would expect a large effect if words were sometimes read as ideographs. For another, judgments of which of two printed numbers is numerically the greater are influenced by the irrelevant physical sizes of the numbers when they are printed ideographically (i.e. as numerals) but not when they are printed alphabetically (Besner and Coltheart, 1979). These points are not conclusive, but they are suggestive: perhaps ideographs will require an additional pathway not shown in Figure 10.1. Whether this will be so or not, we do need pathway A to account for our ability to understand and pronounce exception words, so pathway A must exist.

Pathway C must exist too; if it did not, the only route from print to pronunciation would be via the lexicon, and so we could not pronounce letter strings which lack lexical entries, i.e. we could not pronounce non-words. Since we can, pathway C exists.

Finally, pathway B must also exist. We are able to answer correctly questions requiring semantic decisions about pseudo-homophones – does *phocks* sound like a kind of animal? Since the lexical entry for *fox* cannot be accessed from the letter-string *phocks* by using a visual code, answering this kind of question must depend upon phonological recoding followed by lexical access, i.e. must depend upon pathway B.

Thus experimental investigations aimed at discovering which of these pathways exist are unnecessary. We can pronounce non-words, exception words and ideographs, and we know that *phocks* sounds like an animal; therefore pathways A, B and C must all exist.

The question we should be asking is not whether these pathways exist, but in what circumstances each is used. For example, lexical access based on pre-lexical phonological recoding (pathway B) is something that normal readers *can* accomplish; but is this ever how lexical access during normal reading is achieved? It need not be; as Coltheart *et al.* (1977) pointed out, it may be that pathway B is always slower in operation than pathway A, so that even if both pathways are functioning during normal reading, access to the meaning of a word is always achieved via pathway A.

Thus I will turn now to a discussion of experiments which provide some information about which pathway normal adult readers actually use in a variety of simple reading tasks. The three tasks mainly to be discussed will be *lexical decision* (deciding whether a single letter-string is a word or not), *semantic categorization* (deciding whether a single letter-string represents a word belonging to a pre-specified semantic category or not) and *phrase evaluation* (deciding whether a group of letter-strings represents a meaningful phrase or not).

Lexical decision

The 'No' response is slower and less accurate when a non-word is phonologically identical to some English word (e.g. *ile, fraze*) than when it is not (e.g. *ife, fruze*) (Rubenstein *et al.*, 1971; Coltheart *et al.*, 1977; Gough and Cosky, 1977; Patterson and Marcel, 1977). Thus pathway B influences lexical decision making. However, this is a result obtained with non-words, and it is not inconsistent with the possibility that pathway A *always* works more rapidly than pathway B. It could be argued that only when pathway A cannot access a lexical entry does enough time elapse to permit effects due to pathway B to influence behaviour. So this result does not tell us whether or not, when a letter-string is a word, lexical access ever depends upon pathway B. In making this point, Coltheart *et al.* (1977) argued that what should be done was to look for evidence of phonological recoding on the 'Yes' response in lexical decision tasks.

This was done by Coltheart, Besner, Jonasson and Davelaar (1979). Regular words have two pathways to their lexical entries, A and B. Exception words have only one, A. If, for regular words, access via pathway B *ever* occurs prior to access via pathway A, this would mean that lexical access would on the average be faster for regular words than for exception words. On the other hand, if pathway B always lagged behind pathway A, then lexical access would always depend on pathway A, equally for regular words and for exception words. So one can investigate whether pathway B plays a part in lexical access by determining whether the time needed for lexical access (as measured by 'Yes' latency in a lexical decision task) is on the average faster for regular words than for exception words. Coltheart *et al.* (1979) found no trace whatsoever of an advantage in speed or in accuracy for regular words over exception words. This suggests that in the lexical decision task, lexical access, when it occurs, *always* occurs via pathway A. Only when access to a lexical entry is impossible (i.e. when the stimulus is a non-word) can pathway B affect behaviour.

There are a number of interesting avenues to explore here. One of these is represented by some unpublished work by Meyer and Gutschera (1975). They carried out a lexical decision experiment under two different conditions. In task S (for 'spelling') the subject was asked to judge whether letter-strings were or were not words. In task P (for 'pronunciation') the subject was asked to judge whether letter-strings were *pronounced* like words or not. Some of the letter-strings were pseudo-homophones, and so required a 'No' response in task S but a 'Yes' response in task P. What is interesting about this work is that task P *requires* the subject to use pathway B, since it is only by such means that he can respond correctly to pseudo-homophones. The results of this lexical decision experiment are discussed at length by Coltheart (1978); they provide no reasons for rejecting the view that the 'Yes' response in lexical decision experiments under 'normal' (i.e. task S) conditions are made solely by using pathway A.

Semantic categorization

Meyer and Gutschera (1975) carried out a semantic categorization experiment which was analogous to their lexical decision experiment. The stimuli were either category members, pseudo-members, or non-members: for example, for the category *fish*, a member would be *trout*, a pseudo-member *soul*, and a non-member *book*. Again, both task S and task P were used, i.e. the correct response to a pseudo-member was 'No' for task S and 'Yes' for task P.

Although these lexical decision and semantic categorization experiments are analogous, there is a crucial difference between them. When responding 'Yes' to a pseudo-homophone in a task P lexical decision task, the subject *must* use pre-lexical phonological recoding, since the item he is dealing with, being a non-word, has no lexical entry which is non-phonologically accessible. This is not so when responding 'Yes' to a pseudo-member in a task P semantic categorization task, since here the item in question is always a word. There are two different ways in which a subject could respond 'Yes' to the question *sounds like a fruit? – pair*:

(a)   pre-lexical phonological recoding of *pair* and use of this code for access to the lexical entry of its homophone *pear*, i.e. use of pathway B;

(b)   *visual* access to the lexical entry for *pair*, retrieval from this entry of the phonological code of the word, and use of this code to access the lexical entry for *pear*, i.e. use of pathway A.

This distinction here is the vital but often neglected distinction between pre-lexical and post-lexical phonology. Pronouncing a non-word must depend upon pre-lexical phonology; pronouncing an exception word or an ideograph must depend upon post-lexical phonology; but pronouncing a regular word can be accomplished in either of these two ways (this is how the naming-latency advantage for regular words is usually explained) and when a subject uses the phonological code of the word *pair* to answer the question *sounds like a fruit? – pair*, we cannot tell whether it is a pre-lexical or a post-lexical code that he is using.

This chapter began by discussing the evidence indicating that deep dyslexics cannot utilize phonological representations of printed letter-strings. It is now evident that we should consider whether what they are lacking is pre-lexical phonology, post-lexical phonology, or both. The answer appears to be both. If they possessed pre-lexical phonology, they could pronounce non-words and regular words; but they are impaired on both of these tasks. If they possessed post-lexical phonology, they could pronounce all words (even if unable to pronounce non-words), but they cannot. Thus both forms of phonology are impaired.

To return to Meyer and Gutschera: methods are available for determining the importance of pre-lexical and of post-lexical phonology in their experiment. Since exception words have incorrect pre-lexical phonology, any phonological effects with such words must be post-lexical. Alternatively, since non-words cannot have post-lexical phonology, any phonological effects with non-words must be pre-lexical.

The former method was used by Midgley-West (1978). She

repeated Meyer and Gutschera's semantic-categorization experiment (using task S and task P) with one modification: half the words in each of the conditions were exceptions and half were regulars. The first important result here was that 'Yes' responses to pseudo-members in the P condition (i.e. responses to the items of the type *sounds like a kind of fruit?* – *pair*) were much faster for regular than for exception words. This indicates that subjects were applying GPC rules to the test words in the P task, i.e. were using pre-lexical phonological recoding. However, these rules were not used in the S task, which is the one which resembles normal reading, because neither the 'Yes' response to members nor the 'No' response to pseudo-members or non-members was influenced by whether the test word in the S task was a regular word or an exception. These findings indicate, then, that skilled readers know and can use GPC rules to obtain phonological representations of printed words in certain circumstances (the P task) but that in the condition which resembles normal reading (the S task) there is no evidence that lexical access is ever anything but visual – no evidence that a phonological code is used for lexical access. An identical conclusion was reached above when the results of lexical decision experiments were being considered.

Phrase evaluation

Baron (1973) asked subjects to judge whether short printed sequences of words made sense or not. He used three types of sequence: phrases (e.g. *tie the knot*) pseudo-phrases (*tie the not*) and non-phrases (*ill him*) and two instructional tasks, task S and task P, as defined above.

The crucial comparison here is between pseudo-phrases and non-phrases in task S. If pseudo-phrases are more difficult to reject than non-phrases, then phonological encoding is influencing behaviour. Baron found no differences in the mean RT of 'No' responses in these two conditions; however, although error rates were very small, subjects wrongly responded 'Yes' more than twice as often to pseudo-phrases as to non-phrases, a difference which was significant. This error effect clearly shows that some phonological encoding *was* occurring in this experiment, and it is therefore unfortunate that Baron's error results have usually been ignored by subsequent authors, so that his work is usually quoted as providing no evidence for phonological encoding during reading. For example, 'Baron (1973) demonstrated that subjects had no more difficulty in deciding that a phrase was nonsense when it sounded sensible than when it didn't' (Levy, 1979); and 'It appears that a phonemic representation was not consulted in making this meaning decision (Baron, 1973)' (Levy, 1978). If subjects did sometimes evaluate Baron's phrases in terms of their phonology, then errors should occur; but there is no obvious reason why slow but correct responses should occur. If they did, one would need to postulate some additional mechanism (e.g. visual re-checking) to explain the effect. Thus the error effect is the natural one to expect if some phonological recoding is occurring, which makes its neglect even more incomprehensible.

Baron's experiment has been repeated and extended by Doctor (1978), for two reasons: firstly, to see whether the finding of an error effect but no RT effect can be reproduced, and secondly to see whether any phonological effect observed is pre-lexical or post-lexical. She achieved the latter by including non-word pseudo-phrases such as *he throo the ball*. If subjects have difficulty with the non-word pseudo-phrases, then they must be recoding these into phonological form prior to lexical access; if their pseudo-phrase difficulties are confined to all-word pseudo-phrases, these difficulties must be arising post-lexically. Examples of the items used by Doctor, together with the mean RT of correct responses and the error rate for each item type, are shown in Table 10.1.

TABLE 10.1 *Mean RTs and error rates for the six sentence types used by Doctor (1978)*

Sentence examples	Correct response	Mean correct RT in secs	Mean error %
We stand in the queue	Yes	1.20	9
We wait in the queue	Yes	1.17	15
We weight in the queue	No	1.39	27
We grate in the queue	No	1.50	14.5
We wate in the queue	No	1.18	11
We grait in the queue	No	1.22	6.5

The Civic Quarter Library

Item(s) borrowed on:

11/05/06
01:46 pm

n:Developmental dyslexia
0580422
Date: 25/5/2006,23:59

n:Deep dyslexia
0305408
Date: 25/5/2006,23:59

Telephone (0113) 283 3106

Please retain this receipt

Comparison of all-word pseudo-phrases with all-word non-phrases showed that Baron's finding was reproduced exactly: the two types of item did not differ significantly in mean RT, but subjects made significantly more errors on the pseudo-phrases than on the non-phrases.

This effect was not observed with non-word phrases: here responses to pseudo-phrases and to non-phrases did not differ in speed or in accuracy. Furthermore, 'No' responses were much faster to non-word pseudo-phrases and non-phrases than to all-word pseudo-phrases and non-phrases.

The following interpretation of these findings is suggested. The subject begins by accessing lexical entries for individual letter-strings using a visual code, i.e. pathway A. If any letter-string does not generate lexical access, then a 'No' response is immediately made, because, since the phrase contains a non-word, it cannot make sense. This stratagem enables fast 'No' responses to be made to non-word items.

If all letter-strings are words and hence all achieve lexical access, the subject's task is then to determine whether the phrase as a whole is meaningful. Even if the method by which a subject actually makes such determinations remains obscure, it might nevertheless be argued that the individual words of a phrase or sentence need to be held in some form of buffer storage whilst the processes by which the meaningfulness of the set of words as a whole is decided are applied to the words. A number of proposals along these lines have recently been made, e.g. by Kleiman (1975), who suggested that semantic integration of a set of words into a phrase or higher order unit depends upon holding the set of words in some form of short-term buffer storage, a form of storage in which information is represented in a phonological code. If so, then when a subject is attempting to comprehend a phrase or sentence he will need to retrieve from each accessed lexical entry the word's phonological code, and it is a representation of the phrase in terms of a sequence of phonological codes which exists in the buffer memory and is operated upon when the subject is attempting to determine whether the phrase is meaningful. How this determination is actually made is as yet a mystery; nor is it clear why the subject does not *always* give an incorrect 'Yes' response to all-word pseudo-phrases. However, if whatever the subject does to deal with such phrases (e.g. 'visual re-checking') is not error-free, or not always employed, then this will induce errors on pseudo-phrases but not on non-phrases, which is the effect observed by Doctor and by Baron. It should be noted that Doctor also found that genuine phrases which contained homophones produced significantly more incorrect 'No' responses than genuine phrases which did not: thus phonological ambiguity does tax whatever process is used for evaluating phrases, which is consistent with the claim that this process uses phonological representations of words.

Résumé

Work on lexical decision, semantic categorization and phrase evaluation has been discussed. In conditions which correspond to normal reading (task S conditions with words), effects which should have occurred if pre-lexical phonological recoding were contributing to performance were absent. The only situation in which a clear phonological effect was observed was when subjects were asked to judge the meaningfulness of a short piece of text. Here the phonological effect was post-lexical, and it was argued that the effect arose because short-term storage of words is needed in the phrase-evaluation task and such short-term storage uses a phonological code.

Articulatory suppression and reading

One experimental method which has sometimes been used to investigate the roles of phonological encoding in reading is to interfere with the reader's ability to use his articulatory apparatus. Eighty years ago this was done by inserting objects into the reader's mouth (see, for example, Vago, 1968); now it is done by asking him to articulate some irrelevant message.

The pertinence of this method is by no means obvious. If a subject is asked to pronounce a printed letter-string, he must do so first by *obtaining* an articulatory representation of the string, and then by *executing* the articulatory instructions contained in that representation. The second of these stages obviously requires the use of the articulatory apparatus, but the first does not. One might claim, then, that occupying the articulatory apparatus with some other, irrelevant, task will prevent the second stage from occurring; but why should it affect the first? Yet it is the first stage, the derivation of a phonological representation from a printed letter string, which is of importance in theoretical treatments of reading.

Even if we put this objection aside, problems remain for work using this kind of technique. If one wishes to study the role of phonological encoding in reading by using a technique which suppresses articulation of the text being read, one needs to be sure that the effects produced by the technique are in fact due to the suppression of articulation, and one also needs to be sure that the primary task being carried out by the subject is a reasonable facsimile of reading. In recent work such as that of Kleiman (1975) and Levy (1977, 1978, 1979) such assurances appear to be lacking.

Kleiman's suppression technique required the subject to repeat aloud a sequence of auditory digits presented at a rate of eighty-four digits per minute or faster. This shadowing task slowed the subject's judgments of whether or not two printed words rhymed much more than it slowed his judgments of whether they were visually similar or his judgments of whether they were synonymous. Judgments of whether a sentence was semantically acceptable or not were also greatly slowed by concurrent shadowing. Kleiman assumed that the degree to which a task was slowed by shadowing was an indication of the degree to which it required phonological encoding, since he was using shadowing to impede articulation. However, this is not all that shadowing involves; it is a demanding task which also requires speech perception, for example. It turns out that when one uses a task which, while blocking articulation, does little else, one finds that suppression of articulation has no effect on reading comprehension. Baddeley (1979) found that the time taken by subjects to decide whether printed sentences were true or false was not affected at all by asking them to count rapidly from one to six over and over again while reading. However, if a mental load were added to this simple articulatory task, by requiring the subjects to repeat a memorized random digit sequence rather than the overlearned sequence one to six, then judgments of the truth of the printed sentence did become slower. Thus it seems clear that the effects obtained by Kleiman (1975) were due not to interference simply with articulation but to competing demands upon 'spare processing capacity' (whatever that might be).

This point is further demonstrated by the work of Smith (1976).

She had subjects judge the truth of printed sentences and also the validity of printed syllogisms. In both cases, subjects were just as fast at the task when they were continuously articulating (repeating 'hiya' aloud as fast as they could) as when they read with no interfering condition. Articulatory suppression did not increase error rates in the sentence verification task. It did so in the syllogism task, but this effect was not specific to reading, since in one of two experiments it also occurred with auditory presentation of syllogisms.

In experiments by Levy (1977, 1979), subjects were given a set of six sentences, followed by a single test sentence to which they had to respond 'Yes' if it were identical to one of the original six and 'No' if it were not. One way in which a subject might tackle this would be to read the original six sentences, and, having understood them, to store a representation of their meanings, against which the test sentence could be checked. However, Levy's subjects could not do this, because on 50 per cent of 'No' trials, the test sentence was identical in meaning to one of the original six sentences; thus using semantic coding in memory would produce many errors. Using storage of the meanings of individual words would be even worse, since on the remaining 50 per cent of 'No' trials, the test sentence was identical to one of the original sentences except for an interchange of position of two words. Thus this task required the subject to store verbatim rather than semantic sentence representations if he were to succeed at all, and in this sense what was being investigated was rote memory, not reading. Hence it is not surprising that the results obtained were very similar to those obtained in earlier experiments explicitly dealing with rote memory: articulatory suppression impaired performance when material was presented visually, but not when it was presented auditorily.

In contrast, in subsequent experiments (Levy, 1978) semantic encoding and storage were encouraged, because the subject's task was to decide whether the test sentence did or did not have the same *meaning* as one of the original test sentences. Now performance was not affected by articulatory suppression, in either modality (visual or auditory).

The various experiments just described, and others by Simmonds, referred to in Baddeley (1979), indicate that provided one's technique for suppressing articulation does this and nothing else, and provided the primary task given the subject is close enough to a reading comprehension task, then suppression of articulation has no effect on the reading comprehension of skilled readers. (It might be another story with children or poor readers.) However, because we do not understand what effects articulatory suppression *could* have, it is not entirely clear what we should conclude from the absence of effects of articulatory suppression on reading comprehension.

One attempt at specifying the possible effects of articulatory suppression is that of Baddeley and co-workers, within the framework of the theoretical concept of working memory. Working memory consists of two components: an articulatory loop (AL), which re-circulates phonologically-encoded information, and a central executive (CE) which controls such circulation and carries out a variety of executive tasks. The CE component can store information; the supplementary storage capability offered by the AL component can free some of the CE space for other storage or processing. Thus AL assists, but is not essential for, storage in working memory.

Although one might suppose that articulatory suppression would interfere with the operation of the AL component itself, the data refute such a view. Phonological effects on memory (effects due to phonological similarity of items and to phonological complexity of items), which are considered to reflect the operation of AL, are abolished by articulatory suppression when presentation is visual, but they occur even under articulatory suppression when presentation is auditory (Baddeley, 1979). Therefore, one cannot claim that what articulatory suppression does is impair or abolish AL itself, since if this were the case, one should obtain the same effects of articulatory suppression whether modality of input was visual or auditory. Instead, there must be some process, process X, which:

(a)   is used to encode visual information into the AL;
(b)   is not needed when information is presented auditorily;
(c)   is abolished by articulatory suppression.

Baddeley (1979) expressed this view by suggesting that the AL is 'a system, perhaps involving motor speech programmes, which can be primed either by articulation, or by hearing a particular sequence of speech sounds. On this view, sub-vocal articulation is a means of priming the system, but it is not the sub-vocalization itself that holds the phonemic information.'

Process X is defined by the three properties, (a), (b), and (c), listed above, and this definition is sufficiently precise for us to ask the following question: whilst it is evident that process X is responsible for phonological effects in working-memory experiments with visual presentation, is process X the process which is responsible for phonological effects in reading experiments?

As noted earlier, phonological effects in reading experiments can be pre-lexical or post-lexical effects. Thus the above question is actually two questions. The first question is, does pre-lexical phonological recoding require process X? The second is, does post-lexical phonological recoding require process X? Since, by definition, concurrent articulation abolishes process X, one can investigate these questions by investigating what effects concurrent articulation has upon (a) pre-lexical phonology and (b) post-lexical phonology.

The first of these issues can be investigated by experiments in which subjects judge whether a pair of non-words have the same or different pronunciations. Non-words are used to ensure that the phonological representations upon which the judgments are based cannot be obtained from the lexicon; thus it must be pre-lexical phonology which is being used. The question is, can subjects judge that *bue* and *bew* have the same pronunciation, whilst *bue* and *bem* do not, under conditions of articulatory suppression? A second task, equally appropriate, is to ask subjects to decide whether or not a non-word is pronounced exactly like a member of a semantic category or not; does *phocks* sound like an animal? If articulatory suppression abolishes pre-lexical phonology, this task will be impossible when articulation is suppressed.

A pure test of post-lexical phonology is more difficult to devise. One possibility is judging how many syllables there are in two-digit numerals. Another possibility is a rhyming task where all the words are exception words. A third possibility is judging whether picture-pairs have rhyming names.

These experiments remain to be done. In my opinion, both the pre-lexical and post-lexical phonological tasks can be performed during concurrent articulation – at least, I seem to be able to do them. If this is so, then the system (or systems) responsible for phonological effects in reading experiments is (or are) different from the system responsible for phonological recoding of visually-presented material in experiments on working memory, in that the latter system does not operate during concurrent articulation, whereas the former does. From this it follows that studying the effect of concurrent articulation upon reading cannot at present tell us anything about the role or roles of phonological encoding during reading. This point may be made in another way: since articulatory suppression does not affect reading comprehension, one may conclude, as Baddeley (1979) did, that 'the articulatory loop is not necessary for either reading or comprehending simple sentences'; but this conclusion implies nothing about whether reading comprehension does or does not depend upon phonological encoding (pre-lexical, post-lexical, or both) if it is the case that phonological encoding does not require the activity of the articulatory loop, i.e. if phonological encoding can still occur during articulatory suppression.

This would be one way of resolving the apparent conflict between the results of Baddeley (1979) and those of Baron (1973) and Doctor (1978). If phonological effects with visually presented material reflect the activity of the AL, and the AL is not used in reading, as Baddeley (1979) argues, then phonological effects should not occur in reading; yet Baron (1973) and Doctor (1978) have found such effects. The conflict would no longer remain a conflict if the system responsible for phonological recoding in working-memory experiments could not be equated with the system responsible for phonological effects in reading experiments.

An alternative way of resolving this apparent conflict would be to propose that the system responsible for phonological effects in reading experiments does not *assist* reading, but merely hinders reading, whenever it has any effect at all. The system may be a re-checking procedure based on phonological recoding, called into play only when a 'No' response is contemplated in the Baron and Doctor experiments; or it may be a relatively slow phonological recoding system which can exhibit effects only when the fast visual-access system does not yield evidence favouring a 'Yes' response. In either case, abolishing the phonological system via articulatory suppression would not impair performance, yet without articulatory suppression phonological effects due to this system would be evident on 'No' trials.

At present it is impossible to evaluate these various possibilities, since we do not know what relationship there is between phonological encoding as it is operationally defined in working memory experiments and phonological encoding as it is operationally defined in experiments on lexical access. One method of *rapprochement* here would be to take techniques traditionally applied in studying working memory and to use them for investigating lexical access. For example, how would articulatory suppression influence the various phonological effects which can be observed in experiments on lexical decision, semantic categorization, and phrase evaluation? Several years ago, I tried an experiment of this sort in collaboration with Jon Jonasson, Derek Besner and Eileen Davelaar: we investigated whether non-words which sound identical to English words would still cause difficulties in a lexical decision task when the subject was concurrently vocalizing (saying 'Double, double, double . . .' as fast as he could). We found that the 'No' response to such non-words was now no slower than the 'No' response to non-words which did not sound identical to English words. However, although articulatory suppression did abolish the RT effect here, it did not abolish the error effect: pseudo-homophonic non-words still generated twice as many errors as non-pseudo-homophonic non-words. We are still thinking about this.

Analogously, one could investigate whether the difficulties caused by sentences such as *I no you are right* in phrase-evaluation tasks depend upon the use of the AL by determining whether such effects remain or are abolished when articulatory suppression is used.

The work of Martin (1978) is relevant here. She studied Stroop interference with two techniques. One was card-sorting: cards were sorted as rapidly as possible into six piles depending upon the ink colour of the stimulus on the card. The stimulus itself was either XXXXX (control condition), the name of the ink colour (congruent condition), or a colour name different from the ink colour (conflict condition). The congruent condition produced faster sorting than the control condition, which in turn was faster than the conflict condition. When subjects suppressed articulation by saying 'bla' continuously while sorting, the facilitating effect of congruency was reduced relative to the control condition (where concurrent articulation had no effect on performance) and the effect of incongruent words on sorting time was eliminated completely.

The second technique used by Martin was two-choice reaction time. Subjects classified the ink colour of green or brown stimuli by an appropriate button press. Here the congruent and control conditions yielded the same RT, and concurrent articulation did not affect either RT. In the conflict condition, RT was slower than in the control condition, and the size of this interference effect was reduced by concurrent articulation.

This experiment involves both concurrent articulation and a lexical-access effect, since the difference between the congruent and conflict conditions can only occur as a consequence of lexical access. Unfortunately, these experiments raise more questions than they answer. Martin assumed that the effect of concurrent articulation is to prevent pre-lexical phonological recoding, and hence to prevent lexical access based on such recoding; and she interpreted the effects of concurrent articulation on Stroop interferences as due to the prevention of lexical access. However, this interpretation raises the following problems:

(a)   Concurrent articulation abolished Stroop interference *completely* in the first experiment; this implies that lexical access must *always* depend upon pre-lexical phonological recoding, a view which conflicts with virtually all the evidence cited in this chapter.

(b)   If lexical access does always depend upon pre-lexical phonological recoding and such recoding is abolished by concurrent articulation, why did a congruency effect occur in Martin's first experiment even with concurrent articulation?

(c)   Why was there no congruency effect in her second experiment even without concurrent articulation?

Even if these puzzles are ignored, it should be noted that with Stroop stimuli it is usually argued that on the average the ink colour of the word is 'processed' more slowly than the word itself – hence the word interferes with the ink colour more than vice versa. If phonological recoding is a relatively slow activity, the need to wait until ink colour is processed might provide enough time for phonological recoding to be completed, and this might result in a contribution to the Stroop interference effect, a contribution which might be eliminated by concurrent articulation. Such a pattern of results could occur even if under normal circumstances visual access is invariably faster than phonological access; hence this pattern of results would not imply that reading ever depends upon phonological access. By this reasoning, however, *some* Stroop interference should remain, even with concurrent articulation, since visual lexical access should still occur. However, there was no interference (though as noted above it is difficult to reconcile this result with much of the evidence discussed in this chapter). Of interest here is a finding reported by Gough and Cosky (1977): colour naming interference is just as great when items are non-word pseudo-homophones of colour words (*grene*, *bloo*) as when they are genuine colour words (*green*, *blue*). This result is highly consistent with Martin's conclusions, though of course it is also consistent with the claim that visual access is always faster than phonological access, since one can argue that the need to wait for ink colour to be processed gives enough time for phonological recoding to be completed.

This discussion of work using the articulatory suppression technique has been lengthy yet inconclusive. It has, however, been necessary, since the technique has been used in recent years to investigate phonological encoding effects in reading, and indeed conclusions have been advanced concerning these effects on the basis of experiments using this technique. Such conclusions are premature, since we do not know what the effects of articulatory suppression are. If one can judge under articulatory suppression that *bew* and *bue* sound identical, whilst *bem* and *bue* do not, then articulatory suppression does not prevent pre-lexical phonological recoding; if so, the failure of articulatory suppression to impair reading comprehension would not imply that pre-lexical phonological recoding does not contribute to reading comprehension. The general point to be made is that, unless one *first demonstrates* that a specific hypothetical component of the reading process (e.g. pre-lexical phonological recoding) is abolished by articulatory suppression, any effect of articulatory suppression upon the reading process itself will be uninterpretable, since its source will be unknown.

Conclusions

The experimental work discussed in this chapter suggests that the role of phonological encoding in skilled reading, whether it is pre-lexical or post-lexical encoding, is at best slight. The failure to demonstrate any effects of regularity on lexical access times (in lexical decision and semantic categorization tasks) implies that lexical access in skilled readers relies exclusively on a visual code, even though phonological encoding is occurring (as evidenced by the effects of pseudo-homophonic non-words in lexical decision tasks). If so, a brain injury which abolished the ability to carry out pre-lexical phonological encoding would not impair lexical access at all in skilled readers, and hence would not impair their ability to understand the meanings of single printed words. Since in naming latency experiments regular words are named slightly more rapidly than exception words (Baron and Strawson, 1976; Gough and Cosky, 1977; Coltheart *et al.*, 1979), abolition of pre-lexical phonological recoding might slightly increase naming latency for regular words, but it would not lead to an *inability* to pronounce any words. In general, this work suggests that a loss of pre-lexical phonological recoding would have only minor and subtle effects: differences in naming latency between regular and exception words would be abolished; the difficulties caused in lexical decision experiments by pseudo-homophones would disappear; it might be impossible to pronounce non-words aloud (though here an analogy strategy might allow much pronunciation). There is no evidence from studies of skilled readers that loss of pre-lexical phonology would lead to specific difficulties in dealing with inflected words, abstract words, low-frequency words, or function words, nor any evidence that such loss would lead to the occurrence of semantic errors. Thus it is very doubtful whether one can attribute any of these symptoms of deep dyslexia to the loss of pre-lexical phonological recoding. Certainly, neuropsychological theories of reading such as those of Geschwind (1965), according to which reading comprehension occurs *only* after a pre-lexical phonological recoding, can be rejected outright on the basis of the work with normal readers (and for other obvious reasons as well – for example, on a purely phonological theory of lexical access, we could never distinguish between printed homophones, which we obviously can do; we know the different meanings belonging to *sail* and *sale*, and those belonging to 2, too and to, too). A slight but unfortunate complication here is that nearly all experimental work on reading deals either with highly skilled readers or with children who have recently learned to read; deep dyslexics usually belonged to neither category of reader before the onset of their disorder. If we had some experimental work on how the man in the street reads, we would be in a stronger position to relate deep dyslexic symptomatology to experimental work on reading.

As for the role of post-lexical phonology in normal skilled reading, this is less clear. One possibility is that a word-buffer using a phonological code is needed when continuous text is being comprehended. To take this view one has to be prepared to argue that neither input to this buffer from print, nor the maintenance of the buffer, is affected by concurrent articulation. I have suggested that this argument can be put forward, since no one has yet shown that going from print to phonology is prevented by concurrent articulation, nor that buffer storage of the resulting phonological representations is prevented by concurrent articulation. If the results of Baron (1973) and Doctor (1978) are taken as illustrating that comprehension of text requires the use of a word-buffer containing post-lexically derived phonological representations of words, then a brain injury which prevented the use of post-lexical phonology would impair comprehension of continuous text (without affecting comprehension of single words).

This buffer-storage view may well be a fruitful approach to specifying the role of phonology in reading. Zaidel (1978) studied the auditory comprehension of the disconnected left and right hemispheres, and found that as phrase length increased from one to four words, the performance of the right hemisphere deteriorated sharply, whilst the performance of the left hemisphere remained good. This result presumably reflects the poor short-term memory of the right hemisphere. When the experiment was repeated with *printed* phrases, the same thing happened: the ability of the right hemisphere to comprehend the printed phrase declined as phrase length increased. This is consistent with the view that short-term memory is used in the comprehension of continuous text. Tzeng, Hung and Wang (1977) used a Chinese version of the phrase evaluation task, asking Chinese subjects to judge whether a sentence printed in Chinese characters made sense or not. This task was performed more slowly when the characters in a phrase were phonologically similar than when they were not. This must be a post-lexical phonological effect (since pre-lexical phonological recoding of ideographic text is in principle impossible) and it presumably reflects the use of post-lexical phonological codes in short-term memory, indicating that short-term memory was being used for reading comprehension in this task, as has been suggested earlier in this chapter. Since Hitch and Baddeley (1976) found, in a verbal reasoning task with printed items, that concurrent articulation did not affect performance, even with passive sentences (which should rely particularly heavily on buffer storage for comprehension), it is beginning to become evident that concurrent articulation does not influence the form of short-term memory used for reading comprehension, even though this form of memory utilizes a phonological code.

A consequence of loss of post-lexical phonology would be an inability to pronounce correctly any printed stimuli to which grapheme-phoneme correspondence rules cannot be applied, or cannot be applied successfully: ideographs such as numerals and abbreviations, and exception words. Deep dyslexics do not show this kind of disability; if anything, their ability to pronounce numerals and abbreviations is relatively spared (see for example Goldstein, 1948) and there is no evidence that they are more accurate at pronouncing regular words than exception words. The data discussed in this chapter offer no evidence to suggest that loss of post-lexical phonology would lead especially to semantic errors or to derivational errors: nor should such loss cause selective difficulties in pronouncing function words, abstract words, or low-frequency words.

In general, then, the evidence suggests that the roles of pre-lexical and post-lexical phonological recoding are negligible for adults' comprehension of single printed words, and so loss of the ability to perform such recoding would have negligible effects on comprehending single words. It may be the case that post-lexical phonological encoding is needed for the text comprehension during reading, though this has by no means been demonstrated; if it is so, then loss of post-lexical phonology would lead to impaired comprehension of continuous printed text. Even where loss of phonology would be expected to have some effects on reading performance, there is no reason to suppose that any of these effects would correspond to any of the specific symptoms of deep dyslexia. If this conclusion is correct, then one cannot argue that any of these symptoms are secondary consequences of a primary phonological disability; instead, semantic errors, derivational errors, and function word, abstractness and frequency effects are independent of, and equivalent in status to, the phonological-disability effects.

References

Baddeley, A. D. (1979) Working memory and reading. In P. A. Kolers, M. E. Wrolstad and H. Bouma (eds), *Processing of Visible Language*, New York: Plenum.

Baron, J. (1973) Phonemic stage not necessary for reading. *Quarterly Journal of Experimental Psychology, 25,* 241–6.

Baron, J. and Strawson, C. (1976) Use of orthographic and word-specific knowledge in reading words aloud. *Journal of Experimental Psychology (Human Perception and Performance), 2,* 386–93.

Benson, D. F. and Geschwind, N. (1969) The alexias. In P. U. Vinken and G. W. Bruyn (eds), *Handbook of Clinical Neurology,* vol. 4. Amsterdam: North Holland.

Besner, D. and Coltheart, M. (1979) Ideographic and alphabetic processing in skilled reading of English. *Neuropsychologia, 17,* 467–72.

Bloomfield, L. (1942) Linguistics and reading. *Elementary English Review, 19,* 125–30.

Bower, T. G. R. (1970) Reading by eye. In H. Levin and J. P. Williams (eds), *Basic Studies in Reading.* New York: Basic Books.

Coltheart, M. (1978) Lexical access in simple reading tasks. In G. Underwood (ed.), *Strategies of Information Processing.* London: Academic Press.

Coltheart, M., Davelaar, E., Jonasson, J. T. and Besner, D. (1977) Access to the internal lexicon. In S. Dornic (ed.), *Attention and Performance,* VI. Hillsdale: Lawrence Erlbaum.

Coltheart, M., Besner, D., Jonasson, J. T. and Davelaar, E. (1979) Phonological recoding in the lexical decision task. *Quarterly Journal of Experimental Psychology, 31,* 489–507.

Doctor, E. (1978) Studies of reading comprehension in children and adults. Unpublished Ph.D. thesis, Birkbeck College, University of London.

Fudge, E. (1970) Phonological structure and 'expressiveness'. *Journal of Linguistics, 6,* 161–88.

Geschwind, N. (1965) Disconnexion syndromes in animals and man. *Brain, 88,* 237–94 and 585–644.

Gibson, E. (1970) The ontogeny of reading. *American Psychologist, 25,* 136–43.

Gibson, E. and Levin, H. (1975) *The Psychology of Reading.* Cambridge, Mass.: MIT.

Goldstein, K. (1948) *Language and Language Disturbances.* New York: Grune & Stratton.

Gough, P. B. (1972) One second of reading. In J. P. Kavanagh and I. G. Mattingly (eds), *Language by Eye and by Ear.* Cambridge, Mass.: MIT.

Gough, P. B. and Cosky, M. L. (1977) One second of reading again. In J. N. Castellan, D. B. Pisoni and G. P. Potts (eds), *Cognitive Theory,* Vol. 2. Hillsdale: Lawrence Erlbaum.

Hécaen, H. and Kremin, H. (1976) Neurolinguistic research on reading disorders resulting from left hemisphere lesions: aphasic and 'pure' alexia. In H. Whitaker and H. A. Whitaker (eds), *Studies in Neurolinguistics,* vol. 2. New York: Academic Press.

Hitch, G. and Baddeley, A. D. (1976) Verbal reasoning and working memory. *Quarterly Journal of Experimental Psychology, 28,* 603–21.

Huey, E. B. (1908, reissued 1968) *The Psychology and Pedagogy of Reading.* Cambridge, Mass.: MIT.

Kleiman, G. M. (1975) Speech recoding in reading. *Journal of Verbal Learning and Verbal Behaviour, 14,* 323–39.

Kolers, P. (1970) Three stages of reading. In H. Levin and J. P. Williams (eds), *Basic Studies in Reading.* New York: Basic Books.

Levy, B. A. (1977) Reading: speech and meaning processes. *Journal of Verbal Learning and Verbal Behaviour, 16,* 623–38.

Levy, B. A. (1978) Speech processing during reading. In A. M. Lesgold, J. W. Pellegrino, S. D. Fokkema and R. L. Glaser (eds), *Cognitive Psychology and Instruction.* New York: Plenum Press.

Levy, B. A. (1978) Speech analysis during sentence processing: reading and listening. *Visible Language, 12,* 81–101.

Marshall, J. C. and Newcombe, F. (1973) Patterns of paralexia: a psycholinguistic approach. *Journal of Psycholinguistic Research, 2,* 175–99.

Martin, M. (1978) Speech recoding in silent reading. *Memory and Cognition, 6,* 108–14.

Meyer, D. E. and Gutschera, K. (1975) Orthographic versus phonemic processing of printed words. Presented at the Psychonomic Society Meeting, Denver, Colorado.

Meyer, D. E., Schvaneveldt, R. W. and Ruddy, M. G. (1974) Function of graphemic and phonemic codes in visual word recognition. *Memory and Cognition, 2,* 309–21.

Midgley-West, L. (1978) Unpublished experiments, Birkbeck College, University of London.

Patterson, K. (1977) What is right with phonemic dyslexic patients? Colloquium, University College London.

Patterson, K. (1978) Phonemic dyslexia: errors of meaning and the meaning of errors. *Quarterly Journal of Experimental Psychology, 30,* 587–601.

Patterson, K. and Marcel, A. J. (1977) Aphasia, dyslexia, and the phonological coding of written words. *Quarterly Journal of Experimental Psychology, 29,* 307–18.

Rubenstein, H., Lewis, S. S. and Rubenstein, M. A. (1971) Evidence for phonemic recoding in visual word recognition. *Journal of Verbal Learning and Verbal Behaviour, 10,* 647–57.

Saffran, E. M. and Marin, O. S. M. (1977) Reading without phonology: evidence from aphasia. *Quarterly Journal of Experimental Psychology, 29,* 515–25.

Shallice, T. and Warrington, E. K. (1975) Word recognition in a phonemic dyslexic patient. *Quarterly Journal of Experimental Psychology, 27,* 187–99.

Smith, F. (1971) Understanding Reading. New York: Holt, Rinehart & Winston.

Smith, M. C. (1976) Evidence for speech recoding when reading for comprehension. Paper presented to the Psychonomic Society Meeting, St Louis, Missouri.

Tzeng, O. L., Hung, D. L. and Wang, W. S.-Y. (1977) Speech recoding in reading Chinese characters. *Journal of Experimental Psychology: Human Learning and Memory, 3,* 621–30.

Vago, V. (1968) The peripheral accompaniments of mental activity. Unpublished M.Sc. thesis, Monash University Melbourne, Australia.

Venezky, R. L. (1970) *The Structure of English Orthography.* The Hague: Mouton.

Wijk, A. (1966) *Rules of Pronunciation for the English Language.* Oxford University Press.

Zaidel, E. (1978) Lexical structure in the right hemisphere. In P. Buser and A. Rougeul-Buser (eds), *Cerebral Correlates of Conscious Experience.* Amsterdam: Elsevier.

11 Surface dyslexia and beginning reading: a revised hypothesis of the pronunciation of print and its impairments

Tony Marcel

1 Introduction

Two of the categories into which acquired reading impairments have been classified by Marshall and Newcombe (1973) are surface dyslexia and deep dyslexia. These syndromes, especially the latter, have been discussed extensively in this volume. However their cardinal distinguishing characteristics as conceptualised by most people so far may be summarised as follows. When attempting to read single words, the nature of the errors made by deep dyslexic patients appears to be determined at least in part by the semantic and syntactic nature of the target word and semantic and syntactic processing of it. The nature of the errors made by surface dyslexic patients appears to be determined largely by spelling-to-sound characteristics of the target word. Deep dyslexic patients can hardly read non-words, if at all, and their errors often reflect some degree of comprehension of the written target. Any comprehension in surface dyslexics appears to be based on the reader's oral response.

The main concern of this chapter is a particular aspect of the conceptual notions in terms of which these impairments have been discussed by people who have recently dealt with them. That aspect is the distinction of two ways of pronouncing written letter-strings, and can be encapsulated by reference to Figure 11.1.

This diagram does not aspire to represent the particular views of any of the individual contributors to this volume. However it seems

I am grateful to Max Coltheart for helping me to clarify the notions expressed in this paper. Their ultimate inadequacy is my fault. I am also grateful to Estelle Doctor for discussing her data with me, and to Tim Shallice for discussing the ideas.

fair to say that most of them subscribe to one aspect of the structural and information-flow model of reading the figure represents. This is that the pronunciation of a word may be achieved in either of two ways. The first method is lexical. The written word is recognised visually as an entry in a visual input lexicon which contains the orthographic descriptions of known words. Its articulation is generated, much as it would be in spontaneous speech, by retrieving its phonology as a whole. The second method is entirely non-lexical. The letter-string is segmented into graphemic units. These units are converted into phonemes by grapheme-phoneme rules (see Colt-heart, 1978), which are then combined for articulation. Other aspects of Figure 11.1 are not immediately critical, but will be discussed in as much as they relate to specific models.

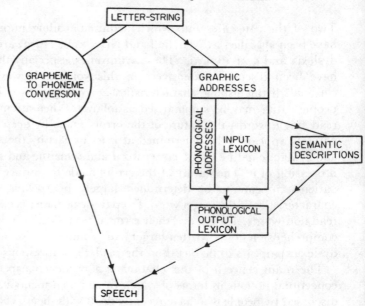

FIGURE 11.1 Modal structural model for reading and impairments

According to the ideas outlined with reference to Figure 11.1, deep dyslexia (Marshall and Newcombe, 1973) or phonemic dyslexia (Shallice and Warrington, 1975; Patterson and Marcel, 1977) involves two malfunctions: (a) a severe impairment to, or even loss of, the ability to convert graphemes to phonemes without lexical involvement, and (b) lack of the connections which normally exist between entries in a visual input lexicon, which contains the visual specifications for recognising words, and their corresponding phonological entries in an output lexicon for speech production. Reading in such patients relies on (i) access from a graphic representation of the written letter-string to an entry in the input lexicon, (ii) thence to a semantic representation of that word's meaning, and (iii) thence to an entry in the output lexicon which will meet the semantic specification.

The predominantly accepted version of surface dyslexia (Marshall and Newcombe, 1973) is that there are two impairments minimally necessary to account for the reading of patients: (a) an impairment of access to the input lexicon from graphic input, and (b) a partial impairment or distortion of the process of grapheme-phoneme conversion. Semantic errors (*little* → 'small') never occur, and if the reader shows comprehension it is almost always of the error rather than the target (*listen* → /lɪstən/ → 'the boxer'), though sometimes the word fails to be recognised even when pronounced correctly. Therefore some component of the route from the graphic representation of the letter-string to the visual input lexicon to semantics is assumed to be impaired. An impairment to access to the input lexicon is preferred to proposing an impairment to either (a) access from input lexicon to semantics, or (b) connections between entries in the input and the output lexicon. Although it has not been made explicit, one must suppose that the reasons for such a preference are as follows. If there was only impairment from the input lexicon to semantics, words ought to be pronounced correctly. If there was only impairment from input to output lexicons, words ought to be correctly understood even if mispronounced, which they are not. Instead of proposing an impairment to both 'routes' it is more economical to propose an earlier impairment which will preempt both the routes which depend on it. Note that this account is in terms of impairments to connections or conversions, rather than to the structures themselves. This is how Marshall and Newcombe deal with acquired dyslexias in their 1973 paper.

The notions expressed above provide a problem. In deep dyslexia, severe grapheme-to-phoneme impairment exists without necessarily involving grapheme-to-lexical impairment. However in surface dyslexia grapheme-to-lexical impairment does seem to implicate impairment to grapheme-to-phoneme conversion. Are the two routes from print to pronunciation doubly dissociable or not?

I would like to offer a view of the process of pronouncing written letter-strings which differs in emphasis from that discussed above and prototypically depicted in Figure 11.1. It will give a different picture primarily of surface dyslexia, but also of deep dyslexia and phonological alexia. This account bears some similarities to the emphasis in Shallice and Warrington's view of surface dyslexia presented in this volume. It attempts to eschew the notion of a completely non-lexical process of grapheme-to-phoneme conversion. In so doing it will be proposed that the surface dyslexic is functionally equivalent to a beginning reader in what he or she lacks and in the strategy used to cope.

2 Dissatisfaction with current accounts of surface dyslexia

2.1 Current accounts

Before raising some problems associated with conceptions of surface dyslexia it is worthwhile briefly rehearsing the available views. Marshall and Newcombe's discussion of surface dyslexia assumes an information-flow model of reading which is slightly ambiguous, or at least under-specified (Marshall and Newcombe, 1973, Figure 1 and discussion, pp. 188 and 191). The problem is that they say that 'both phonological and semantic addresses must . . . be associated with individual visual addresses' (p. 188), which seems to imply a whole-word or at least morphemic correspondence between visual and phonological addresses. Yet they say on page 191 that if the pathway from visual to semantic addresses is unavailable, 'the subject will have no option but to read via putative grapheme-phoneme correspondence rules (pathway bd)'. Since 'pathway bd' is the link between visual and phonological addresses, this implies that the visual address is segmented or segmentable into graphemes. The problem with their account is that no distinction is made, or discussed, between obtaining whole-word phonology from unique visual addresses and obtaining the phonology from segments of the visual addresses. What is crucial for our present purposes is that Marshall and Newcombe imply that if a visually presented word cannot be pronounced via its meaning, then its phonology is derived by grapheme-phoneme rules, i.e. (a) that phonology is achieved via algorithmic rules, and (b) that these are at the segmentation level of the phoneme. The importance of this formulation is that it implies that pronunciation achieved thus is in no way constrained by or dependent on lexical factors, that is, what the subject knows about the appearance and pronunciation of individual words. The mis-pronunciations of individual words is then attributed to difficulty with the conditional and contextual aspects of grapheme-phoneme rules.

This theme is taken up and made more explicit by Coltheart (1978). Coltheart's concept of grapheme-phoneme conversion is a procedure which is entirely independent of lexically held visual specifications for words, and is even pre-lexical. He expresses the grapheme-phoneme correspondences in terms of phonemes and as algorithmic contingent rules or 'productions'. For example, 'For vowel + consonant + final E, the vowel is long'; 'G or C are soft before E or I, otherwise hard'. In addition, the procedure of parsing a letter-string into graphemes appears to be viewed as an in-dependent stage. Coltheart proposes that the reading of surface dyslexics provides evidence of the psychological reality of grapheme-phoneme procedures as conceptualised by him. But this is a peculiar argument. Their independent psychological existence would be indicated if they operated *successfully* in someone who could be supposed to have no access to lexical knowledge or processing. But one can hardly argue for their independent existence in such a person when they *fail* to operate successfully. It appears that Coltheart's view of surface dyslexia is that indicated in the intro-duction:

(a)   lack of lexical access, at least for words which are read incorrectly and misunderstood,
(b)   failures in parsing the letter-string into appropriate graphemes, and
(c)   misapplication or failure to apply certain grapheme-phoneme rules.

Although Morton and Patterson make no comment on surface dyslexia, their model developed to account for deep dyslexia (Chapter 4, this volume) invites, indeed permits only a certain view of surface dyslexia. They postulate three routes from print to pronunciation: (a) completely non-lexical grapheme-to-phoneme rules, as in Patterson and Marcel (1977) and Coltheart (1978); (b) direct connections between corresponding entries in input and output logogen systems (or lexicons); and (c) from input logogens to the semantic system and thence to output logogens activated by the semantic specifications. Shallice and Warrington (Chapter 5, this volume) suggest that to obtain the oral reading errors of surface dyslexia, Morton and Patterson's model requires that both the route from input to output logogens and the route from input logogens to semantics be inoperative. However this is not necessarily so. In Morton and Patterson's model structural units rather than routes between them can be impaired. Further, grapheme-to-phoneme conversion is derived from the representation of the graphic array which precedes input logogens. Therefore all that is required is that visual input logogens or access to them be inoperative. Shallice and Warrington's error is due to projecting their own concepts onto Morton and Patterson, i.e. (a) that phonological recoding proceeds from visual word-forms and that these are equivalent to visual input logogens, and (b) it is only the routes (arrows in diagrams) which can be impaired – a 'disconnection' view.

In fact the simplest account of surface dyslexia according to the revised logogen model would be (a) that visual input logogens or access to them are impaired, and (b) that grapheme-to-phoneme rules are malfunctioning. One point about Morton and Patterson's model merits comment. Since input logogens correspond to root morphemes and not words, it is only the phonology of root morphemes that can be accessed in the output lexicon from the input lexicon. Any bound morphemes have to be transmitted by another route and re-added at the output logogen later. But if this is so, how is stress assignment carried out? Consider the following derivations: télegraph, telegráphic, telégraphy. It is not just that the stress shifts depend on the particular bound morpheme, but that they are internal to the root morpheme(s). Further, such shifts cannot just be rules which are universally applied once a bound morpheme is added. In spite of Chomsky and Halle (1968), certain shifts depend on the specific word involved. While the shift in reláte-rélative is the most frequent for the specific syllables and morphemes involved, colláte-collátive is an exception. This kind of knowledge must be lexically stored. The point of this digression is to emphasise the problems encountered if the *only* phonology accessed lexically is that of root morphemes. Patterson (Chapter 14, this volume) points out other problems with the root morpheme view of the lexicon in connection with derivational reading errors in deep dyslexia.

Schwartz, Saffran and Marin (Chapter 12, this volume) essentially hold a view equivalent to Morton and Patterson's and Coltheart's. They separate a lexical route for retrieving phonology from one which uses spelling-to-sound rules.

Shallice and Warrington's position in this volume is somewhat different, but it is difficult to be sure of their view since they do not explicate a specific model. It appears that the 'visual word-form' is equivalent to what I have called an entry in the visual input lexicon. Shallice and Warrington postulate two extremely interesting characteristics of this stage. Firstly, this unit itself parses (multiply) a letter-string into components which range in size from graphemes, through syllables, to whole words (though no mention of morphemes is made), and categorises these components. This categorisation, in the case of word-sized segments (Shallice, personal communication), gives direct access to meanings, without any further intervening stage or stored representation. Secondly, it appears that (though it is not explicitly stated) phonological recoding is based on the parsings produced by the visual word-form stage. Phonology is derived not only from graphemes but also from syllables and short whole-words. The actual pronunciation of any letter-string depends not on rules but on the frequency with which a parsed letter combination occurs with a particular pronunciation in known words. Note that this formulation does not postulate a grapheme-phoneme translation process which is independent of descriptions which yield lexical access.[1]

Shallice and Warrington's account of surface dyslexia is that the direct route from visual word-form to semantics is impaired. Whether this is supposed to be so for all words or just some subset is not clear. To the extent that it is the *route* which is said to be damaged, we must suppose that this applies to all words. Some words may be understood correctly because they are pronounced correctly, others may just happen to survive the damaged route. To the extent that it is the semantics of specific words which are lost or inaccessible (as in Warrington's patient, A.B.) the impairment will apply to only those words. At any rate Shallice and Warrington argue that this damage only permits the patients to read 'phonologically'. Since they do not conceive of whole-word correspondences as a general facility (i.e. from input to output lexicon) nor of morphemic correspondences, all that is left intact is their own version of phonological recoding. In less severe cases this process is supposed to be manifested as it normally functions, but without any semantic influence (e.g. cónvert or convért). In more severe cases the pronunciations are increasingly biased to the most frequent correspondences between letter-string segments and phonology. Shallice and Warrington assert that in the latter case it would operate on the basis of 'one letter-one syllable'. However, as I will argue later on, the most frequent correspondences are not equivalent to 'one letter-one syllable'. In summary Shallice and Warrington's position is that the central characteristic of surface dyslexia is impairment to the route from visual word-form to semantics, leading them to label the syndrome 'semantic dyslexia'. Since they do not differentiate grapheme-phoneme conversion from lexically derived phonology, what the principal damage leaves is what they call 'phonological reading'. As they describe it, this process reduces in its essential form to a syllabary biased by frequency of individual print-to-sound mappings.

In sum then, those people who have been concerned with acquired dyslexias all treat oral reading in surface dyslexia as non-lexical. Coltheart, Marshall and Newcombe, Morton and Patterson, and Schwartz, Saffran and Marin view this in terms of grapheme-to-phoneme rules which are partially malfunctioning. Shallice and Warrington view it in terms of a device sensitive to graphemes and syllables but which translates on the basis of frequency of each existing correspondence. Alternative views to those presented above of how printed letter-strings might be pronounced have been proposed (see Baron, 1977; Glushko, 1980; and Coltheart, 1978, for a review). But these have all been directed only at the normal population. These alternatives will be discussed insofar as necessary in section 3.2 below. However, I wish now to show how the views presented above are inadequate to deal with the data they aspire to account for.

2.2 Problems for current accounts of surface dyslexia

As noted above, all current accounts, except possibly Shallice and Warrington's, ascribe surface dyslexia to an entirely non-lexical system and characterise that system in terms of algorithmic grapheme-to-phoneme rules. In this section these views will be confronted with the characteristics of surface dyslexia as reported by Marshall and Newcombe (1973) and it will be argued that the patients' reading cannot be adequately described as either entirely non-lexical or as mediated by malfunctioning grapheme-to-phoneme rules.

The main source of data on surface dyslexia is the corpus collected by Holmes (1973) and reported by Marshall and Newcombe (1973). Another potential source is Shallice and Warrington's report (Chapter 5, this volume). Unfortunately, Shallice and Warrington's presentation of their data is extremely cursory and restricted to percentages of words read from small lists. Furthermore, both they and Marshall and Newcombe fail to render the pronunciations in phonetic symbols and we are left with the problem of interpreting their own glosses in terms of the alphabet. Thus, for example, was 'rissend' pronounced /ri:send/ or /rɪsend/, what was the stress assignment, and were there pauses, e.g. between *ri* and *send*? This data is contained in Holmes's thesis. Since the present remarks are addressed to Marshall and Newcombe's descriptions, primary reference will be made to what they present. Data as presented in Holmes's thesis will be invoked separately. The two issues raised here are lexical involvement and the functioning of grapheme-phoneme rules.

A Lexical involvement

Various characteristics of the reading of both the patients, J.C. and S.T. described by Marshall and Newcombe suggest some lexical involvement.

1 Concrete nouns were more likely to be read correctly than abstract nouns,[2] nouns were more likely to be correct than adjectives and adjectives than verbs. In addition the more frequent the word and the shorter, the more likely was it to be read correctly. This evidence of course may only reflect the possibility that certain word classes are more frequent or that the more frequent and shorter a word, the more likely it is to be spelled in such a way that minimal grapheme-phoneme rules will yield an appropriate pronunciation. Alternatively, it may reflect a greater probability of loss of visual input entries or specifications for less frequent words and for certain form classes of word. But the effect of syntactic form class is reminiscent of the reading capabilities of deep dyslexic patients and suggests an effect which is at least lexical if not beyond. These effects

of the nature of the target word are suggestive but not critical. While they suggest that lexical impairments are not in *access to* but rather *within* the lexicon, they may only mean that lexical impairment is not total but selective. We will return later to the reason why certain types of word are more susceptible than others.

2 More important are effects to be found in the erroneous responses. Those errors in which the responses were words tended to be nouns more than any other form class and they tended to be more frequent than the target word. In addition verbs were sometimes nominalised (refresh → refreshment, govern → government). All these are lexical tendencies. Further, in both patients only about 25 per cent of all errors were neologisms. That is, there was a strong tendency to produce words as responses. Thus not only does there seem to be some constraint to utter meaningful or at least known speech segments, there is a bias to produce certain syntactic forms. While this is probably a property of an output lexicon rather than an input lexicon, it nonetheless suggests that the production of phonology in these patients is not independent of the lexicon or logogen system. It is to be noted that in Morton and Patterson's paper (Chapter 4, this volume) grapheme-phoneme conversion leads to the response-buffer, not to the output logogens.[3]

B Grapheme-phoneme involvement

The second issue is whether patients read via malfunctioning grapheme-phoneme rules. Several aspects of the data make this unlikely.

1 There are many instances where the phonetic values given to graphemes is inconsistent from one word to another. In J.C.'s case, *barge* → 'bargain', but *guest* → 'just'. In this case the rule of E softening G does not just fail but if anything is reversed. *Insect* → 'insist', but *incense* → 'increase'. Here we cannot claim reversal of 'C hard unless followed by E', since in *niece* → 'nice' the rule of E is maintained. In S.T.'s case, *gauge* → 'jug', but *gaol* → 'gold'. If grapheme-to-phoneme rules were failing to be applied, we would at least expect some regularity. Again, if grapheme parsing was failing or if phoneme assignment was failing, why does only one vowel of a digraph get treated and why is the particular vowel inconsistent: (a) g*u*est → j*u*st, but ga*u*ge → j*u*g (*u* pronounced irrespective of ordinal position); (b) n*i*ece → n*i*ce, but b*oi*l → b*o*wl (first vowel pronounced irrespective of identity).

If we are to describe these cases as failures of grapheme-phoneme rules, then the way in which they fail appears to be ad hoc according to each example. Of course we could say that failure of the procedure consists precisely in quasi-random application of the rules. But then we are left with the question of why quasi-random application of grapheme-phoneme rules should result so often in a real word being produced.

2 Many examples of misreadings cannot be accounted for by application of grapheme-phoneme rules, functioning or not, and certainly not by Marshall and Newcombe's (1977) notion of 'one letter–one phoneme'.

(a)   In the case of *incense* → 'increase' and *barge* → 'bargain', Coltheart and Marshall and Newcombe both describe this simply as failure of the rule 'G and C soft before E or I, otherwise hard'. But if this was all that was wrong then why was *incense* not pronounced /ɪnkens/, where did the /r/ come from and why did the /n/ disappear? Where has the last syllable /ən/ come from in *barge* → 'bargain'?

If the rule of 'E softens C' was not being applied, why do we get *lace* → 'lass', rather than the responses 'lack' or 'lake'?

(b)   If there was a rule of one letter–one phoneme, why is there such inconsistency in phonological realisations of individual letters? Why is final E not given a phonetic value? Why is only one vowel often given a value in vowel digraphs (*violent* → 'volent', *boil* → 'bowl')?

(c)   Why are whole syllables deleted (*banishment* → 'banment')?

(d)   Why are syllables added, both in consonant clusters (*applaud* → 'appollo', *pigsty* → 'pigisty'), where apparently the added vowel is not merely a schwa, and in verb nominalisation (*govern* → 'governor')?

(e)   In some cases it is hard to see how a reduced or simplified set of grapheme-phoneme rules would yield the response. In the case of *insect* → 'insist', not only is the *e* given a value it hardly ever takes singly (/ɪ/), but the stress is shifted from the first to the second syllable which is very unusual for two-syllable words. In fact, what we might have expected from grapheme-phoneme rules insensitive to context would have been 'incest'.

In sum, the notion of failed or misapplied grapheme-phoneme rules cannot alone account for the data.

2.3 Similarities to young readers

Something which, surprisingly, nobody seems to have commented on is the striking similarity between the attempts to read single words by surface dyslexic patients and the attempts made by beginning readers.[4] Two phenomena spring to mind quite readily. One is that children will often guess words with two constraints – that most of the letters should be accounted for phonetically and that the guess is probably in the child's spoken vocabulary. More often than not the beginning of the target and response have a closer similarity than the end (Shankweiler and Liberman, 1972). Indeed the child often gives a good phonological rendering of the beginning of the word and appears to give up, guessing some lexically adequate ending. This is more noticeable, the longer the word. MacKinnon (1959) has described the conditions associated with this phenomenon of 'blocking'. The second phenomenon is related to this and is that the child laboriously attempts to sound out the elements of the word in order, often making several attempts. Certainly those children who have been taught a phonics strategy (not necessarily grapheme-phoneme rules) will produce what looks like the result of partially failed or misapplied grapheme-phoneme rules, which do not take account of context and which certainly fail on 'exception' words. Examples can be found in MacKinnon (1959), Goodman (1967) and Barr (1975). Unfortunately most oral reading errors have been collected from attempts on text rather than single words and so the children's errors are semantically influenced by the context (see Biemiller, 1970; Weber, 1968). However a small corpus of attempts to read single words has been gathered by Doctor (1978), and this permits us to examine the correspondence between the attempts of ordinary children and people classified as surface dyslexics. Doctor's responses were gathered from eight children of each age of 5, 6, 7, 8, 9, and 10 years old. The target words consisted of 100 words from the Schonell test and her own list of 24 words which varied orthogonally on orthographic regularity and familiarity. (Frequency norms for children do not exist.) Two cautions are necessary. First, Barr (1975) has shown that children's oral reading is affected by method of instruction. Doctor's children had all been taught by 'eclectic' methods. Second, Marshall and Newcombe's characteris-ations of errors are not necessarily accepted by the present author and a redescription will follow from views expressed below. However, for purposes of comparison their descriptive categories will be used. The comparison between Marshall and Newcombe's examples from patients and Doctor's examples from children appears in Table 11.1.

It can be seen from this table that ordinary children produce attempts which correspond to those of surface dyslexics. There are also other characteristics of Doctor's results which show similarities. Familiarity (which will be taken as functionally equivalent to frequency) played a significant role. In terms of the stimulus words, familiarity was overall a better predictor of ability to pronounce a word than spelling-sound regularity. Indeed it was only when a word was unfamiliar that regularity had an effect. In addition, although no analysis was conducted, in several cases Doctor interprets the responses in terms of their being more frequent than the stimuli. For example, with regard to *gaol* she says 'having decided that the initial G was a /g/, most children reversed the vowels and pronounced the more common word /gəʊl/. A few younger children chose the even more common /gɜːl/' (p. 257).[5] Another similarity was in the predominance of known words as opposed to neologisms as responses. Doctor says: '*Gone* was pronounced as /grəʊn/. The child selects the regular (here, wrong) pronunciation of the vowel but in order to prevent a nonsensical response, he inserts a letter to make a real word' (p. 257). The comment here is very revealing. If what the child is doing is to interpret the letter-string in terms of his (phonological) vocabulary of known words, then a description in terms of grapheme-phoneme rules is far from adequate as an account of the behaviour. It is interesting to see the problems such an account provides for Doctor. She says:

> the regular initial *c* of *ceiling* should have been pronounced as
> /s/, but because *ei* was sometimes pronounced as /e/ and some-
> times as /ɪ/ the *c*'s pronunciation was affected. The children
> used the rule insofar as they pronounced the *c* as an /s/ when
> they pronounced the vowel as /e/, and as a /k/ when they
> pronounced it as /ɪ/. Another error was to sound out the *ei* as
> the diphthong /eɪ/ which resulted in 'sailing'.

To call the above 'using the rule' is somewhat bizarre, since the 'rule' applies both to *e* and *i* when they follow *c*. A much more satisfactory account is that the reason why the phonology of the *c* is affected is that the child has no lexical entry corresponding to /keliŋ/

TABLE 11.1 *Examples of reading errors from Marshall and Newcombe (1973) and Doctor (1978)**

Marshall and Newcombe's (1973) categories and examples	Examples from Doctor (1978)

Visual confusions
spy → 'shy'   father → 'ɑftə'
polite → 'police'   funny → 'frʌŋ'

Partial failures of grapheme-phoneme rules

Misapplication
disease → 'decease'   orchestra → 'ɔtʃestrə'
choir → 'chore'   shepherd → 'ʃef'

Voiced → unvoiced
resent → 'rissend'   diseased → 'dəsisd'
of → 'off'   plausible → 'plɒsibɫ'

Silent grapheme phoneticised
island → 'izland'   gnome → 'gɒnəm'
listen → 'liston'   campaign → 'kʌmpeigən'
reign → 'region'   gawky → 'gəweiki'

Failure of postsyllabic E to diphthongise vowel
bike → 'bik'   take → 'tæk'
unite → 'unit'   gnome → 'gnɒm'
lace → 'lass'   stroke → 'strɒk'

Insensitivity of G and C to succeeding vowel
recent → 'rikunt'   ceiling → 'kɪlɪŋ'
incense → 'increase'   fascinate → 'fæskɪnɪt'
guest → 'just'   gawky → 'dʒəʊki'
logic → 'lugus'   barge → 'bɒg'

One element of vowel digraphs ignored
niece → 'nice'   road → 'rɒd'
violent → 'volent'   people → 'pɒpəɫ'
reapply → 'reply'   saucer → 'sʌkə'
boil → 'bowl'   mouse → 'mɒs'

Insertion of vowel in consonant clusters
applaud → 'appollo'   soloist → 'sɒlɪsɪt'
monarch → 'monarutch'   mongrel → 'mɒnɪgæl'
pigsty → 'pigisti'   gross → 'gɒrəs'

Stress shift (to first syllable)
devóur → 'dáyver'   canary → 'kǽnəri'†
implý → 'úmply'   heroic → 'hérək'†
begín → 'béggin'   imagine → 'íməgən'†
omít → 'ómmit'   applaud → 'ǽpləd'†

TABLE 11.1 *continued*

Marshall and Newcombe's (1973) categories and examples	Examples from Doctor (1978)
Loss of syllable	
banishment → 'banment'	beginning → 'biɪŋ'
exaggerate → 'aggerate'	ceiling → 'seɫ'
	people → 'pɒp'
Consonants misplaced	
naturally → 'anterally'	plausible → 'pʌblɪʃ'
syllable → 'sibbali'	susceptible → 'sʌspektibɫ'

* Marshall and Newcombe give their responses in English orthography, Doctor transcribed her responses in phonetic alphabet.

† Stress in Doctor's corpus inferred from ə and non-neutral vowels.

N.B. One further characteristic, on which neither Marshall and Newcome nor Doctor comment, but which is evident from examination of responses, is that for both patients and children the first segments of words are far less susceptible to error than medial and terminal segments.

or to /sɪlɪŋ/, but he does have entries for /kɪlɪŋ/ and/or /seɪŋ/. The role of grapheme-phoneme rules is secondary and is in terms of the constraints of how a *c can* be pronounced. What primarily determines what he says is a function of what he has in his lexicon. Indeed an interesting metaphor for what appears to be going on is what many people do when they play 'Scrabble'. With certain constraints on the order, they try to produce candidate utterances which will account for as many letters as possible, rejecting non-words. This notion of strategy will be returned to later, as will further examples from Doctor's corpus. The question which the next section will attempt to answer is: what are the basic mechanisms and their state which produce the attempts of the children and the patients?

3 A sketch of a print-to-pronunciation hypothesis

3.1 The basic process

In this section a brief attempt will be made to outline an approach to how letter-strings, both words and non-words, are pronounced. A full justification of what is postulated will not be made. Nor will the many existing alternatives be discussed, mainly for reasons of space. The issue is whether it will account for surface dyslexia and some of the relevant phenomena in the oral reading of single words by normal people. The components of the model are illustrated in Figure 11.2.

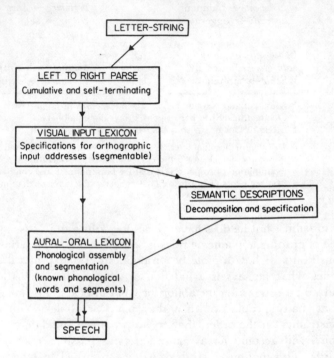

FIGURE 11.2 Modified model for oral reading

1 A letter-string is represented as individual letters in spatial order. Each letter is described in terms of which letter it is, visually but conceptually, i.e. irrespective of upper-/lower-case. This does not necessarily involve the name of the letter, merely the alphabetic abstraction. In the case of script a heterarchical problem solving process may be necessary, involving hypotheses derived from the visual input lexicon and semantic descriptions.

2 Entries in the visual input lexicon contain specifications to accept known words and morphemes. These specifications are in

terms of a left-to-right description of letters in ordinal positions. Thus they would be of the form:

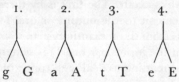

It seems to have been assumed on no good grounds that the only graphemic representation which gives visual access to lexical entries is based on a 'whole word gestalt' description, which depends on the total visual appearance of the word. There are two types of evidence against this being the only means of visual access to the lexicon. Firstly, how could script be recognised if this were the case? Secondly there is the evidence of deep dyslexic patients, who can only access the lexicon visually from print and can not *directly* convert print to phonology. Saffran and Marin's (1977) patient was able to read words whose normal printed form was distorted tHuS, thu^s or t+h+u+s. Patterson (personal communication) has presented words to the deep dyslexic P.W. by laying cards, each with one letter on it, on top of one another one at a time. This did not prevent him reading the words spelled by the letters, although he cannot name letters. If access specifications for lexical entries are indeed in the form of spatially ordered concatenations of single letters, then there is little reason why they cannot also be segmented.

3 Each of the addresses in the visual input lexicon has at least two pointers. One of these leads to a semantic description (or descriptions in the case of homographs and polysemous words). The other is to an entry or combination of entries (e.g. Liver+pool, but see below) in the output lexicon or speech vocabulary which is dubbed 'the aural-oral lexicon' in Figure 11.2.

4 The nature of semantic descriptions and semantic processing is irrelevant for present concerns, except that they will determine in critical cases the pronunciation of homographs (lead) and stress assignments (cónvert/convért).

5 It is convenient to deal with parsing of the letter-string and retrieval of phonology together. In normal 'skilled' readers there is little reason why the following two methods should not yield the pronunciation of both words and non-words. Difficulties and criticisms will be discussed after exposition. (a) If an entry in the

visual input lexicon is accessed, i.e. by a known word or morpheme, its pronunciation is retrieved as a whole as a result of two processes, though both may not always occur. The first is by direct access or look-up from the input lexicon to the output or oral lexicon. The second is via specifications from the semantic system which has been accessed from the entry in the input lexicon. This semantic route is required in normal textual reading to deal with contextual influence on the pronunciations of homographs such as *lead* (/led/ or /lid/). Something which will be returned to is that, while the pronunciation may be accessed as a whole, it must be segmentable. If it were not, we could plainly never obtain blend errors in speech as reported by Fromkin (1973) of the form 'momentaneous' (momentary + instantaneous). Such blends appear to be produced by semantic specifications accessing two lexical entries, whose phonology always blends at a common phoneme at an equivalent morphemic point. (b) The parsing of the letter-string is achieved by two processes, both of which normally operate. The first is a cumulative exhaustive procedure. The second, of which context-sensitivity is a result, is the operation of morpheme-sensitive specifications in the visual input lexicon. The first mechanism operates on the letter-string as follows. As each letter is encountered in a left-to-right (simultaneous) scan it is marked as a possible segment. As each new letter is encountered it is added to the previous letters and a series of ever larger segments are marked, with the previous bracketings remaining. Thus for 'revise', the following segmentations would be yielded (prior to the operation of the second mechanism): (r) . . , [(r) e] . . , . . , [([([(r) e]v)i]s)e]. Although bracketing is centred on the first letter, a segment such as (vis) or (vise) would be yielded because once *r* and *e* are bracketed together what remains is a potential segment.

The influence of orthographic specifications in the input lexicon will be twofold. If the specification for a segment represented as a lexical address is met, then the criterial segment in the letter-string is marked. But bracketing internal to that segment is not overridden. Thus in *revise*, the outside brackets of [(r)e] would be marked. Note that bound morphemes such as *re-* are contained in the visual input lexicon. The external motivation for this is that in many cases such bound morphemes, especially prefixes, perform a semantic function, and must therefore have access to semantics. However in the case of *revise*, whatever the case historically, *-vise* is not a root morpheme in present day English. Therefore the status of *re-* is dubious in *revise*.

This leads to the second influence of lexical specifications. This is to override or delete candidate bracketings. In the case of *read*, the potential bracketing of (*re*) would be overridden since -*ad* is not a segment which exists as a lexical address, and the most satisfactory lexical 'account' of the letter-string is to treat it as (*read*). Better examples are *relate*, *ream*, and *resin*, where the segment left by *re*- is a morpheme but the morphemic combination makes little lexical sense. Lexical overriding has the consequence in *ream* of establishing *ea* as a single-grapheme digraph, and in *resin* of shifting the stress assignment and voicing of the *s* (see below). Thus context sensitivity in parsing of a letter-string may *result* in producing graphemes, but it *arises from* the matching of successively larger candidate segments to existing lexical addresses. Context sensitivity would then consist of three things: (a) the bracketing of segments which correspond to morphemes will be marked, (b) later addition of letters can override previous bracketings, and (c) as more satisfactory accounts in terms of morphemes or words are yielded they can override bracketings.

This parsing process, which is sensitive to lexical constraints, should yield the minimum 'satisfactory' number of segments and should allow the pronunciation of all known words. With non-words or unknown words the pronunciation will be a function of two factors: (1) that segmentation most economically accounted for by known letter combinations and morphemes, or that segmentation found in most words of that consonant and vowel structure, and (2) the pronunciation found for each segment in the largest number of lexical cases. Thus in most cases, the letter combination -*int* is pronounced /ɪnt/. Stress assignment should follow from the most frequent stress effect that those segmented syllables or morphemes have in words of the same number of syllables.

3.2 *The segmentation and pronunciation of non-words*

So far we have dealt mainly with the pronunciation of letter-strings which can be segmented into morphemes. Two aspects of non-words need to be dealt with. Firstly there are non-words which we have no trouble pronouncing but which contain letter combinations which do not occur in any known words. One example is *kwib*, where *kw*- does not occur in any English word. The other aspect of non-words is where they may contain letter combinations which rely on context sensitivity for their segmentation and pronunciation. An example is *phoce*, where *p* and *h* have to be bracketed together and where terminal *e* influences the pronunciation of both the *o* and the *c*. Both of the cases exemplified above provide problems of segmentation and pronunciation.

Let us deal first with the problem of single letters. Coltheart (1978) argues that the notion of a phonological lexicon which contains the pronunciation of each entry in a visual input lexicon does not explain how non-words are pronounced. But this is only true if we could not (a) segment the criterial visual address in the input lexicon into letters or graphemes, and (b) segment speech codes into phonemes. There is no reason why we could not do (a), at the same time as being sensitive to the totality of the orthographic address, especially if the address were in the form of individual letters ordinally arranged. Indeed unless this were possible we could not find situations where real words could be treated as non-words and pronounced accordingly. Midgley-West (1977) has a good example of this where after 24 non-words, *wolf* was presented and pronounced as /wɒlf/. However, in order for graphemic segmentation to have any meaning phonologically, phonemic segmentation is a prerequisite. Now, it is important to remember that phonemic segmentation is by no means a primary linguistic activity; it has to be learnt. It is something which many children find extremely difficult to grasp (Mattingly, 1972; Savin, 1972), and who therefore cannot learn Pig Latin. I have also witnessed many adults at adult literacy classes who after reading or even repeating *cat, hat, fat, sat,* cannot read *dat* or, given /d/ aurally, say /dæt/. Coltheart says 'it could scarcely be argued that the phonological lexicon contains entries for every possible pronounceable non-word'. Well, yes it does – *potentially*, insofar as it can be segmented. If the phonological lexicon under discussion is the same as that which produces speech from semantic specifications, then it is extremely probable that it represents speech in phonemic terms, even if it is difficult to gain conscious access to the code. The evidence for this lies in transposition errors in speech production. In the example 'That's what *T*omsky was *ch*alking about' (Garrett, 1976), what are transposed are phonemes. If such errors arise from a later stage than the lexicon, it is hardly likely (though it is possible) that the lexicon has passed on a code in larger segments than phonemes, which is then broken down into phonemes, only to be reassembled later into larger units once again. If, as this suggests, the output lexicon is phonemically segmentable, then it could mediate the pronunciation of non-words by segmentation and synthesis. Indeed what else is it to converse in secret languages than to segment and synthesise non-words from known words (lexical entries) and vice versa?

In view of the above, let us consider the pronunciation of *kwib*. The initially parsed segmentation of $[([(k)w]i)b]$ will not be overridden by any lexically stored segments. Therefore each letter, as it appears in words, will be accessed as a segment in the input lexicon. The most frequent pronunciation of each segment or letter (in the equivalent position in a word) will then be retrieved. Thus when there are no segments that can be dealt with other than as individual letters, the system will operate like a grapheme-to-phoneme converter. However, while at first sight this may look like grapheme-to-phoneme conversion its operation is by recourse to lexical knowledge.

Coltheart's (1978) concept of grapheme-phoneme conversion requires that grapheme parsing is carried out before and independently of phoneme assignment. He says that 'there is no procedure which, applied to all English words produces a correct parsing of every word into its constitutent functional spelling units without any use of lexical knowledge'. In the present conception functional spelling units in normal skilled readers are segmented precisely by lexical means. The two claims made above, that both spelling-unit segmentation and retrieval of phonology for non-morphemic letters or letter groups are lexical processes, can be illuminated by digressing to the influence of spelling-sound regularity on pronunciation.

3.2.1 Pronunciation of regular and irregular words and non-words

According to the present theory, words may be pronounced both by the phonology being retrieved for the whole letter-string specified as an entry in the input lexicon, and from the segments parsed by their matching segments, however small, in the input lexicon. Indeed if both processes operate then latency differences which have been found by Baron and Strawson (1976) for orthographically regular and exception words are generated as follows. Each segment as it is parsed will automatically activate each of its pronunciations as found in different words. The correct pronunciation results from the treatment of the whole letter-string which overrides prior segments.

But alternative pronunciations derived from non-final segmentations may provide conflicting phonology. Regular words are those whose segments have a smaller number of alternative pronunciations. Indeed the most regular words are those whose pronunciation derived from their segments agrees with that derived from the whole word. As Coltheart says, 'when there is more than one legitimate assignment of a phoneme to a particular functional spelling unit, the *regular assignment* is that which occurs in the largest number of those words containing the functional spelling unit'. Thus there will be less conflicting phonology to override for regular words than for irregular words. This generates the longer pronunciation latency found for exception than regular words (Baron, 1977).

A non-word is pronounced by exactly the same mechanisms. It will be parsed by the parser and input-lexical specifications will mark those segments which occur in known words. (Thus the initial bracketing of *ph* will be marked.) The only difference is that a complete lexical specification will not be met and so the segmentations will not be overridden in non-words (as the *ph* bracketing would be overridden in *shepherd*). The segments which are marked will activate all their potential pronunciations and that which is found in most words will 'win'. Non-words will take longer to pronounce because there is no existing pronunciation from a complete orthographic specification, and no complete specification to override segments. Thus non-words should receive 'regular' pronunciations. Glushko (1980) has provided evidence for this kind of model and against the dual-route (lexical versus grapheme-phoneme) model of pronunciation. His evidence is that non-words like *tave*, whose graphemes are phonologically inconsistent in words (as in *have*), take longer to pronounce than non-words like *taze*, whose graphemes have a consistent phonology in all the words in which they occur (as in *haze*). If non-words were pronounced via non-lexical grapheme-phoneme rules this should not occur. Glushko also found two interesting phenomena in the pronunciation of words. Words whose pronunciation is regular (*wave*) but whose graphemes are pronounced irregularly in other words (*have*) took longer to pronounce than words whose graphemes are pronounced consistently (*wade*). Thus what appears to be crucial is not whether a word is regular but whether its graphemes have competing pronunciations. This cannot be handled by a model which achieves pronunciation by only whole-word methods or non-lexical rules.

Glushko's other observation leads to the same conclusion. Exception words like *tomb* were sometimes mispronounced in accord with other exception words like *comb* (i.e. /tom/). This could not occur if the only source of conflict were from a rule-based orthographic mechanism.

3.2.2 Return to segmentation

The data discussed above bears upon the problems introduced at the beginning of section 3.2 of segmentation into non-morphemic spelling units. Glushko's data suggests that the letters *ave* in *tave* are dealt with lexically, i.e. by reference to their occurrence *together* and *in the equivalent position* in known words. There is little reason to suppose that the initial *t* is dealt with otherwise. Thus specifications in the visual input lexicon can be segmented into what amount to graphemes. Grapheme-to-phoneme conversion will in fact be accomplished by lexical retrieval of phonology.

There still remains the problem created by *oce* in *phoce*. The problem is that *oce* does not occur terminally in any English word. If it does not occur lexically then it is hard to see how it is pronounced 'correctly', without some other source of context-sensitivity. But this is also a problem for non-lexical grapheme-phoneme conversion. An entirely speculative answer is that such letter combinations are dealt with by analogy (Baron, 1977). Suppose that on failure to find any word in the input lexicon ending in *-oce*, words are accessed which end in *-ace* and *-ote*. The appropriate pronunciations for the *o* and the *c* could be retrieved and combined. Presumably this would predict longer pronunciation latencies for such non-words. Further speculation along these lines however needs to await data.

4 A new account of surface dyslexia and beginning readers

The data of beginning reading and surface dyslexia can be derived from the present model by supposing a single type of incompleteness and a general strategy adopted by the reader. All that is required is that beginning readers have not yet acquired orthographic specifications in the input lexicon for some words and that surface dyslexics have lost those specifications for some words. The strategy is to assume that the printed letter-string is a word, that is, what is pronounced should be phonologically recognised by the reader as a word he knows.

In beginning readers the lower the frequency of a word the less likely is it to have acquired an orthographic lexical address. In adults it is not unreasonable to suppose that if lexical entries are lost, low frequency items will more readily suffer. Given what we know about deep dyslexia, neither is it implausible to suppose that, in terms of content or 'phonological' words, certain form-classes are more susceptible than others. An alternative explanation of syntactic class effects in surface dyslexia is that, in terms of early teaching methods, concrete nouns would have been learnt before abstract nouns in reading and would have primacy over adjectives and verbs. The plausibility of this is suggested by Lukatela *et al.*'s (1978) demonstration that the effects of the orthography of what is first learnt in reading can last over periods of at least twenty years.

The consequences of the absence of the lexical specification for a whole word would be twofold. First, its pronunciation could not be retrieved as a whole and would therefore rely on parsed segments. Second, primary bracketings in the parsing of the letter-string would not be overriden by lexical knowledge (e.g. the *re* in *recent* would remain bracketed), nor would later letters override previous bracketings. The eventual phonology would then be a result of two factors: the most frequent phonology for segments parsed thus, and more importantly the constraint that the result is an entry in the aural-oral lexicon. Of course the second factor would not always overrule the first before a candidate response is made.

To test this view, it would have to account for all the responses made by surface dyslexic patients and beginning readers. It might be argued that it allows alternative glosses to be given to individual responses. But this is certainly no more ad hoc than the way the grapheme-phoneme account has to be used, and should at least provide more comfortable accounts and for more of the attempts. The most appropriate and tractable course to take at present is to return to some of the phenomena which were problematic for the grapheme-phoneme approach, to illustrate the processes said above to be operating in surface dyslexia, and to work through a few examples in detail.

To return first to some of the problematic phenomena noted in section 2.2, two of the problems were the inconsistency of the phonology assigned to graphemes and the omission and insertion of phonemes with respect to the target string. Examples of the former were *insect* → 'insist', *incense* → 'increase', *niece* → 'nice', *gauge* → 'jug', *gaol* → 'gold'. Examples of the latter were *barge* → 'bargain', *reapply* → 'reply'. All of these can be seen as a product of three successive processes: (1) context-insensitive left-to-right parsing, (2) the most frequent pronunciation(s) of each segment being retrieved, and (3) modification to make the result acceptable to a phonological lexicon. To understand the responses all three processes must be taken into account. However it is possible to illustrate the predominance of each process in individual examples.

The first process is the parsing of the letter-string. One result of lack of orthographic lexical addresses is that letter-segmentations early in the string are not overridden by letters later in the string. This has four obvious effects: (1) removal of the effect of *e* and *i* on *c* and *g*; (2) removal of the effect of final *e* on vowels preceding the consonant before the *e*; (3) removal of the effect of vowels in digraphs for synthesis or diphthongisation; (4) silent letters are given a phonetic value (*reign* → 'region', *colonel* → 'col-on-el'). The other result of the lack of lexical addresses is that morpheme segments are not overridden. Thus: *island* → 'is+land', *begin* → 'beg+in', *monarch* → 'mon+arch', *unite* → 'unit', *placebo* → 'place+bo', *disease* → 'dis+case', *resent* → 're+send'.

The second process is the retrieval of the most frequent pronunciation for a segment. Thus the hardened *c* in *recent* → /rɪkənt/ is the most frequent rendering of *c* when its segmentation is not overridden by (*cent*). In *disease* → /dɪsiːz/, /dɪs/ is the most frequent rendering of the segment (*dis*). In *reapply* → /rɪplaːɪ/, /ri/ is the most frequent rendering of (*rea-*). In *scintillate* → /skɪntɪleɪt/, /sk/ is the most frequent rendering of the non-overridden segment (*sc*). In *choir* → /tʃɔr/,/tʃ/ is the most frequent rendering of (*ch*).

Thirdly there is the attempt to make (aural-oral) lexical sense. This can be achieved in two ways. One is by choosing an appropriate phonetic value for a letter or segment that can take more than one phonetic value. Thus *insect* → 'insist', *phase* → 'face'. The other is to delete, insert, or change one or more phonemes. Thus: *incense* → 'increase', *barge* → 'bargain', *applaud* → 'appollo', *broad* → 'broke, braid', *gaol* → 'gold', *mouse* → 'must', *attractive* → 'active', *gradually* → 'grandly', *campaign* → 'camping'. It must be remembered that making the stimulus a word means making it into a word that exists in the subject's vocabulary or one that is more probable in his/her vocabulary. Another example of the attempt to make lexical sense of the stimulus is making a series of attempts in response. Thus *broad* → 'broke, break, braid, brode'; *route* → 'rote, rut-th, rout'. This strategy is discussed by Holmes (1973) exactly as attempts to make sense of the stimulus.

While each of the above processes may produce a response it is to be emphasised that all of the processes operate. Thus responses may be, and most probably are, the result of each process operating on the result of the previous one (s). When errors are produced by more than one process one has to resort to glossing, and a 'clean' account cannot be given of every example. However, the present notion does no worse if not better than the standard model.

All of the forementioned classes can be found abundantly in Doctor's (1978) corpus from young normal readers. The only exception is the last, that of trying a series of responses, since she did not permit or record more than one or the first attempt. Two further aspects of the reading responses in the two groups merit comment. First, apparent stress shifts can be seen as having two sources. Many of the examples where stress is classified as being on the first syllable would be the perceptual result (for the experimenter) of each segment being pronounced as it is parsed. Other examples of stress shift result from recognition of one morpheme in the word where the whole word specification is absent. As Holmes puts it (1973, p. 100), 'The explicit reaction to the configuration *tent* in *patent* is a pointer to the problem of *constable* too; if J.C. recognizes a part of a word he evidently finds it difficult not to give that part full stress'. Second, the omission of syllables and the misplacing of consonants, which occur in both groups, can be seen as attempts to produce acceptable morphemes by juggling with the components in what I have called the Phonological Assembly System. This is rather important. Not only because it is hard to account for with a grapheme-phoneme algorithm, even a partially failing one. More importantly because it emphasises the role of an active strategy on the part of the reader.

Let us return to three examples from Holmes' (1973) corpus. Shallice and Warrington (Chapter 5, this volume) characterise *disease* → 'decease' as 'misapplication of valid correspondence rules', and *resent* → 'rissend' as 'partial failure' of rules. How does the currently proposed process deal with them? The process is a left-to-right scan marking plausible morphemes and retrieving the most frequent phonology for those segments. To take *disease*, the scan brackets (*d*), then (*di*), pronounced /dɪ/, then (*dis*) which is a known morpheme which does not change the pronunciation of (*di*) and is pronounced most often /dɪs/. Moving further we would have (*dise*) which would alter the pronunciation, but is not a recognisable segment. If (*dis*) is left marked the next acceptable whole segment is (*ease*). If the phonology of a segment is retrieved when the segment is marked and if the candidate pronunciation(s) are not overridden by subsequent context or by lexical acceptance of the whole string, then the phonology of the two segments will be produced as retrieved, i.e. /dɪs/ + /iːz/. The same process will work for *resent* to produce /ri/ + /sent/. If indeed this was pronounced with a final *voiced* consonant, /d/ (Holmes, 1973), then the morpheme account is even stronger, since none of the partial failures of grapheme-phoneme conversion predict this. Lastly take *placebo*→ 'place+bo'. A letter-to-phoneme account would predict hardening of the *c* and/or sounding of the *e*. But, as long as 'place' exists in the input lexicon, then left-to-right self-terminating parsing would yield the observed result.

Finally, a brief comment on developmental dyslexia is appropriate. In Holmes' (1973) study the four boys aged 9 to 13 who showed similar reading behaviour to the two adult patients are described as dyslexic. Yet their reading is certainly not qualitatively different from that of the normal beginning readers in Doctor's (1978) study. The behaviour of beginning readers has been characterised here as a result of having not yet acquired orthographic specifications for certain words. Is it possible that the boys classified as dyslexic in Holmes' study had merely not yet learnt the appropriate specifications rather than had a disability? The teachers' notes cited by Holmes (Appendix II) are revealing in this connection. In all four cases it appears that with the appropriate teaching the boys made great progress. If the problems of 'developmental dyslexics' of this type are not insuperable, then maybe those of traumatic dyslexics of this type are not either.

5 Implications for deep dyslexia and phonological alexia

Clearly the formulation expressed in Figure 11.2 and the processes described in sections 3 and 4 have implications for characterising other forms of reading impairment. The two principal classes of reading disorder to which this is applicable are deep dyslexia and phonological alexia. Deep dyslexia is characterised at length in this volume and a discussion of the criterial attributes is to be found in papers cited in section 1 of this chapter. In terms of Figure 11.1 of this chapter it is characterised by at least two impairments, one to grapheme-phoneme conversion and one to either or both of (a) the lexical retrieval of phonology (input to output lexicon) and (b) certain parts of the semantic system (see Shallice and Warrington, Chapter 5, for discussion). Phonological alexia has been described by Shallice and Warrington and Beauvois and Dérouesné (1979). It is characterised by the inability to read non-words but the relatively unimpaired ability to read words. Certainly word-class effects are not evident in such patients. In terms of Figure 11.1, this syndrome is caused by impairment to the grapheme-phoneme conversion route.

Now in Figure 11.2 the grapheme-phoneme route has been done away with as a separate entity. So how does one describe these syndromes functionally? In fact deep dyslexia becomes much simpler to describe. We no longer have to say that both intra-lexical and extra-lexical routes to phonology have been impaired. The inability to read non-words and the existence of certain errors are both implied by an impairment to retrieval of phonology from orthographic descriptions, for which route a single (lexical) mechanism exists. If the lexical means of retrieving phonology (the connection between visual input lexicon and aural-oral lexicon) for words is lost, then the means of retrieving phonology for non-words is also lost. If the route which makes use of semantic descriptions remains intact, it will permit certain words to be read and allow semantic and derivational paralexias, but will not permit responses to non-words. This simplification of course does not affect the postulation of additional impairments to the semantic system or visual input addresses themselves which have been discussed by Shallice and Warrington (this volume) and Patterson (1978).

But if non-words and words are read by the same mechanism, how can phonological alexia occur? Quite simply by the fact that although phonology is *retrieved* in the same way, the *segmentation requirements* with regard to the letter-string and phonology are different for words and non-words. If the complete orthographic input specifications for words are extant, then the phonology of words can be retrieved, but if either the orthographic string or the phonological representations in the output lexicon cannot be segmented, then non-words cannot be read accurately, if at all. If the ability to segment is lost it would only necessarily affect the reading of non-words. Since it is not needed for known words, their reading should remain intact. Indeed Shallice and Warrington's phonological alexic patient, B.T.T., is relevant to this. They say that she tended to read nonsense syllables as real words (e.g. *bef*→ 'beef', *fod* → 'food'). This is exactly what would be expected if output phonology could not be segmented. Dérouesné and Beauvois's (1979) distinction between impairments at the graphemic and the phonological stages would map rather well onto segmentation impairments at the two stages. A test of this idea is to examine the ability of phonological alexic patients to perform tests of phonetic segmentation, such as that used by Liberman *et al.* (1977), or by Marcel (1979), and of graphemic segmentation. One test which might reflect graphemic segmentation is that used by Beauvois and Dérouesné, and consists of printing the letters in reverse order of a word which can normally be read. Another test would be to see if patients could separate out of words those segments which comprised morphemes or other whole words (e.g. *recent, postage*). If these types of tests do show that phonological alexic patients have segmentation difficulties, then their problem can be seen as equivalent to one encountered by beginning readers, but which is different from that which characterises surface dyslexia. The ability to segment phonetically is a prerequisite for acquiring the principle of alphabeticisation (Rozin and Gleitman, 1977; Liberman *et al.*, 1977). To this extent both surface dyslexia and phonological alexia would represent 'regression'. But on an optimistic note, regression would not be in terms of development, but in terms of what is learnt.

6 Conclusion

In conclusion, dissatisfaction with accounts of surface dyslexia have motivated an alternative model of pronouncing written words. In this model two methods of retrieving phonology have been collapsed into one method which is lexical and the ability to pronounce non-words relies on segmentation of lexical orthography and phonology. The problem raised in the introduction was that the standard 'two-route' model predicted a double dissociation of reading impairments in deep and surface dyslexia, which is not the case. The solution to that problem in the present model is that the impairments in the two 'syndromes' arise at different points in the processes. Finally the contrast between the two kinds of model raises the issue of the psychological reality of grapheme-phoneme rules. We may have the ability to use rules to derive a pronunciation. But the mere fact that our conscious explanation of how we deal with a new word or a non-word is in terms of rules does not mean that that is how we do it.

Notes

1 At the time when I originally formulated the views in this chapter, I was unaware of Shallice and Warrington's proposal. My proposal in what follows bears strong similarities to their view but also differs somewhat in my view of parsing and visual input specifications.
2 In the case of Warrington's patient, A.B., it was concrete nouns which gave the most trouble, presumably due to his agnosia. However, this only reinforces the point that the problem is not restricted to a 'peripheral' process.
3 It would be grossly unfair to Morton's model if one did not adduce at this point data discussed by Holmes. At least two of her subjects made great use of the strategy of uttering a series of responses, wherein variants are generated within a phonological 'frame' until one attempt is auditorily recognised as an acceptable word (for *different:* ['dif . . . 'dif . . . di'fens . . . di'f . . . 'end . . . di'fend . . . di'fendens . . . di'fend . . . de'fens . . . de'fons] . . . 'difference'). These cases can clearly be interpreted as non-lexically produced articulation, where an ultimate response which is a word is chosen on the basis of an auditory input lexicon. This strategy will be discussed later. It should be noted, however, that it does not reduce the importance of the lexical tendency of single-word responses, which do implicate lexical involvement.
4 In fact, Holmes (1978) has compared surface dyslexic adult patients with children in the context of the notion of 'regression'. However, her comparison is with children classified as 'developmental dyslexics', not with the normal beginning reader.
5 I am obliged to Estelle Doctor for giving me permission to cite results and text from her thesis.

References

Baron, J. (1977) What we might know about orthographic rules. In S. Dornič (ed.), *Attention and Performance,* VI. Hillsdale, N.J.: Lawrence Erlbaum.

Baron, J. and Strawson, C. (1976) Use of orthographic and word-specific knowledge in reading words aloud. *Journal of Experimental Psychology: Human Perception and Performance, 2,* 386–93.

Barr, R. (1975) The effect of instruction on pupil reading strategies. *Reading Research Quarterly, 10,* 555–82.

Beauvois, M.-F. and Dérouesné, J. (1979) Phonological Alexia: three dissociations. *Journal of Neurology, Neurosurgery and Psychiatry, 42,* 1115–24.

Biemiller, A. (1970) The development of the use of graphic and contextual information as children learn to read. *Reading Research Quarterly, 6,* 75–96.

Chomsky, N. and Halle, M. (1968) *The Sound Pattern of English.* New York: Harper & Row.

Coltheart, M. (1978) Lexical access in simple reading tasks. In G. Underwood (ed.), *Strategies of Information Processing.* London: Academic Press.

Dérouesné, J. and Beauvois, H. F. (1979) Phonological processing in reading: data from alexia. *Journal of Neurology, Neurosurgery and Psychiatry, 42,* 1125–32.

Doctor, E. A. (1978) Studies on reading comprehension in children and adults. Unpublished Ph.D. thesis, Birkbeck College, University of London.

Fromkin, V. A. (ed.) (1973) *Speech Errors as Linguistic Evidence.* The Hague: Mouton.

Garrett, M. F. (1976) Syntactic processes in sentence production. In R. J. Wales and E. C. T. Walker (eds), *New Approaches to Language Mechanisms.* Amsterdam: North Holland.

Glushko, R. J. (1980) The organization and activation of orthographic knowledge in reading aloud. *Journal of Experimental Psychology.*

Goodman, K. S. (1967) Reading: a psycholinguistic guessing game. *Journal of the Reading Specialist,* 259–64, 266–71.

Holmes, J. M. (1973) Dyslexia: a neurolinguistic study of traumatic and developmental disorders of reading. Unpublished Ph.D. thesis, University of Edinburgh.

Holmes, J. M. (1978) 'Regression' and reading breakdown. In A. Caramazza and E. B. Zurif (eds), *Language Acquisition and Language Breakdown: Parallels and Divergencies.* Baltimore: Johns Hopkins.

Liberman, I. Y., Shankweiler, D., Liberman, A. M., Fowler, C. and Fischer, F. W. (1977) Phonetic segmentation and recoding in the beginning reader. In A. S. Reber and D. L. Scarborough (eds), *Toward a Psychology of Reading.* Hillsdale, N.J.: Lawrence Erlbaum.

Lukatela, G., Savić, M. D., Ognjenović, P. and Turvey, M. T. (1978) On the relation between processing the Roman and Cyrillic alphabets: a preliminary analysis with bi-alphabetic readers. *Language and Speech, 21,* 113–41.

MacKinnon, A. R. (1959) *How do children learn to read?* Vancouver: Copp Clark.

Marcel, A. J. (1979) Phonological awareness and phonological representation: investigation of a specific spelling problem. In U. Frith (ed.), *Cognitive Processes in Spelling*. London: Academic Press.

Marshall, J. C. and Newcombe, F. (1973) Patterns of paralexia: a psycholinguistic approach. *Journal of Psycholinguistic Research, 2,* 175–99.

Marshall, J. C. and Newcombe, F. (1977) Variability and constraint in acquired dyslexia. In H. A. Whitaker and H. Whitaker (eds), *Studies in Neurolinguistics*, vol. 3. New York: Academic Press.

Mattingly, I. G. (1972) Reading, the linguistic process and linguistic awareness. In J. F. Kavanagh and I. G. Mattingly (eds), *Language by Ear and by Eye*. Cambridge, Mass: MIT.

Midgley-West, L. (1977) Unpublished experiments. Birkbeck College, London University.

Patterson, K. E. (1978) Phonemic dyslexia: errors of meaning and the meaning of errors. *Quarterly Journal of Experimental Psychology, 30,* 587–601.

Patterson, K. E. and Marcel, A. J. (1977) Aphasia, dyslexia and the phonological coding of written words. *Quarterly Journal of Experimental Psychology, 29,* 307–18.

Rozin, P. and Gleitman, L. R. (1977) The structure and acquisition of reading. II: The reading process and the acquisition of the alphabetic principle. In A. S. Reber and D. L. Scarborough (eds), *Toward a Psychology of Reading*. Hillsdale, N.J.: Lawrence Erlbaum.

Saffran, E. M. and Marin, O. S. M. (1977) Reading without phonology: evidence from aphasia. *Quarterly Journal of Experimental Psychology, 29,* 515–26.

Savin, H. B. (1972) What the child knows about speech when he starts to learn to read. In J. F. Kavanagh and I. G. Mattingley (eds), *Language by Ear and by Eye*. Cambridge, Mass.: MIT.

Shallice, T. and Warrington, E. K. (1975) Word recognition in a phonemic dyslexic patient. *Quarterly Journal of Experimental Psychology, 27,* 187–99.

Shankweiler, D. and Liberman, I. Y. (1972) Misreading: a search for causes. In J. F. Kavanagh and I. G. Mattingley (eds), *Language by Ear and by Eye*. Cambridge, Mass.: MIT.

Weber, R.-M. (1968) The study of oral reading errors: a survey of the literature. *Reading Research Quarterly, 4,* 96–119.

12 Fractionating the reading process in dementia: evidence for word-specific print-to-sound associations

Myrna F. Schwartz, Eleanor M. Saffran and Oscar S. M. Marin

How does the fluent adult reader go from print to sound? We, along with many others, assume two primary mechanisms. The first is *lexical*, involving recognition of the printed item as a word with a characteristic pronunciation. The second is *non-lexical*: a phonological code is derived directly from the graphemic information, presumably by the application of sound-spelling rules to letters or groups of letters. This distinction is discussed further in Chapters 4 and 10.

In postulating a lexical pathway from print to sound, we account for the ability to read aloud words which do not conform to the spelling rules of English, or which are ambiguous with regard to these rules (e.g. read, live, bow). Furthermore, such a mechanism provides the basis for our understanding of deep dyslexia, the retained capacity for pronouncing written words – but not non-words – in brain-damaged subjects who have lost the ability to translate graphemes into phonemes.

The character of deep dyslexia has in turn influenced the form of the reading model. Since these patients, who are reading exclusively by the lexical route, tend to make semantic errors in reading aloud, it is reasonable to suppose that lexical reading involves the mediation of a semantic representation. But does it *necessarily*? In fact, this question is tautologous if we restrict ourselves to the linguists' definition of 'lexicon', in which semantic and phonological components of word knowledge are stored together. But once these components are separated conceptually, as they are, for example in

This research has been supported by N.I.H. grants AG01152 (M. F. Schwartz) and NS13992 (E. M. Saffran).

Morton's logogen system (Morton, 1970), then it becomes meaningful to ask whether in the normal reader (although not in the deep dyslexic) there operates a more direct lexical mechanism, one which proceeds directly from visual word form (visual input logogen) to a stored representation in a phonological lexicon (output logogen). (For suggestions along this line, see Baron, 1977; and see Morton and Patterson; Shallice and Warrington; Chapters 4 and 5 this volume.)

There is little which addresses this question in the experimental literature on normal reading; but data from pathology may once again be instructive. For example, Warrington (1975) has reported that patients who suffer a moderate loss of semantic knowledge have disproportionate difficulty in pronouncing written exception words, as compared with words that conform to the spelling rules of English. This is precisely what one would expect on the view that (a) exception words are read via the lexical route; and (b) this route depends upon the mediation of the (impaired) semantic system. On the basis of this observation, Shallice and Warrington (Chapter 5) tentatively conclude that there exist no word-specific print-to-sound associations.

We have data, gathered in the course of a three year case study of anomic dementia,[1] which contradicts this view. The general details of this study are reported elsewhere (Schwartz, Marin and Saffran, 1979). Of relevance to the question of reading mechanisms is the following set of claims:

1   That over the course of the 30-month long study, the patient, W.L.P., suffered the progressive breakdown in the scope and specificity of semantic knowledge which could be brought to bear in the comprehension of language, both spoken and written;
2   That at a time when semantic knowledge was severely compromised and she was unable to access phonology for the purpose of naming or making reference, W.L.P. retained the ability to read words aloud;
3   That her oral reading was not accomplished solely by the application of spelling rules (although she was capable of applying these rules for the successful pronunciation of pseudo-words). Because W.L.P. was able to read aloud exception words not conforming to regular spelling patterns – words with meanings she did not know – this case would seem to provide strong

evidence for the role of word-specific print-to-sound associations in reading.

1 Pronunciation vs. comprehension of written animal names

Initially, the reading data were obtained incidentally in the assessment of W.L.P.'s semantic loss. Since W.L.P. could read aloud with facility, we utilized this capacity to circumvent potential memory limitations in other tasks. Thus, in an early investigation of W.L.P.'s comprehension of animal names, we presented the target name visually and asked her to read the word aloud before matching it to one of four depicted animals.

W.L.P.'s matching performance was random; she correctly identified the pictorial referent on only six of the 40 trials. In contrast, her oral reading was near perfect; she required correction on only two occasions, both times having misplaced primary stress (/buz zard′/; /rhino cer′os/). In general W.L.P. read fluently and without effort, frequently appending comments that emphasized the discrepancy between her ability to pronounce the target, and to comprehend it (e.g. 'hyena . . . hyena . . . what in the heck is that?').

In Table 12.1 are listed the animal names used as targets in this matching task. There were 40 items in all, half of them very familiar (at least 30 occurrences per million, Thorndike & Lorge, 1944), the other half less so (less than 6 per million). Note that some of these stimuli, in particular those of lower frequency, have pronunciations which are not unambiguously specified by their orthography (i.e. by the rules which relate graphemes to phonemes).

What did W.L.P. know about these words which she could read aloud but not match to referents? We explored this question with a simple category-sorting procedure. W.L.P. was given a deck of 80 index cards, each containing the name of an animal, color, or body part (Table 12.1), and was asked to place each card 'in the pile where it belongs'. The four piles were labeled, from left to right, 'an animal', 'a color', 'a part of my body', 'something else'. The results of this sorting test are presented in Table 12.2. W.L.P.'s performance is best with terms designating parts of the body. With color words, and animal names, she is consistently correct only with the more common exemplars. With less common terms, her ability to identify superordinate category falls precipitously.

TABLE 12.1 *Category-sorting task (written stimuli)*

Animals		Colors	Body parts
High frequency (>30/million)			
bear	elephant	black	ear
bee	goat	blue	eye
bull	horse	brown	finger
cat	lamb	gray	foot
chicken	lion	green	heel
cow	owl	orange	knee
deer	pig	pink	mouth
dog	rabbit	purple	nail
duck	sheep	red	nose
eagle	tiger	yellow	tongue
Low frequency (<30/million)			
alligator	kangaroo	amber	abdomen
baboon	leopard	auburn	ankle
buzzard	llama	beige	chin
crocodile	octopus	crimson	elbow
gazelle	ostrich	ebony	hip
giraffe	panther	fuchsia	kidney
gopher	raccoon	lavender	thigh
gorilla	rhinoceros	magenta	thumb
hippo	tortoise	maroon	torso
hyena	zebra	turquoise	wrist

Thorndike & Lorge (1944).

TABLE 12.2 *W.L.P.'s category sorting, April, 1975*

	Sorting response			
	animal	body part	color	other
Animal names				
high frequency (n=20)	16	0	0	4
low frequency (n=20)	7	0	1	12
Body parts				
high frequency (n=10)	0	7	0	3
low frequency (n=10)	0	8	0	2
Color names				
high frequency (n=10)	0	0	9	1
low frequency (n=10)	0	1	1	8

TABLE 12.3 *Production vs. comprehension of animal names: W.L.P., March through April, 1975*

	Oral reading	Matching to category label	Matching to pictorial referent [a]
High frequency names			
bear	✓	✗	✗
bee	✓	✗	✗
bull	✓	✓	✗
cat	✓	✓	✗
chicken	✓	✓	✗
cow	✓	✓	✗
deer	✓	✓	✗
dog	✓	✓	✓
duck	✓	✓	✗
eagle	✓	✗	✓
elephant	✓	✗	✗
goat	✓	✓	✗
horse	✓	✓	✓
lamb	✓	✓	✗
lion	✓	✓	✗
owl	✓	✗	✗
pig	✓	✓	✓
rabbit	✓	✓	✗
sheep	✓	✓	✗
tiger	✓	✓	✗
Low frequency names			
alligator	✓	✓	✗
baboon	✓	✗	✗
buzzard	buz zard'	✓	✗
crocodile	✓	✗	✗
gazelle	✓	✗	✗
giraffe	✓	✓	✓
gopher	✓	✗	✗
gorilla	✓	✓	✗
hippo	✓	✗	✓
hyena	✓	✓	✗
kangaroo	✓	✗	✗
leopard	✓	✗	✗
llama	✓	✗	✗
octopus	✓	✗	✗
ostrich	✓	✗	✗
panther	✓	✗	✗
raccoon	✓	✗	✗
rhinoceros	rhino cer'os	✓	✗
tortoise	✓	✗	✗
zebra	✓	✓	✗

[a] From a set of four alternatives.

In Table 12.3, these data are contrasted with W.L.P.'s oral reading performance. The high frequency animal names are sorted and read correctly (although they are matched to referents at a level of accuracy no greater than chance).[2] The disparity between pronunciation and comprehension emerges clearly, however, with the low frequency items. Twelve of these 20 items were not recognized as referring to animals, yet all were read correctly.

2 W.L.P.'s pronunciation of regular spellings and exception words

Our case study of W.L.P. spanned a period of 30 months, from February 1975 to July 1977. The study of animal names described above was conducted early in that period, in April 1975. Over the next two years there occurred a steady deterioration in W.L.P.'s understanding of referential terms (see Schwartz *et al.*, 1979, for details). As her condition worsened, it became increasingly apparent that her oral reading – which remained fluent – could not be semantically mediated.

Was her reading then dependent upon the rules which related graphemes to phonemes? Several observations suggested not: her success in pronouncing exception words like 'tortoise' and 'leopard' (Table 12.3); the rarity of phonological errors in reading; the speed and fluency of her reading. These stand in sharp contrast to descriptions of brain-damaged subjects who are in fact dependent on non-lexical recoding mechanisms in reading (so called 'surface' dyslexics, see Marshall and Newcombe, 1973; Shallice and Warrington, Chapter 5, this volume).

In order to determine whether W.L.P. was, as we suspected, utilizing lexical knowledge in reading, we had her read aloud a list of 52 high frequency words, consisting of 26 pairs matched for spelling pattern but differing in pronunciation (e.g. cost-post). For each pair, the consistent application of a spelling rule would result in a pronunciation error on one of the items of the pair. Overall, then, a reader dependent upon spelling rules could be expected to make pronunciation errors on at least half of the items.

This list was administered to W.L.P. on three occasions. In March of 1976 she read all the words correctly but one ('bury' was pronounced /burey/ as in 'fury'). In September, six months later, she was still pronouncing 85 per cent of the words correctly, and in January of 1977, 77 per cent. To achieve this performance, W.L.P. had to be capable of lexical reading, i.e. she had to have recognized the stimuli as words which have characteristic pronunciations. Did the orthography influence her reading at all? To determine this, we dichotomized the test words according to whether or not they conformed to spelling rules.[3] Forty-four of the words could be so classified; these words, and W.L.P.'s responses to them, are itemized in Table 12.4.

TABLE 12.4 *W.L.P.'s oral reading*

Regular words				Exception words			
	3/1/76	9/22/76	1/21/77		3/1/76	9/22/76	1/21/77
food	✓	✓	✓	blood	✓	✓	plud
cow	✓	✓	✓	blow	✓	✓	blough (as in bough)
bone	✓	✓	✓	one	✓	✓	✓
jury	✓	✓	jerry	bury	burey (as in fury)	✓	✓
bead	✓	✓	✓	bread	✓	✓	✓
road	✓	✓	✓	broad	✓	✓	✓
bother	✓	✓	buther	brother	✓	✓	✓
howl	✓	✓	✓	bowl	✓	✓	✓
charge	✓	✓	✓	character	✓	char ak'tor (as in charcoal)	✓
limb	✓	lime	limp	climb	✓	✓	✓
cloth	✓	✓	✓	both	✓	✓	bawth
home	✓	✓	✓	come	✓	kome	✓
cost	✓	✓	✓	post	✓	✓	✓
penny	✓	✓	✓	deny	✓	denny	denny
go	✓	✓	✓	do	✓	✓	✓
down	✓	✓	✓	own	✓	owen	✓
ear	✓	✓	✓	wear	✓	✓	✓
each	✓	✓	✓	earth	✓	✓	✓
allow	✓	ah lo'ah	ah'lo (as in hallow)	fellow	✓	✓	✓
flower	✓	✓	✓	flow	✓	flower	flower
food	✓	✓	✓	foot	✓	✓	food
floor	✓	✓	flower	flood	✓	✓	✓

Is is clear that W.L.P.'s reading was indeed influenced by spelling patterns. Regular words were read more accurately than exception words, and the majority of her errors can be construed as misapplication or over-generalization of grapheme-phoneme rules. Nor was this effect restricted to this particular word list. From J. Baron we obtained a new list of exception words, chosen because they both violated spelling rules and resisted pronunciation by analogy (Baron, 1978). These words were presented to W.L.P. along with corresponding stimuli which did obey the spelling rules. Once again the influence of spelling pattern was evident in her superior reading of regular over exception words, and in her occasional over-regularizations (Table 12.5). However, it is W.L.P.'s successes, rather than her failures, which are most informative. On Baron's list, as on our own, W.L.P. succeeded in reading approximately three-quarters of the exception words. If one accepts the premise that her correct pronunciations could not have been specified by her knowledge of word meanings, then this success with exception words constitutes strong evidence for the role of word specific print-to-sound associations.

Discussion

In light of the severity of her semantic loss, W.L.P.'s success in reading exception words is most impressive. In early 1977, when she could still pronounce fluently words like 'blood', 'doll', 'liquor', 'watch', 'dollar', 'flood', 'police', 'shoe', 'sweat', and so on (Tables 12.4 and 12.5), W.L.P. was unable to match the most familiar object names to their referents; not could she sort object names with others from the same superordinate category (although she could do so with pictures of the objects themselves). The most reasonable account of W.L.P.'s successful pronunciation of these exception words is to suppose that the visual word form (visual input logogen) activated in some direct fashion an associated representation in a phonological lexicon (output logogen).

It is interesting to note that there was no comparable access to this phonological lexicon for purposes of naming or making reference. W.L.P. was severely anomic even at the outset of our testing program. She rarely produced paraphasias of either the semantic or literal type. She asserted repeatedly that she had 'forgotten' the words for which she sought; nor was her search aided by phonological prompting by the listener. This situation progressed to the point where, in early 1977, the only reference term that remained in her speaking vocabulary was 'shopping-center'. In

TABLE 12.5 *Baron's reading list: W.L.P., 9/15/76*

Regular words		Exception words	
tooth	✓	blood	✓
cape	✓	cafe	caf
maker	✓	water	✓
along	✓	among	✓
soft	✓	both	bawth
float	✓	broad	bred
open	✓	once	✓
swoop	swip	sword	sword (as in *swore*)
whip	✓	whom	hume
hunter	✓	honest	✓
cheap	✓	sweat	✓
motor	✓	woman	✓
goes	✓	does	✓
boost	✓	flood	✓
corn	✓	word	✓
toll	✓	doll	✓
divine	✓	marine	marin
summit	✓	sugar	✓
holy	✓	honor	✓
couch	coach	touch	✓
hose	✓	lose	loose
suck	✓	sure	sewer
tone	✓	gone	✓
alike	ay light'	elite	e light' (as in *delight*)
foul	foal	tour	✓
crew	✓	sew	✓
liquid	✓	liquor	✓
honey	✓	hour	✓
pinch	✓	pint	pint (as in *hint*)
advice	advance	police	✓
holder	✓	dollar	✓
toes	✓	shoe	✓
sink	✓	ninth	ninth (as in *pin*)
match	✓	watch	✓
hand	✓	want	✓
fuse	fuz	busy	✓
wheel	✓	whole	✓
bone	✓	gone	✓
treat	✓	great	✓

contrast to the situation in reading, then, there appears to be no comparable 'direct' route for naming objects, or pictures; at least none was operating in W.L.P. It is our view that naming and referring always require the mediation of a conceptual/semantic network, and for W.L.P. such mediated access to the phonological lexicon was not possible (Schwartz *et al.*, 1979).

Returning to reading: the presence of over-regularizing errors in W.L.P.'s reading corpus, and her superior performance on regular spellings over exception words affirms the psychological reality of spelling rules in oral reading (Baron, 1978; Baron and Strawson, 1976). Furthermore, there is the suggestion in W.L.P.'s data that, over time, these rules may have come to play an increasingly important role in her performance (Table 12.4, and see Warrington, 1975). We have no definitive account of this pattern; it may perhaps represent the onset of deterioration within the phonological lexicon, or perhaps the tendency toward piecemeal recoding of the graphemic input. In any case, it is remarkable that the rule-bound non-lexical pathway to phonology, which we know from deep dyslexia to be vulnerable to lesions within the left hemisphere, should resist the ravages of the diffuse, degenerative pathological process which affected W.L.P. and compromised so profoundly the lexical/semantic aspects of both productive and receptive language. Elsewhere we have presented evidence that her syntactic competence was also in large measure spared, again in sharp contrast to aphasics with left hemisphere lesions (Schwartz *et al.*, 1979). It is our contention that these functional dissociations may reflect differences in basic neural organization underlying these separable components of language function.

Notes

1 More precisely, this was a case of pre-senile dementia in a woman aged 62, presenting with prominent language pathology against a background of generalized and progressive memory loss. Neurological examination revealed no evidence of focal pathology, but was rather consistent with bilateral, diffuse involvement of the cerebral hemispheres. Computerized brain tomography revealed a moderate degree of generalized cortical atrophy.

2 On subsequent explorations along these lines we systematically manipulated the set of picture distractors and learned that W.L.P.'s performance was not as indiscriminate as it appeared to be here. That is, presented with the name of a small, pet-like animal (e.g. dog), she

would often match it to a picture of a different pet-like animal (a cat or squirrel), but rarely to an animal out of that subclass (i.e. a horse or a cow).

3 We are grateful to Max Coltheart for assisting us in this classification.

References

Baron, J. (1977) Mechanisms for pronouncing printed words: use and acquisition. In D. LaBerge and S. J. Samuels (eds), *Basic Processes in Reading: Perception and Comprehension*. Hillsdale, N.J.: Lawrence Erlbaum.

Baron, J. and Strawson, C. (1976) Use of orthographic and word-specific knowledge in reading words aloud. *Journal of Experimental Psychology: Human Perception and Performance, 2,* 386–93.

Marshall, J. C. and Newcombe, F. (1973) Patterns of paralexia. *Journal of Psycholinguistic Research, 2,* 175–99.

Morton, J. (1970) A functional model for memory. In D. A. Norman (ed.), *Models of Human Memory*. New York: Academic Press.

Schwartz, M. F., Marin, O. S. M. and Saffran, E. M. (1979) Dissociations of language function in dementia: a case study. *Brain and Language, 7,* 277–306.

Thorndike, E. L. and Lorge, I. (1944) *The Teacher's Word Book of 30,000 Words*. New York: Teacher's College.

Warrington, E. K. (1975) The selective impairment of semantic memory. *Quarterly Journal of Experimental Psychology, 27,* 635–57.

13 'Little words – No!'

John Morton and Karalyn Patterson

This is a study of one patient, P.W. (born 1908), a retired civil servant who had a stroke in 1965. This patient has been described at length in Patterson (1978, 1979) and Patterson and Marcel (1977).

The outstanding features of P.W.'s condition are:

1 *Spontaneous speech.* P.W. is a classic and severe agrammatic aphasic. His severity rating on the Boston Diagnostic Aphasia Test (Goodglass and Kaplan, 1972), which encompasses a range from 0 (most impaired) to 5, is 1; and his profile is that of Broca's aphasia.

2 *Speech comprehension.* His auditory comprehension is impaired (and even severely so given syntactically complex utterances) but adequate for conversation.

3 *Phonological manipulations.* A prototypic deep dyslexic, P.W. cannot do any non-lexical phonological coding of written language.

4 *Reading.* Performance varies with word type, but a broad sample of content words (nouns, adjectives, verbs) yields about 50 per cent correct responses when P.W. reads single words aloud. About half of his paralexic reading responses are semantic (e.g. *upset* → 'quarrel').

When invited to read, on one occasion, his response was 'Big words – Yes! Little words – No!' and it is on the 'little words' that this paper focuses. Previous work on function words with P.W. has shown the following:

1 *Reading aloud.* P.W. correctly read only 8 per cent of a list of 60

function words (Patterson, 1979). In addition he had a higher proportion of omissions than in response to content words. This general weakness on function words is a well established feature of the deep dyslexic literature. Thus G.R. read two out of 111 function words correctly (Marshall and Newcombe, 1973), K.F. read 11 per cent of his function words (Shallice and Warrington, 1975) and V.S. read 29 per cent correctly (Saffran and Marin, 1977).

2 *Comprehension.* P.W.'s comprehension of function words appears to be very poor. On auditory presentation of the Token Test he scored four out of fifteen (Patterson and Marcel, 1977). In a variety of other simple tests on prepositions he scarcely scored better than chance (Elvin and Hatfield, 1978). We are not aware of previously published results for other patients with deep dyslexia.

3 *Lexical decision.* On the basis of his reading performance, it might have been thought that function words were rather like nonsense syllables to P.W. However Patterson (1979) has demonstrated that P.W. is able to discriminate function words from non-words in a lexical decision task. He correctly accepted 60 out of 60 function words, making only two false-positive errors on the 60 non-words. Since the non-words closely resembled function words (e.g., *thise, thore, whar, weth*), we must assume that the system responsible for categorisation of visually presented words operates as accurately for function words as for any other.

4 *Auditory-visual matching.* A function word was presented visually and three function words were read out for him to select the correct match. He scored 58 per cent correct (Patterson, 1978), which is better than chance, but very poor.

In this paper we explore further his reading aloud of function words and introduce some new tasks aimed at exploring his comprehension processes.

Reading aloud

Over the last 18 months we have often presented him with lists of function words to read. These trials have been with a number of motives: comparison of function words with words of different classes; attempts to increase both his reading and his comprehension of function words; and concentration on a small set of words which were cued indirectly (Morton and Patterson, 1977). We have collated all these data and present the results in Table 13.1. The words have been divided into more or less classical grammatical divisions, without too much concern over words which could be members of two or more classes. The errors have been classified into omissions and a variety of other headings which are here illustrated.

TABLE 13.1

Word class	(n)	Correct	Omission	Function word paralexia			Paralexia (not function word)
				Semantic	Visual	Other	
Prepositions and conjunctions	(105)	0.36	0.11	0.05	0.20	0.17	0.10
Adverbs and quantifiers	(129)	0.21	0.14	0.12	0.05	0.23	0.24
Interrogatives	(16)	0.31	0.37	0.06	0.13	0.06	0.00
Auxiliary verbs	(57)	0.11	0.33	0.05	0.14	0.26	0.10
Personal pronouns	(82)	0.22	0.26	0.22	0.10	0.04	0.16
Relative pronouns	(17)	0.00	0.65	0.00	0.12	0.00	0.23
Total	(406)	0.23	0.21	0.10	0.12	0.17	0.17
Cued words	(207)	0.40	0.14	0.06	0.08	0.12	0.20

(a) Semantically related function-word paralexia

me	→	'I'
often	→	'sometimes'
where	→	'whither'
usually	→	'sometimes'
us	→	'we'
before	→	'front of'
we	→	'me and you'

(b) Visually similar function-word paralexia (note: these are sometimes the result of a particular reading strategy whereby initial or final letters are covered over until some other word is revealed)

his	→	'is'
beside	→	'because'
us	→	'is'
our	→	'or'
about	→	'out'
where	→	'she' (via the intermediate 'her', so in fact this is a visual paralexia followed by a semantic one)

(c)   Other function-word paralexia

both	→	'perhaps'
between	→	'sometimes'
nor	→	'and'
the	→	'and'

Because there are not a great many of the following types and there is limited space in Table 13.1, these are not presented separately in the table. But to give the full flavour of his reading responses . . .

(d)   Semantic paralexia – not function word

beneath	→	'downstairs'
none	→	'negative'
if	→	'query'
both	→	'two'
she	→	'woman'
her	→	'girl'

(e)   Visual paralexia – not function word (and see note for (b) above)

must	→	'musk'
yet	→	'yak'
what	→	'hat'
again	→	'gain'
through	→	'rough'
when	→	'hen'

(f)   Visual-then-semantic paralexia – not function word

> *when*   → 'chick'
> *when*   → 'cockerel'
> *their*   → 'throne'
> *their*   → 'earl'

Cued-words. One class of function words has been examined separately. These are words for which P.W. has cues to help him to read them. He has accumulated these cues over the years in an exercise book which he occasionally consults. We have added to this set and examined his performance with them (Morton and Patterson, 1977). The cues are of three main kinds:

1   Homophones

> *been*   → bean   → 'been'
> *through* → threw → 'through'
> *would* → wood → 'would'

2   Syllabic decomposition

> *even*   → even(song)   → 'even'
> *after* → after(noon) → 'after'
> *from*   → from(age)   → 'from'

3   Phrase decomposition

> *the*   → (God Save) the (Queen)   → 'the'
> *off*   → (they're) off!   → 'off'
> *here* → (hear) hear!   → 'here'

The cued words are listed separately in Table 13.1 where it can be seen that the cues are moderately effective so far as his ability to read function words aloud is concerned. Many of his failures on this set arise from paralexias on the intervening word (e.g. *generally*, for which his cue is General Lee, led to the response 'colonel'; *even*, for which his cue is even(song), → 'sunset') or from appropriate decomposition followed by inappropriate selection (e.g. *after* → 'noon').

In Table 13.1 the outstanding features are (a) the appalling performance with relative pronouns and auxiliary verbs, (b) the frequent semantic paralexias with personal pronouns, and (c) the overall high level of function word paralexias (0.39). This value might be in part a function of the homogeneity of the lists. In a heterogenous list of mixed function and content words, the number of function word paralexias to function words was 10/38 = 0.26. That his overall level of correct reading of function words is higher in Table 13.1 (0.23) than previously reported (0.08) is, we assume, attributable to the fact that both we and P.W.'s speech therapists have been hammering him with these words.

Comprehension

Comprehension of single words: the triad method

It was the occasional occurrence of semantic paralexias in reading function words which alerted us to the possibility that P.W. had more comprehension of these words than revealed by any tasks to date. After one or two false attempts, we settled on a two-alternative forced choice task where he had to indicate which one of two alternative words went with a third word, all presented visually. He was tested on a number of separate occasions, with the nature and extent of the tests varying as we gradually came to understand what we were doing. Oddly enough, *he* seemed to understand what we were doing; we do not mean that he necessarily understood it consciously but rather that he needed minimal instructions. The instruction essentially directed 'choose which one of these two words goes with this third word' together with some easy examples like:

> man
> > boy
> woman

We present the data below, by type of word and type of judgement required and with examples. It should be noted that a total of twelve judgements of one type does not usually mean that there were twelve *different* triads of that type. Some specific triads were repeated over the various sessions.

Personal pronouns					Correct
(a) *number* e.g.	me us	we	him them	theirs	10/12
(b) *gender*	him her	he	he she	hers	11/12
(c) *person within number*	me him	he	us them	our	9/14
(d) *person across number*	I he	we	they we	she	6/8
(e) *case*	he him	her	my me	our	9/18

Prepositions and adverbs					Correct
(a) *space*	beside apart	next to	over under	up	25/31
(b) *time*	now then	later	before after	since	13/18
(c) *frequency*	every few	all	always seldom	rarely	16/20

Demonstratives[1]					Correct
(a) *locational*	that this	these	near far	that	2/8
(b) *number*	this these	that	those that	many	12/12

Interrogatives				Correct
who	person	which	thing	14/17
why		why		

Conjunctions				Correct
(a) *logical* *number*	except	instead	one	12/14
	with	together		
(b) *logical* *function?*	if	therefore	because	3/6
	though	however		

Part-of-speech				Correct
this	that	if	by	3/10
thus		under		

Summary of triad data

This technique shows that P.W. can extract quite a lot of information from written function words. The judgements he made reasonably well involved (a) the gender of pronouns; (b) prepositions and adverbs specifying space; (c) prepositions and adverbs specifying frequency; (d) interrogatives; and (e) anything concerning number, whether it be pronouns, demonstratives or conjunctions of logical number. He could not perform judgements based on part-of-speech or case; also, though the amount of data is small, it appears that he could not handle locational demonstratives or conjunctions of logical function. We do not claim to have predicted this pattern, nor entirely to know how to account for it, but the following summary suggests itself: P.W. seems to understand the semantic content of function words, but not the syntactic content. Words specifying gender, space and frequency provide substantive information apart from any role they play in or form they are required to take by their sentential context. It is not clear that the same can be said for variables like case and part-of-speech. Thus we invoke the traditional split between lexical/semantic knowledge and syntactic ability (Caramazza and Berndt, 1978; Marin, Saffran and Schwartz,

1976). Not only does this distinction broadly characterise much of the general reading performance of deep dyslexics and both the speech production and comprehension of Broca's aphasics; it even seems to be germane within the class of function words. Further we note that these results and our interpretation of them are a counter instance to the statement that function words '. . . are not believed to have a specific semantic representation' (Caramazza and Berndt, 1978, p. 910).

Comprehension of single words: other techniques

1   Ordering of words specifying quantity and frequency
We gave P.W. two tests each consisting of seven words which could be ordered from 'least' to 'most'. The seven words were printed on slips of paper and presented to him altogether, in jumbled order. For the quantity words, his ordering was:

   none   one   few   some   several   many   all

One of the authors would also produce this order, and the other would reverse *some* and *several*, but in any case we call P.W.'s performance quite good. For the frequency words, his ordering was:

   never   once   seldom   usually   sometimes   often   always

We disagree with his placement of *usually*, but again consider his performance adequate.

2   Associating word pairs
Eight pairs of function words like *in-out, above-below, on-off* were printed on slips of paper, one word to a slip. The sixteen bits of paper were given to P.W. altogether, in jumbled order. He was asked to put them into appropriate pairs (we gave him *yes-no*, which was not one of the test pairs, as an example). He did this at first correctly and then after some thought dissolved three pairs and incorrectly re-paired them as *now-before, above-then*, and *after-below*. On another session he got six correct pairs easily, but slowly and incorrectly joined *now-after* and *then-before*. In this test, time-relevant words appeared to cause him difficulty.

3   Picture-word assignments
This test involved simple drawings of two or three objects in some spatial relationship to one another, together with two or three

printed words describing the position of each object. All of the drawings and words are shown in Figure 13.1. For the test, P.W. was given one picture at a time, plus the corresponding two-three words on slips of paper, and asked to assign the words to the pictures. This test was done on five separate occasions (only four for the last picture), and performance is also shown in Figure 13.1. As in the previous test, *before-after* seems especially problematic for P.W. Otherwise, performance was perfect.

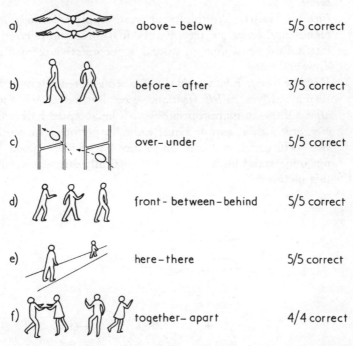

a)   above - below   5/5 correct

b)   before - after   3/5 correct

c)   over - under   5/5 correct

d)   front - between - behind   5/5 correct

e)   here - there   5/5 correct

f)   together - apart   4/4 correct

FIGURE 13.1 Pictures, words and performance for the test of picture-word assignments

4 Judgements of appropriateness

Using three pictures (which appear in Figure 13.2), we asked P.W. to say which of a list of function words could appropriately be used to describe the positions of the pictured objects. There were 17 words: *above, below, before, after, right, left, over, under, up, down, beside, between, through, across, around, beneath, behind.* Each was printed on a slip of paper. With one picture in front of P.W., the 17 words were presented one at a time in a random order. He was to look at each word silently and respond 'yes' if it was appropriate for the picture and 'no' otherwise. His performance was as follows:

Picture 1 (airplanes): By our reckoning, seven of the 17 words are appropriate; he responded positively to six of these but rejected *beneath*. He also accepted two inappropriate words, *right* and *before*.

Picture 2 (houses): We think four words apply here, *right*, *left*, *between* and *beside*; he accepted the first three and rejected the last. Of the remaining 13 words, he incorrectly accepted *up*, *down* and *under*.

Picture 3 (cars): Five words could be considered relevant; he responded 'yes' to *left*, *right* and *before*, but 'no' to *behind* and *after*. Of the 12 inappropriate words, he accepted half (*up*, *down*, *over*, *under*, *above*, *below*). Thus, while his performance on the first two pictures was not bad, on picture 3 it was very poor. We do not understand his acceptance of vertically oriented words for this picture.[2]

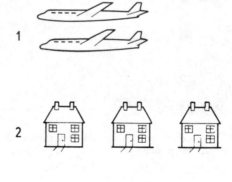

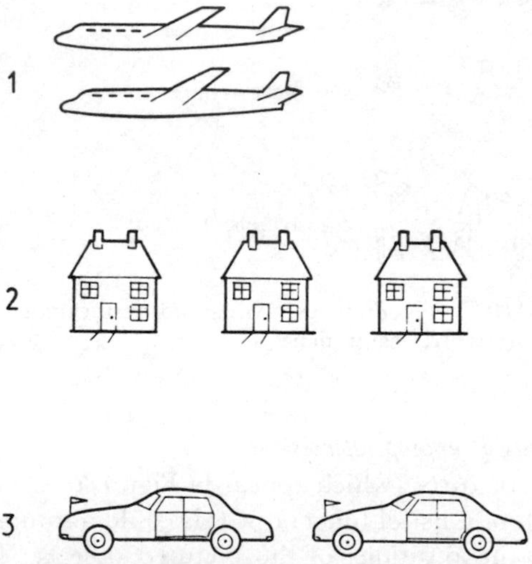

FIGURE 13.2 Pictures for the test of judgements of appropriateness

Comprehension of words in context: prepositions

In a kind of version of the Token Test (De Renzi and Vignolo, 1962), three objects (cup, saucer and pen) were placed on the table, and written instructions of the form *Put the saucer on the cup* were presented to P.W. one at a time. There were 18 such sentences; we wish to discuss a coherent set of 12 which involved six specified relationships (*on, over, under, below, in front of, behind*) and in effect six matched pairs. That is, the set included both *cup on saucer* and *saucer on cup*, both *pen behind cup* and *cup behind pen*. The order of presentation was of course randomised, and the position of the objects was re-set to neutral after each instruction had been carried out.

For these 12 instructions, P.W.'s performance reflected the correct *dimension* of spatial relationship in 11/12 cases; but only once was his response correct. In other words, he consistently reversed the relationship expressed by the sentence. This is scarcely random, and we infer that his performance was rule-governed – but by the wrong rule. It appears that he assigned the spatial semantics of the preposition to the second noun (i.e. the noun in the same constituent). We have no idea whether the rule has any simple motivation or whether it would generalise to other sentence types. To ascertain whether it would even be consistent, we repeated the test on another session. This time all 12 of his responses preserved the correct dimension; four responses were correct and eight had the relationship backwards. If anything, our problem here is to account for the four correct responses! A variety of factors could be influencing his performance, but we might note that he seems unaffected by a pragmatic preference for *cup on saucer*. Thus, for all three of the instructions *put the cup on the saucer, put the saucer under the cup* and *put the saucer below the cup*, he put the saucer on the cup.

Comprehension of words in context: pronouns

1   Action descriptions

The two authors and P.W. sat round a table with a pile of sugar cubes in front of each. The test material consisted of sentences like 'I give one to her' and 'He gives one to you'. Initially we read a set of eight such sentences aloud and asked P.W. to effect the action described by the sentence. He did this correctly for 7/8 sentences.

Then we put a set of eight written sentences in front of him, one at a time, and though we once again read them aloud we instructed him to perform the actions as though he were saying the sentences. Again he was 7/8 correct. His error was on *'they give one to me'*, for which he only transferred a cube from K.P. to P.W.; this is not wrong but is incomplete by our implied rules. Initially we assumed that he understood both the semantics of *give* and the pronoun referents. However, recalling that he had performed consistently but incorrectly as a result of a strategy with the prepositions, we then felt that we had accepted his performance too readily. Clearly, a more adequate test would involve a random choice between *give* and *take* as the verb for each sentence. On a subsequent session, therefore, we gave him 16 sentences, eight with *give* and eight with *take* (e.g. *I take one from her*). This time the sentences were presented visually and were not read aloud. On all except one of the items, he treated the subject nouns as donor; that is, for both *I give one to him* and *I take one from him* he transferred a sugar cube from P.W. to J.M. Thus his performance was incorrect for half of the sentences. But his treatment of the pronouns was consistent and error-free. It looks, then, as though P.W. treats *give to* and *take from* as at least approximately synonymous. Indeed, in their underlying transactional meaning, they do refer to the same concept (see Collins and Quillian, 1972, p. 317 for a discussion of this using *buy* and *sell* as examples). The difference between them could be seen as syntactic rather than semantic, and thus P.W.'s difficulty with these expressions would relate to his general dissociation between syntactic and semantic abilities.

2   Grammaticality judgements

P.W. was asked to judge whether each of 16 sentences was acceptable. The eight grammatical sentences were of the sort *They give it to us* and *I gave it to him*; examples of the ungrammatical sentences are *Me gave it to him* and *He gave it to we*. On separate sessions the test was done with visual and auditory presentation, and the results are shown in Table 13.2. He refused to judge three of the visually presented sentences (response = 'pass'). If we assign these equally to the 'yes' and 'no' categories (one each for grammatical and a half each for ungrammatical stimuli), we can calculate approximate d'

(visual) = 1.53 and d' (auditory) = 1.35. This hardly represents brilliant performance but it is not at chance. He thus seems to have some information about the appropriate case of pronouns though he cannot do case judgements in the triad task. Zurif, Caramazza and Myerson (1972) describe anterior aphasics as having agrammatic intuitions about language. In general, we would accept this as characteristic of P.W.; but his grammaticality judgements are perhaps a bit better than this notion would predict.

TABLE 13.2

	Visual presentation			Auditory presentation	
	'Yes'	*'No'*	*'Pass'*	*'Yes'*	*'No'*
Grammatical	4	2	2	6	2
Ungrammatical		7	1	2	6

Summary

In spite of his very impoverished ability to read function words aloud, P.W. apparently has a great deal of lexical/semantic information about them. We are thus inclined to believe that they are treated no differently from content words by the logogen system or the semantic part of the cognitive system. There is however a severe loss of syntactic ability, and to the extent that a judgement required about an individual function word is biased toward its syntactic function, P.W. will be impaired on that judgement. His ability to compute precisely-correct meanings for sentences is, of course, disrupted by his syntactic impairment. He can generate rules for interpretation, but they do not necessarily correspond to those of the language; and if they do, it could at this stage be attributed to luck rather than residual syntactic ability. There is a hint from the grammaticality judgements that his ability to parse sentences is partly functional (see also Andreewsky and Seron, 1975). But it seems that the parser cannot make information available to other parts of the system, in particular the linguistic processor (see Figure 4.3, p.115). Our results do not 'explain' the deep dyslexic's difficulty with function words, but they go some way toward specifying it.

Notes

1 We are aware of the oddity of performance on these next two classes, and hope that it reflects more than our confusion about what constitutes a 'type of judgement'. We had rather thought that the locational demonstrations would behave like prepositions and adverbs of space, but they seem not to do; perhaps he is treating them more as relative pronouns than demonstratives. This topic needs further work.

2 An interesting phenomenon occurred here and in several other tasks as well, which we should note though we cannot explain it. Words like *up, over* and *before* in contrast to *down, under* and *after* have a property akin to markedness; and whatever this property is, P.W. seems to be sensitive to it. In the appropriateness test, though we did not ask him to specify which object in the picture was described by an acceptable word, he often voluntarily pointed to an object. For his incorrect acceptances on the cars picture, all were in accordance with this 'markedness' concept (at least with our intuitions about it). Thus he pointed to the front car for *up, above* and *over*, and to the car behind for *down, below* and *under*.

References

Andreewsky, E. and Seron, X. (1975) Implicit processing of grammatical rules in a classical case of agrammatism. *Cortex, 11*, 379–90.

Caramazza, A. and Berndt, R. S. (1978) Semantic and syntactic processes in aphasia: a review of the literature. *Psychological Bulletin, 85*, 898–918.

Collins, A. M. and Quillian, M. R. (1972) How to make a language user. In E. Tulving and W. Donaldson (eds), *Organization of Memory*. New York: Academic Press.

De Renzi, E. and Vignolo, L. A. (1962) The token test: a sensitive test to detect receptive disturbances in aphasics. *Brain, 85*, 665–78.

Goodglass, H. and Kaplan, E. (1972) *The Assessment of Aphasia and Related Disorders*. Philadelphia: Lee and Febiger.

Elvin, M. and Hatfield, F. M. (1978) Comprehension by agrammatic patients of prepositions and prepositional phrases. *I.A.L.P. Congress Proceedings*, B. Egg (ed.), vol. 2. Copenhagen: Speciale-Paedagogisk Forlag.

Marin, O. S. M., Saffran, E. M. and Schwartz, M. F. (1976) Dissociations of language in aphasia: implications for normal function. *Annals of the New York Academy of Sciences, 280*, 868–84.

Marshall, J. C. and Newcombe, F. (1973) Patterns of paralexia: a psycholinguistic approach. *Journal of Psycholinguistic Research, 2*, 175–99.

Morton, J. and Patterson, K. E. (1977) The internal and external dictionaries of a deep dyslexic patient. Paper presented to the International Neuropsychology Society, Oxford, July 1977.

Patterson, K. E. (1978) Phonemic dyslexia: errors of meaning and the meaning of errors. *Quarterly Journal of Experimental Psychology, 30,* 587–601.
Patterson, K. E. (1979) What is right with 'deep' dyslexic patients? *Brain and Language, 8,* 111–29.
Patterson, K. E. and Marcel, A. J. (1977) Aphasia, dyslexia and the phonological coding of written words. *Quarterly Journal of Experimental Psychology, 29,* 307–18.
Saffran, E. M. and Marin, O. S. M. (1977) Reading without phonology: evidence from aphasia. *Quarterly Journal of Experimental Psychology, 29,* 515–25.
Shallice, T. and Warrington, E. K. (1975) Word recognition in a phonemic dyslexic patient. *Quarterly Journal of Experimental Psychology, 27,* 187–99.
Zurif, E. B., Caramazza, A. and Myerson, R. (1972) Grammatical judgements of agrammatic aphasics. *Neuropsychologia, 10,* 405–17.

14 Derivational errors

Karalyn Patterson

Two of the cardinal features of deep dyslexic reading are the occurrence of derivational paralexias and the existence of a part-of-speech effect. Although these features do, or at least can, implicate the morphemic structure of the words in question, relatively little is known about the patients' ability to deal with words of varying morphemic structure. This chapter presents data on several tasks in which the derivational or morphemic form of the word stimuli was varied. Typically the manipulations involved regular suffixes such as -ed, -er, -ing. The issues to be addressed and the techniques of addressing them are:

1 Is there any orderly pattern to be discovered in the patients' derivational paralexias? Several analyses of their oral reading of single words with and without suffixes will be presented.

2 How is recognition of letter-strings as words affected by suffixes, and do these data provide any evidence about the morphological nature of the internal lexicon? Several lexical decision tests will be described, which utilised correctly suffixed words (e.g. *helping*), incorrectly suffixed words (e.g. *darking*) and non-words with English suffixes (e.g. *neaking*).

3 Even if the patients cannot read aloud the correct derivational form of a written word, can they recognise it? A three-alternative forced choice test (visually presented target, auditorily presented alternatives) was performed, with systematic variation of parts-of-speech.

4 Given two derivational forms of the same root morpheme, can the patients identify the appropriate one for a particular context? They were asked to select one of two derivational alternatives to fit in a sentence, given both visual and auditory presentation.

The data presented here are from tests on D.E. and P.W., two deep dyslexic patients who have been seen regularly at Addenbrooke's Hospital, Cambridge for the last several years. Fuller descriptions of these patients are available in Patterson (1978, 1979) and Patterson and Marcel (1977).

1 Reading of words with and without affixes

A corpus of single word paralexic errors has been collected for these two patients (and is presented in Appendix 2 of this book) in which derivational paralexias represent a frequent error category for both patients. All responses which might reasonably be considered to bear a derivational relationship to the target word were so classified, despite the fact that the actual basis of many of these errors may be either visual (e.g. *bit* → 'bite') or semantic (*buy* → 'bought'). Simply classifying them as derivational, in other words, involves some assumptions about the way in which such errors arise, assumptions which may be generally unwarranted or at least inappropriate for some instances in the classification.

About two-thirds of the patients' derivational paralexias occurred when the presented word contained a suffix; the responses can be characterised as suffix deletions (e.g. *soloist* → 'solo'), suffix substitutions (e.g. *projection* → 'projector'), or (rarely) some other change(s) (e.g. *parting* → 'apart'). Averaging across the two patients (who are very similar in this regard), the three types of derivational paralexias to suffixed words occurred in the following proportions: deletions .58, substitutions .38, other .04. Although the most common error to a suffixed word is production of the root morpheme on its own, there are two facts which indicate that the patients are generally aware of suffixes. Firstly, the patient's response is more likely to contain a suffix if the presented word does; secondly, even when deleting a suffix the patient occasionally indicates that he knows something else should be there (D.E. *hardest* → 'hardsomething'; P.W. *smartest* → 'smart-uh').

One-third of the patients' derivational paralexias occurred when the presented word was a free morpheme without a suffix; here the responses involve either addition of a suffix (e.g. *contain* → 'container') or a change in form not involving a suffix such as a change in part-of-speech (e.g. *applaud* → 'applause') or in tense (e.g. *buy* →

TABLE 14.1 *A matrix showing, for each of the 7 types of regular suffixes presented (rows), the proportion receiving each of 9 types of reading responses (columns). Only reading responses in which the base morpheme was produced correctly are included.*

Word produced

Word presented	-ing	-er	-ly	-y	-ed	-est	-tion	other	delete	Total N
-ing	.58	.07	–	.02	.04	–	.02	.02	.25	53
-er	.13	.57	.10	–	–	–	–	–	.20	30
-ly	.09	.05	.48	–	–	–	–	–	.38	21
-y	.07	–	–	.80	–	–	–	–	.13	15
-ed	.09	–	–	.05	.05	–	.09	.09	.64	22
-est	–	.45	–	–	–	.09	–	–	.45	11
-tion	–	–	–	–	–	–	.22	.56	.22	9
Total:	40	27	13	14	3	1	5	8	50	161

'bought'). Suffix additions account for .70 of the derivational errors to single-morpheme words, and the remaining .30 were tense or part-of-speech changes. Since the patients so frequently delete suffixes when attempting to read suffixed words, their addition of suffixes to free morphemes, even though less common, is rather surprising. Given what we know about semantic biases against certain word classes in deep dyslexic reading (for example against abstract words and verbs), one might look for such effects in the derivational paralexias. And indeed many of the patients' suffix additions transform a verb or concept into either an object (*calculate* → 'calculator') or a person (*employ* → 'employers'), thus making the word more concrete/imageable. But it is less easy to see why nouns often become adjectives, as observed previously by Marshall and Newcombe (1973) (e.g. *courage* → 'courageous') and why the suffix -ing is often added (*cough* → 'coughing'); and an occasional suffix addition even seems to reduce concreteness (*admiral* → 'admiralty').

For a closer look at performance on reading words with simple suffixes, and including correct reading responses as well as derivational paralexias, Table 14.1 shows a confusion matrix for the seven regular endings which happen to have been presented frequently enough to warrant inclusion. The proportions given are of course proportions of the row totals, but column totals are also included for complete information. Data for the two patients, whose behaviour in this context is essentially identical, have been combined to increase the number of observations. The alternatives for 'word produced' include the seven suffix forms presented, plus 'delete' (which is self-explanatory) and 'other' which means substitution of a suffix other than the seven being analysed. There were very few 'other' responses, and almost all of them represent substitution of -or for -tion (*projection* → 'projector', *edition* → 'editor'). Table 14.1 indicates the following: (a) All seven of these suffixes are often deleted in reading. (b) Certain suffixes (namely, -ing, -er, -ly, and -y) have a fair chance of being produced correctly, whereas others (-ed and -est) essentially never appear correctly; in fact, these latter two suffixes almost never occur at all in the patients' reading. The paradox of the difference between -er and -est is partially reduced by noting that some -er words were nouns (e.g. *starter*) rather than adjectives (e.g. *fairer*). But even restricting the comparison to adjectives, more -er words were read correctly than -est words. (c) Only two suffixes, -ing and -er, occur with any notable frequency as substitutions.

2 Lexical decision on affixed words

According to a hypothesis which can be called morphological decomposition, words are separated into constituent morphemes prior to lexical access, and lexical units or input logogens correspond only to root or base morphemes. (See Morton and Patterson, Chapter 4 this volume, for the general assumptions and terminology employed here regarding word recognition and production.) Thus the input logogen which transduces between stimulus information and the cognitive system would be exactly the same unit for *walk*, *walked* and *walking*. For normal comprehension, information about affixes must reach the cognitive system by a separate (though largely unspecified) process. And the ability to recognise *darker* as a word but *darking* as a non-word indicates that there must be somewhere a list (or a set of rules by which such a list could be generated) of legitimate affixes or derivational forms for each root. There are some unresolved issues in such an account of lexical access, but several studies of normal subjects claim to provide support for the notion of morphological decomposition. Murrell and Morton (1974) found facilitation in tachistoscopic recognition of a word like *seen* from prior exposure to a morphologically related word (*sees*) but not from a different morpheme of equivalent visual similarity (*seed*). Taft and Forster (1975) took prefixed words (e.g. *rejuvenate*) and non-prefixed words (e.g. *repertoire*) and created non-words from them which were either stems alone (*juvenate* and *pertoire*) or prefixed non-words (*dejuvenate* and *depertoire*). In lexical decision tests, subjects were slower and more error-prone in rejecting non-words derived from the prefixed words (*juvenate* and *dejuvenate*) than non-words like *pertoire* and *depertoire*. Both of these sets of results suggest that words are segmented into roots and affixes prior to lexical access.

An alternative to the decomposition hypothesis, called independence by Mackay (1978) or single unit by its proponents Manelis and Tharp (1977), suggests that lexical access involves the whole word as a single unit; thus each separate derivational form of a word has its own input logogen. In a lexical decision experiment, Manelis and Tharp failed to obtain a difference in reaction time between suffixed words like *darker* and non-suffixed words like *sombre*. A second experiment required subjects to decide whether a previously displayed word (e.g. *snow*) was contained in a test item of one of four types (*snowed, slowed, snowen, slowen*). Manelis and Tharp found a reaction time advantage when the test item was a word, and interpret the results of both experiments as supporting the single unit hypothesis.

Despite this fairly extensive summary of the controversy over decomposition, the aim here is not to evaluate the existing evidence but rather to assess whether data from deep dyslexia can contribute any evidence. Oral reading data from such patients does not help: though suffix deletions and substitutions in reading seem compatible with the notion of morphological decomposition, these phenomena cannot be localised to a pre-lexical stage of word recognition, or even to word recognition (as opposed to production) at all. Lexical decision may be a less equivocal source of evidence, though it too has its ambiguities in this regard: the information upon which lexical decisions are based is not clearly (and may clearly not be) restricted to the input logogens.[1] If the semantic system and/or other aspects of the cognitive system are consulted in lexical decision (which there is in fact reason to suppose, cf. James, 1975; Warrington, 1975; Morton, 1979; Patterson, 1979), then some knowledge or at least assumptions about the operation of these other systems will be required to interpret lexical decision data. But let us have some data to interpret.

The lexical decision tests to be reported were largely inspired by Manelis and Tharp's (1977) experiments on processing of suffixed words by normal subjects. For the first test (A) a list of 70 letter-strings was composed utilising 35 base morphemes, each of which occurred once with an appropriate suffix (e.g. *feared, roomy*) and once with an inappropriate suffix (e.g. *fearest, roomly*). Seven different suffixes were used (the same seven as in Table 14.1 except -or in place of -tion), and although there was some variation in the frequency of appearance of the various suffixes, each occurred equally often as appropriate and inappropriate endings. Each patient was asked to go through a randomly ordered list of the 70 letter-strings, responding (aloud) 'yes' if he recognised a letter-string as a real word and 'no' if he did not. Only accuracy, not reaction time, was measured. The results of the test appear in the top two lines of Table 14.2. D.E.'s performance was poor, though well above

TABLE 14.2 *Lexical decision and reading performance in test A*

	D.E.	P.W.
Lexical decision		
hit rate (35 words)	0.63	0.89
false positive rate (35 non-words)	0.26	0.09
Reading/lexical decision		
35 words		
correct readings	4	9
paralexic readings	17	19
semantic	1	1
derivational	14	16
visual	2	1
other	0	1
'yes but'	0	1
misses	14	6
35 non-words		
correct rejections	27	31
correct readings	0	1
paralexic readings	6	3
'yes but'	2	0

chance (d' = .97); P.W.'s performance was good, though not error-free (d' = 2.58). In a sense both patients performed surprisingly well given that all root and bound morphemes used in the test were separately legitimate, with only the pairing to determine the correct response. Lexical decision performance looks particularly good when it is contrasted with the patients' success in reading the words aloud, which is also shown in Table 14.2. The reading test was done by asking the patients to go through the lexical decision list again, saying 'no' to the non-words and attempting to read the words. As well as providing reading data on the words, this procedure (a) provides another estimate of lexical decision performance, and (b) permits (without requesting) reading responses to non-words. In addition to response categories for correct and paralexic readings of the words, there are two other categories. 'Yes but' refers to letter-strings which a patient identified as legitimate words but to which he could produce no reading response; the label comes from the manner in which D.E. indicated this, saying 'Yes but can't say it'. Misses are words which a patient did not recognise and to which he (following instructions) merely said 'no'.

The results of interest from the reading/lexical decision test can be summarised as follows. (a) The patients are very poor at reading affixed words, many (D.E.) or even most (P.W.) of which they recognise as proper words. (b) A great deal of this reading difficulty is specifically attributable to the affixes: for both patients, an unusually high proportion of their paralexic errors were derivational. In other words, they could often produce the correct base morpheme but not the correct suffix. (c) Although the patients could identify most of the non-words as unacceptable, they tried to read a few of these non-words composed of real base and real-but-illegal suffix. Most of these attempts resulted in 'derivational paralexias'. Five of D.E.'s paralexias to non-words involved substitution of an appropriate suffix (e.g. *highing* → 'higher'); the sixth, more intriguingly, involved substitution of the appropriate base (*lengther* → 'longer'). This test also produced what is, to the author's knowledge, a unique event: P.W. gave a reading response which was a non-word and (unbelievably) was correct, though he clearly did not know about the correctness. To the letter-string *darking*, he said 'darking, no, NO!'. (d) A fact which cannot be ascertained from Table 14.2 is that lexical decision performance on the two versions of the test was reasonably consistent. Of the 35 words, for example, D.E. missed 13 in 'straight' lexical decision, 14 in reading/lexical decision, and there were 12 items in common between these two sets. P.W. missed four words in the first test and rejected all four of these (plus two additional ones) in reading/lexical decision.

There are some additional inferences to be drawn from this first lexical decision test, but as they arise from comparison of performance on this and subsequent tests, they will be discussed after presentation of further results. The second lexical decision test (B) was intended to focus specifically on the effect of real suffixes. D.E.'s performance on test A was rather poor and P.W.'s, though much better than D.E.'s, was perhaps not as good as his own lexical decision performance on non-affixed words (Patterson, 1979; Patterson and Marcel, 1977). To what extent might these decrements be attributable to the ubiquitous presence of real suffixes, independent of the nature of the base letter-string? Unlikely as it seems, might a test with words like *hardest* and non-words like *neakest* produce the same results as test A? A new 70-item list was compiled, composed of 35 legitimate suffixed words and 35 suffixed non-word bases. Each of the suffixes used (-ing, -ed, -est, etc.) occurred equally often on word bases and non-word bases. The procedure was identical to test

TABLE 14.3 *Lexical decision and reading performance in text B*

	D.E.	P.W.
Lexical decision		
hit rate (35 words)	0.74	0.94
false positive rate (35 non-words)	0.17	0.02
Reading/lexical decision		
35 words		
correct readings	10	10
paralexic readings	14	21
semantic	0	5
derivational	12	12
visual	2	0
other	0	4
'yes but'	3	1
misses	8	3
35 non-words		
correct rejections	30	32
paralexic readings	3	3
'yes but'	2	0

A, and the results appear in Table 14.3. Performance on test B was excellent for P.W. (d′ = 3.60) and fairly good for D.E. (d′ = 1.59). Since this represents an improvement over test A levels of discrimination for both patients, the question is at least partially answered: poor performance on test A was not *solely* attributable to the fact that every letter-string had a suffix. But given D.E.'s only moderate performance on test B, the possibility remains that (for him at least) word/non-word discriminability is reduced by the presence of suffixes. Thus one further test (C) was devised, related to tests A and B both in a general and in a specific way.

Generally, the intention of test C was to assess lexical decision and reading performance on word and non-word bases (without suffixes) of the kind used in test B in suffixed form. More specifically, the list of letter-strings in test C included every *base non-word* for which a patient had given a false positive response to the suffixed form in test B. There were only six of these, five arising from D.E.'s performance and one from P.W.'s. A few examples: D.E. had incorrectly accepted the letter strings *firching*, *drowed* and *loundest* as words in test B; test C included the letter-strings *firch*, *drow* and *lound*. Further, every *base word* for which a patient had missed the suffixed form of the word in test A or B was also present in test C. There were 28 of these, 22 from D.E.'s results and six from P.W.'s. For example, D.E. had failed to identify *feared*, *ageing* and *kingly* as legitimate words in test A; so test C incorporated the words *fear*, *age* and *king*. So that the test would not consist primarily of these special cases, additional items were added to a total of 48 words and 48 non-words. The procedure was identical to tests A and B and the results are shown in Table 14.4.

In terms of general level, both patients showed excellent lexical decision performance on test C; this will be discussed further in a moment. As regards the specific comparisons built into this test, for the non-word comparison, P.W. (with only one false positive from test B) provides no relevant information. D.E. correctly rejected the base non-words for five of his six false positives to suffixed non-words in test B: only *lound* was incorrectly accepted. Thus it appears that D.E. is slightly more likely to accept non-words like *firching* than non-words like *firch*. For the word comparison. P.W. correctly recognised the base words for all six of the suffixed words he had missed in tests A and B, and D.E. correctly accepted 19 base words of the 22 words missed in suffixed form. In other words, both patients will

TABLE 14.4 *Lexical decision and reading performance in test C*

	D.E.	P.W.
Lexical decision		
hit rate (48 words)	0.94	0.98
false positive rate (48 non-words)	0.04	0.04
Reading/lexical decision		
48 words		
correct readings	36	34
paralexic readings	7	14
semantic	2	7
derivational	4	5
visual	1	1
other	0	1
'yes but'	2	0
misses	3	0
48 non-words		
correct rejections	45	44
paralexic readings	1	0
'yes but'	2	4

sometimes know that a base morpheme like *fear* is a legitimate word but fail to recognise it as legitimate in an affixed form like *feared*. It should be noted that these conclusions do involve an assumption of reliable performance by the patients. The comparison of D.E.'s response to *firch* today with his response to *firching* three weeks earlier assumes that *firching* would provoke the same response today as it did on the previous occasion. The assumption appears to be a reasonable one on the basis of reliability checks on other lexical decision lists.

To facilitate general discussion of the three lexical decision tests, the most important results are summarised in Table 14.5 (in the form of proportions, since list length was longer in test C than in the other two). Two aspects of the reading data are included in Table 14.5. (1) Proportion correct suggests that suffixes cause enormous reading difficulty for deep dyslexic patients. Given nouns, verbs and adjectives as free morphemes as in test C (e.g. *craft, turn, soft*), the patients read about three-quarters of them correctly. Given the same base morphemes but in suffixed form as in tests A and B (*crafty, turned, softly*), they manage less than one-third correct readings of the

TABLE 14.5 *Comparison of reading performance and word/non-word discriminability in tests, A, B and C*

	D.E.	P.W.
Reading words:		
proportion correct		
Test A	0.11	0.26
B	0.29	0.29
C	0.75	0.71
Derivational paralexias:		
proportion of total		
reading performance		
Test A	0.40	0.46
B	0.34	0.34
C	0.08	0.10
Lexical decision: d'		
Test A	0.97	2.58
B	1.59	3.60
C	3.30	3.80

words.[2] Furthermore, not only do suffixes dramatically reduce the probability that the patient will produce the exact target word presented to him; they even reduce the probability that the patient will produce the correct base morpheme. If reading performance is scored only for presence of appropriate root morpheme (that is, correct readings and derivational paralexias combined), in test C the result is .83 and .81 for D.E. and P.W. respectively; the corresponding figures for tests A and B (taken together) are .57 and .68 for the two patients. (2) The proportion of total reading performance represented by derivational paralexias indicates that suffixes cause a major shift in the pattern of reading. Given free morphemes, of the order of 10 per cent of words will result in derivational paralexias. Given suffixed words, between a third and a half of all words elicit a response of the correct base morpheme but in the wrong derivational form. Another demonstration of the effect of suffixes on the pattern of reading performance results from a comparison of suffixed words with another class of words which are difficult for deep dyslexics, namely abstract words. The proportion of words read correctly from these two classes is roughly equal (see Patterson, 1979 for data on reading of abstract words by these two patients); but the error patterns are dramatically different. Most failures to read abstract words correctly are omissions, with the occasional semantic, derivational or visual paralexia. Most failures to read suffixed words (provided of course that the words are not too abstract!) are derivational paralexias, with the occasional omission, semantic or visual paralexia.

Turning now to lexical decision on suffixed words: the use of d' gives a measure of discriminability between words and non-words, and indicates that discriminability is influenced both by the nature of the base letter-string and by the presence of suffixes. The effect of base strings is shown by the fact that both patients obtained a higher d' in test B (where all items contained suffixes but the non-words had non-word bases, e.g. *hortly*) than in test A (where all items contained suffixes and the non-words had word bases, e.g. *actly*). The effect of suffixes is revealed by the fact that D.E. obtained a higher d' in test C (items without suffixes) than in test B (items with suffixes). (This is possibly true for P.W. as well, but would be difficult to demonstrate since his performance in test B is approaching a ceiling.) As the measure is d', one can conclude that suffixes are affecting discriminability; but just to make it doubly clear that it is not an effect on criterion, it is perhaps worth a reminder that suffixes have opposite effects on words and non-words for D.E. He is more likely to accept a non-word base if it has a suffix but less likely to accept a word base if it has a suffix.

One of the primary purposes of these lexical decision tests on suffixed words concerned their potential implications for the issue of pre-lexical morphological decomposition. Suppose (a) that decomposition (at least for words with regular affixes) does occur prior to lexical access; (b) that lexical decision involves deciding firstly whether the base letter-string is a legitimate morpheme and if so whether it can legitimately take that bound morpheme; (c) that knowledge about legitimate derivational forms is dependent upon a linguistic component of the cognitive system which is to some degree impaired in deep dyslexia. What effects should these suppositions produce in lexical decision? One strong prediction would be a high false positive rate in test A where the non-words were inappropriately suffixed root morphemes like *thicking*. D. E.'s false positive rate in test A was high (.26), higher in fact than his rate of false positives in any of the half-dozen other lexical decision tests he has done. P.W.'s false positive rate in test A was not higher than he has shown in some other tests, but this may merely reflect that his cognitive linguistic system is less impaired than D.E.'s. The difference from test A to B is not large, but both patients did show a higher false positive rate on non-words like *thicking* than on non-words like *neaking* (D.E. 0.26 vs. 0.17, P.W. 0.09 vs. 0.02). Since neither *thicking* nor *neaking* should have an input logogen, it is hard to see how the single unit hypothesis would account for this difference.

A second prediction from this scenario of suppositions is the following: given a word morpheme in both free and suffixed form (e.g. *quick* and *quickly*), a patient might identify both as words, or fail to recognise both, or identify *quick* as a word and miss *quickly* (because his linguistic system could not acknowledge -ly as a legitimate bound morpheme for *quick*) but should never reject *quick* and accept *quickly*. This is in fact a reasonable description of the data. The first two alternatives do obviously occur and are essentially uninteresting; for the latter two (pooled across patients) there were 25 instances of accept-free, reject-suffixed and one instance of reject-free, accept-suffixed. It is not altogether clear what prediction would be generated by an independence hypothesis. If (by this hypothesis) recognition is assumed to be based on the response of a unique input logogen for the whole word, then the hypothesis either (a) should predict more occurrences of reject-free, accept-suffixed than were obtained, or (b) should provide some account of why input logogens for suffixed words are more compromised than those for root words.

Thus far, two predictions from the decomposition hypothesis (or at least a particular version of it) seem reasonably compatible with the data. A third prediction does not fare quite so well, though it may be a stage following decomposition in this account which is in question. If the procedure following segmentation is analysis of the root letter string by the input logogen system, and if failure to obtain a response from a logogen should terminate the procedure and result in a 'no' decision, then suffixes on non-word bases should have no effect. Thus a false positive response should be no more likely to *neaking* than to *neak*. P.W. behaves in accordance with this prediction (0.02 and 0.04 as false positive rates respectively to these two types of non-words); but D.E. is influenced by suffixes on non-words (0.17 and 0.04). Thus it seems that he considers the suffix even if he does not recognise the root; and although this consideration appears to be done separately from analysis of the base, it is not independent of the result of analysing the base. Suffixes on recognised bases make it harder for him to accept the whole letter-string as a word because (by the current description) his linguistic system cannot reliably confirm that -ing (for example) is legitimate on the base *leak*. But suffixes on unrecognised bases make it harder for him to reject the whole letter-string because of his awareness that -ing often accompanies real words, and so *neaking* receives more false positives than *neak*. There seems no way to account for this finding at the logogen level, and thus it does not really address the question of whether input logogens correspond to words or morphemes. Nonetheless, the fact that D.E.'s performance is influenced both by the nature of the base letter-string and by the presence/absence of suffixes does suggest that at some level there is a '. . . functional separation between processing these syntactically important elements and processing lexical root or single-morpheme content words' (Allport, 1977, p. 528).

Very briefly, one additional result relevant to affixed words will be described. The test was lexical decision again, and was a partial replication of Taft and Forster's (1975) Experiment 1 comparing non-words which are the bases of real prefixed words (e.g. *juvenate* from *rejuvenate*) with non-words which do not come from prefixed words (e.g. *pertoire* from *repertoire*). The 40 non-words were taken directly from Taft and Forster (since these letter-strings appear in an appendix to their article); 40 words were assembled of length roughly comparable to the non-words and of frequency roughly comparable to the words from which the non-words derive. This was not a full replication of Taft and Forster's experiment, as only the patients' accuracy and not RT was measured. However, Taft and Forster obtained a difference on both measures between real stems and pseudo-stems (as they call items like *juvenate* and *pertoire*, respectively): their normal subjects produced mean false positive rates of 0.17 and 0.04 to real and pseudo-stems. The comparable figures for D.E. were 0.10 and .05, and for P.W., 0.25 and 0.05. Thus both patients show at least the same direction of difference as normal subjects. To the extent that Taft and Forster's result supports the notion of pre-lexical analysis into constituent morphemes, the patients' performance is in line with this notion.

3 Recognition of derivational forms

Patterson (1978) presents data on a three-alternative forced choice test of visual-auditory word matching. The patients looked at a single printed word and listened to three spoken alternatives: (1) the same word as the visually presented one; (2) the patient's own paralexic reading response to the printed word on a previous occasion; (3) another word related to the printed word in one of the three main ways that paralexias tend to relate to target words, i.e. derivational, visual, or semantic. Though certainly better than chance, the patients were quite poor at choosing the correct match when the paralexic alternative was derivationally related, 0.63 correct for D.E. and 0.50 for P.W. It is not easy, however, to do more detailed analyses of those data in terms of systematic variables like parts-of-speech, since the patients' own responses provided most of the derivational alternatives. Knowing, for example, that there is a strong part-of-speech effect in reading by deep dyslexic patients (Marshall and Newcombe, 1973; Andreewsky and Seron, 1975; Shallice and Warrington, 1975), one might ask whether the same phenomenon would apply to word recognition. As an initial test, 24 word triads were composed, each triad consisting of the noun, adjective and adverb form of a base morpheme. Some examples are *cruelty, cruel, cruelly; hunger, hungry, hungrily*. In the test, the patient looked at one word of the triad printed on a card, listened to the experimenter read the three alternatives, and selected the spoken alternative which he believed to match the printed word. The target

TABLE 14.6 *Three-alternative forced-choice recognition of derivational forms*

	D.E.	P.W.
Number of correct choices overall (out of 24)	13(0.54)	13(0.54)
correct choices of nouns (out of 8)	4	3
adjectives (8)	3	4
adverbs (8)	6	6
total choices of nouns (out of 24)	8	7
adjectives (24)	6	10
adverbs (24)	10	7

word was the noun, adjective and adverb on one-third of the trials each, and also occurred first, second and third among the alternatives on one-third of the trials each. Performance is shown in Table 14.6, at a level better than chance but not impressively so. The results are somewhat disappointing in terms of demonstrating any consistent effects of part-of-speech, either on correct choices or total choices.

This was only a preliminary test, and it is perhaps not surprising that it did not produce major effects. It might have been wiser to vary suffixes systematically rather than parts-of-speech: the adverbs all ended in -ly, but there was a variety of ending types for both the nouns (e.g. *distance, strength, misery, danger*) and the adjectives (*distant, strong, miserable, dangerous*). The test does demonstrate, however (if such demonstration were needed), that the patients' difficulty in reading the correct derivational form is not only or even primarily one of output. One might have hypothesised that the patients 'know' which derivational form of a word they are looking at, and that derivational paralexias arise at the stage of output. It would then seem likely that they should be able to match the written word to the correct (spoken) derivational alternative, which this little experiment shows they do very poorly.

4 Judgements of appropriate derivational form

The tests presented thus far pertain to the patients' ability (a) to assess what constitutes a legitimate (real-word) derivational form, (b) to assess which derivational form is in front of them, and (c) to read aloud the correct derivational form. All of these tests have dealt with words in isolation, and none of the tests has provided much scope for word meaning to play a role. A final experiment in this series, therefore, concerned the ability to use derivational forms in meaningful context. The task was to select one of two derivationally related alternatives to fit in a sentence, and the alternatives were drawn from the patients' own paralexic errors. For derivational paralexias like *rule* → 'ruler' and *directing* → 'directions', sentences were constructed where the correct choice was the original word that had been presented for reading and the incorrect alternative was the patient's original derivational paralexia. The sentences for the paralexias given above, for example, were:

Prince Charles will one day (ruler/rule) the country.
The policeman was (directing/directions) traffic.

Adequate performance in this task presumably requires some comprehension of the sentence; it also requires either (a) an understanding of the difference in meaning between the two derivational forms or (b) an understanding of the difference in grammatical class between the two plus sufficient syntactic knowledge to appreciate which part of speech the sentence needs. It is, in other words, a complex task; and on the basis of previous results from these and other agrammatic patients, one would predict impaired performance (e.g. Caramazza and Berndt, 1978; Patterson 1979; Schwartz, Saffran and Marin, 1978).

The test, which involved 52 sentences, was performed initially with visual presentation; the patients were asked to read each sentence silently and to cross out the wrong word so that the sentence would read correctly. The correct alternative, of course, came first in a random half of the sentences and second in the remaining half. For comparison purposes, the test was performed again about a month later with auditory presentation. In this case, the entire sentence was read twice: 'The policeman was directing traffic', 'The policeman was directions traffic'. Every effort was made to read the two alternatives neutrally, to avoid providing intonation clues as to the correct version.

TABLE 14.7 *Selection of correct derivational form to fit sentence (chance = 0.5)*

	D.E.	P.W.
Proportion correct (out of 52)		
with visual presentation	0.43	0.69
with auditory presentation	0.92	0.94

Performance is presented in Table 14.7, which shows a large discrepancy between the two modalities of presentation. Both patients found the task very difficult when dealing with written sentences; in fact, while P.W. was better than chance at selecting the correct derivational form with visual presentation, D.E.'s performance was at or even slightly below the level of chance. (This is a task where below-chance performance could be meaningful, since the incorrect alternatives were the patients' own derivational paralexias which they might prefer.) With auditory presentation, on the other hand, the patients found it easy to select the correct derivational form in the majority of sentences. D.E. made four errors and P.W. three, in a task on which a person with unimpaired language skills would assuredly perform perfectly. But this level of performance with auditory presentation is surprisingly good for patients who are demonstrably agrammatic in all aspects of language usage. It is not altogether clear how to interpret the auditory superiority in these results. The extent to which deep dyslexic patients generally show better performance with auditory than with visual presentation depends both on the particular patient and the particular task (see Shallice and Warrington, Chapter 5 this volume). In a test of sentence comprehension and semantic memory (the Silly Sentences Test, Baddeley, 1979), D.E. and P.W. are mildly impaired relative to normal subjects (Patterson, 1979); but their performance is similar with visual and auditory presentation. This suggests that the difference obtained in the present task does not reflect an auditory superiority in general sentence comprehension. Also, P.W. shows no auditory superiority in judging grammaticality of sentences like 'He gave it to her' as compared with 'Him gave it to her' (Morton and Patterson, Chapter 13 this volume). Concerning grammatical 'intuitions', therefore, he does not appear to be more skilled at knowing when something sounds right than when it looks right. Given the complexity of the present task it is still difficult to identify the basis for the modality difference. But since so much evidence points to the predominance of semantic over syntactic determinants of performance by patients like these, it will be speculated that auditory input provides the patients with better access to the meaning of words like 'rule' and 'ruler' and thus the difference between them. For syntactically complex sentences, presumably, they would fail on this task in either modality, because the syntactic skills underlying sentence comprehension are (equally?) impaired in both modalities. But for the rather straightforward syntax used here, the patients may understand the sentences well enough to know what meaning will fit; and the meaning of the derivational alternatives may be more available from spoken than from written input.

Summary

Four topics have been addressed in this chapter; by way of summary, here is a brief reminder of those topics, with a note as to what the relevant experiments showed or at least why they were deemed interesting.

1 The first section was primarily to provide a fuller description of derivational paralexias. What sorts of words produce them? (answer: largely words with suffixes); what is the relative frequency of different types of error? (answer: suffix deletions are most common, followed by suffix substitutions); do various suffixes have differential probabilities of being produced? (answer: yes).

2 The bulk of the chapter is taken up with a set of lexical decision experiments on words and non-words with and without suffixes. The experiments do not – and perhaps in principle could not – provide any conclusive evidence on the question of whether root and bound morphemes are segmented prior to word recognition. But the data are compatible with this assumption, or at least with the weaker claim that root and bound morphemes are handled separately 'at some level'. Perhaps in its weaker form the notion seems obvious simply from the observation that deep dyslexic patients make derivational paralexias. On the other hand, since such paralexias resemble their target words both visually and semantically, it has not necessarily been clear that derivational paralexias represent a distinctive class of error. To the extent that root and bound morphemes can be shown to receive separable processing, there is some independent justification for maintaining the derivational classification of paralexias.

3 Section 3 is a brief demonstration of severely impaired performance by the patients in auditory-visual word matching when the alternatives are different derivational forms of the same morpheme. There was no strong indication of a part-of-speech effect in this task.

4 Finally, a task of selecting the correct derivational form in a sentential context provided a large modality effect: the patients showed nearly perfect performance with auditory input but a large deficit with visual input. (In fact, D.E. could not do the task with visual input, scoring at chance.) This result raises some interesting questions regarding both semantic and syntactic skills in the two modalities for agrammatic, deep dyslexic patients.

Notes

1 Indeed, if one takes the position that input logogens correspond to root morphemes, then lexical decision could not be based solely on the logogen system or there would be no way to identify *darking* as a non-word.

2 There is, needless to say, a shift in the distribution of parts-of-speech when moving from base to suffixed forms. In the sets of words used here (which like any words, unless deliberately chosen to be unambiguous with respect to part-of-speech, are difficult to classify: is *landing* a noun or a verb? is *rented* a verb or an adjective?), assuming that a deep dyslexic patient will treat a word as a noun if it is at all possible to do so, slightly more than half of the free morphemes (test C) were nouns while only a quarter of the suffixed words (tests A and B) were nouns.

References

Allport, D. A. (1977) On knowing the meaning of words we are unable to report: the effects of visual masking. In S. Dornic (ed.), *Attention and Performance*, VI. London: Academic Press.

Andreewsky, E. and Seron, X. (1975) Implicit processing of grammatical rules in a classical case of agrammatism. *Cortex, 11*, 379–90.

Baddeley, A. D. (1979) Working memory and reading. In P. A. Kolers, M. E. Wrolstad and H. Bouma (eds), *Processing of Visible Language*. New York: Plenum.

Caramazza, A. and Berndt, R. S. (1978) Semantic and syntactic processes in aphasia: a review of the literature. *Psychological Bulletin, 85*, 898–918.

James, C. T. (1975) The role of semantic information in lexical decisions. *Journal of Experimental Psychology: Human Perception and Performance, 104*, 130–6.

Mackay, D. G. (1978) Derivational rules and the internal lexicon. *Journal of Verbal Learning and Verbal Behavior, 17*, 61–71.

Manelis, L. and Tharp, D. A. (1977) The processing of affixed words. *Memory and Cognition, 5*, 690–5.

Marshall, J. C. and Newcombe, F. (1973) Patterns of paralexia: a psycholinguistic approach. *Journal of Psycholinguistic Research, 2*, 175–99.

Morton, J. (1979) Word recognition. In J. Morton and J. C. Marshall (eds), *Psycholinguistics Series*, vol. 2: *Structures and Processes*. London: Paul Elek.

Murrell, G. A. and Morton, J. (1974) Word recognition and morphemic structure. *Journal of Experimental Psychology, 102*, 963–8.

Patterson, K. E. (1978) Phonemic dyslexia: errors of meaning and the meaning of errors. *Quarterly Journal of Experimental Psychology, 30*, 587–607.

Patterson, K. E. (1979) What is right with 'deep' dyslexic patients? *Brain and Language, 8*, 111–29.

Patterson, K. E. and Marcel, A. J. (1977) Aphasia, dyslexia and the phonological coding of written words. *Quarterly Journal of Experimental Psychology, 29*, 307–18.

Schwartz, M. F., Saffran, E. M. and Marin, O. S. M. (1978) The nature of the comprehension deficit in agrammatic aphasics. Paper presented to the International Neuropsychological Society, February 1978.

Shallice, T. and Warrington, E. K. (1975) Word recognition in a phonemic dyslexic patient. *Quarterly Journal of Experimental Psychology, 27*, 187–99.

Taft, M. and Forster, K. I. (1975) Lexical storage and retrieval of prefixed words. *Journal of Verbal Learning and Verbal Behavior, 14*, 638–47.

Warrington, E. K. (1975) The selective impairment of semantic memory. *Quarterly Journal of Experimental Psychology, 27*, 635–57.

15 Analogies between speed-reading and deep dyslexia: towards a procedural understanding of reading*

E. Andreewsky, G. Deloche and P. Kossanyi

The title of this chapter is, we hope, puzzling; and a puzzle is also an appropriate term for describing our approach, since we are trying to build up a model of the normal human reading system from *pieces* of evidence provided by any means – from any kind of reading behaviour.

Our first claim is that linguistic behaviour can be analysed in terms of underlying procedures for the processing of language. Aphasia being due to some damage of the physical structures supporting language-processing procedures, one may view aphasic behaviour as reflecting the activity of those procedures which have remained intact. Likewise, any *alexic* behaviour reflects some subset of the normal reading procedures. Thus any aphasic or alexic behaviour may provide us with insight into the properties of these underlying procedures.

For example, the deep dyslexic cannot read non-words aloud: that is, he cannot carry out grapheme-to-phoneme conversion using grapheme-phoneme conversion (GPC) rules. Nevertheless, he can read aloud some words, especially content words; when he attempts this task, he often makes semantic errors. The occurrence of semantic errors provides evidence for a component of normal reading mechanisms which may be formalized thus:

$$(1) \quad G \rightarrow S$$
$$S \rightarrow P$$

* This work has benefited from the helpful comments of Mrs M. Desi, M.D. and Mrs G. Chassin, L.C.S.T.
The authors also gratefully acknowledge the kind help of Professor Max Coltheart in pointing out and commenting on several inaccuracies in an earlier version of this paper.

where G is the written form of a word, S is its 'stored meaning' (if any) and P is its uttered form. Thus deep dyslexia suggests the existence of a specific reading process in which utterances are only determined by stored meanings of words, and not by GPC rules: a written form (G) of a word gives rise to an utterance (P) *via* the stored meaning (S).[1]

This specific process is embedded in the normal reading system: it may be isolated not only by pathology, but also by constraining the reading conditions of normal subjects. For example, Allport (1977) reported that when words are presented tachistoscopically and followed by a pattern mask, normal subjects attempting to read these words make semantic errors. Ellis and Marshall (1978) have raised some objections to this conclusion of Allport's. However, other work described by Allport (1977) does suggest that there are conditions under which normal subjects can gain access to some aspects of the meanings of written words without being able to identify the words. A similar conclusion was reached by Andreewsky, Kossanyi and Deloche (1978). They used French non-homophonic homographs such as *fils*: this may mean 'threads' (in which case it is pronounced /fil/) or 'sons' (in which case it is pronounced /fis/). The homograph was presented together with a disambiguating word which was semantically related to one or other of the two meanings of the homograph. Even when the disambiguating word was presented so briefly that it could not be reported, the pronunciation chosen for the homograph indicated that some meaning of the disambiguating word had been accessed. This indicates that semantic features of a word can be accessed before (and, in this case, without) word identification.

These days, two very different systems are being confronted with the task of natural-language processing: the human brain and the computer. Our second claim is that any system dealing with natural-language processing must share certain common properties with any other system capable of this task. There are procedures *inherent* in natural-language processing, and any system capable of such processing requires these procedures. For example, there are linguistic problems inherent in the task of producing P (phonemic output) from G (graphemic input), and any system, be it brain or computer, which seeks to derive P from G must solve these problems.

Consider the following French sentences:[2]

Les poules du <u>couvent</u> <u>couvent</u>. (/le pul dy <u>kuvã</u> <u>kuv</u>/)
(The <u>convent</u> hens are <u>brooding</u>.)
Les <u>portions</u> que nous <u>portions</u>. (/le <u>pɔRsjɔ̃</u> kə nu <u>pɔRtjɔ̃</u>/)
(The <u>portions</u> we were <u>carrying</u>.)
Il <u>est</u> parti vers l'<u>est</u>. (/il <u>e</u> paRti vɛR <u>lɛst</u>/)
(He <u>has</u> gone <u>East</u>.)

The underlined words are uttered in different ways depending upon whether they are nouns or verbs. Thus an 'intelligent' G → P converter *must* perform at least some syntactic analysis prior to utterance. Simply using GPC rules and bypassing syntactic analysis will lead to errors in utterance; this is a requirement whether the task is being performed by a brain or by a computer.

1 General knowledge retrieval

However, the syntactic analysis just mentioned, whilst *necessary* for accurate G → P conversion, is not *sufficient*. This is shown by consideration of the following two French sentences:[3]

Les <u>fils</u> du chirurgien sont en nylon.
(The surgeon's threads are made of nylon.)
Les <u>fils</u> du chirurgien sont en pension.
(The surgeon's sons are in a boarding school.)

Here the underlined word *fils* is a plural noun in both sentences; yet, despite this syntactic equivalence, the word is pronounced /fil/ in the first sentence and /fis/ in the second. In order to produce a correct pronunciation in both cases, a G → P conversion mechanism must have access to general knowledge (in this case knowledge about users of nylon and of boarding school) and must be able to use this knowledge, starting from the written sentence, to retrieve appropriate phonologic information. There must, therefore, be a general-knowledge retrieval process involved in sentence reading; its existence has been deduced from an analysis of the utterance of sentences containing non-homophonic polysemous words. This retrieval process is an essential aspect of the understanding of sentences; it is also an important component of our puzzle.

1.1 An artificial-intelligence (AI) approach

A well-known system for knowledge retrieval is *automatic information retrieval*, a data-based system providing answers to documentation requests. The answers are the papers (or, more often, the paper titles) fitting the documentation request. One example of such a system is MEDLARS. The way in which such automatic information retrieval systems work may provide some insights into the kinds of processing used in general to retrieve knowledge.

The 'knowledge' of an automatic information retrieval system is the stored documents. Attached to each document is a highly specific label: this label consists of *key-words* which are always content words and mostly nouns; they represent the contents of the document. Each documentary request is also assigned this kind of label, representing the key-words in the request. The retrieval process is then a more or less sophisticated procedure, able to match the request label to the stored data-base labels, so as to retrieve those documents best fitting the request.

1.2 Psychological requirements for general knowledge

It was argued earlier that a prerequisite for understanding most sentences is access to stored general knowledge. The examples using polysemous words illustrate this; so does a comparison of the two sentences:

Pierre studies English.
Chomsky studies English.

What we know about Chomsky leads us to understand the word 'studies' differently in these two sentences.

1.3 Retrieval of stored general knowledge

One way in which to generalize relations (1) and (2) from single-word reading to sentence reading, at least in a preliminary way, is to use the notion of 'frame' (Minksy, 1975) in characterizing the retrieval of stored information. This term is defined as follows (Minksy, 1975):

> A frame is a data-structure for representing a stereotyped situation like being in a certain kind of living room or going to a child's birthday party. Attached to each frame are several kinds of information. Some of this information is about how to use the frame. Some is about what one can expect to happen next. Some is about what to do if these expectations are not confirmed . . . Thus, a frame may contain a great many details whose supposition is not specifically warranted by the situation. These have many uses in representing general information, most likely cases, techniques for by-passing 'logic', and ways to make useful generalizations.

Suppose that, to deal with a given sentence G, it is necessary to retrieve the appropriate frame f from stored general knowledge. How might this be done? One could consider the written sentence as an implicit documentation request, as in automatic information retrieval. This request is dealt with by identifying the request keywords $(n_1, n_2, \ldots)$ which then act as the data for the retrieval procedures. It will sometimes be the case that a syntactic disambiguation will be needed when the content words $n_1, n_2, \ldots$ are being identified, so as, for example, in the following sentences:

- G_1 = He *can* leave a *will*.
- G_2 = He *will* leave a *can*.

Understanding a written sentence may thus be formalized as follows:

(3) $G \rightarrow n_1, n_2, \ldots$ (including syntactic disambiguation)
  $n_1, n_2, \ldots \rightarrow f$
  $(G, f) \rightarrow S$

where G is a written sentence, $n_1, n_2 \ldots$ its content words, f is a frame (see definition above), and $(G, f) \rightarrow S$ is the processing of the sentence meaning making joint use of the input string G and the related frame from stored knowledge, f. Thus the *sentence meaning* S is the *product* of these *two components*, by the application of the procedure: ' $\rightarrow$ '.

We will now try to give examples of the reading behaviour of a patient with acquired dyslexia (in this case, deep dyslexia) which may be understood in terms of the implication of general knowledge retrieval processes in sentence reading.

2 Deep dyslexia and general knowledge retrieval

The main characteristics of deep dyslexia are described elsewhere in this volume (Chapter 2, for example) and need only be summarized here. Patients with deep dyslexia utter written content words via their meaning, which is why semantic errors occur and why non-words cannot be read aloud. Content words are much easier to read aloud than function words (or inflections). Disambiguation of syntactic ambiguity occurs and may be evident in the resulting utterance. For example, Andreewsky and Seron (1975) showed that in the sentence:

Le *car* ralentit *car* le moteur chauffe

the first *car* (a noun) was read aloud whilst the second (a conjunction) was not, when a deep dyslexic was trying to read the whole sentence aloud.

Written sentences requiring an appreciation of syntax for their comprehension (such as 'The circle is on [behind, above . . .] the square', or 'The Ford outran the Austin') are generally not understood.

When a deep dyslexic patient was asked to read aloud the sentence

Tu as été en vacances cet hiver.
(You have been on holiday this winter.)

his utterance was:

'Il est question de vacances et d'hiver.'
(It is a matter of holidays and winter.)

There are two important aspects of this example. Firstly, the only words of the written sentence which are reproduced in the spoken utterance are the two content words *vacances* and *hiver*, which reflects the activity: $G \rightarrow n_1, n_2 \ldots$ Secondly, the word *été* means both 'been' (function word) and 'summer' (content word). Its failure to appear in the output reflects the syntactic disambiguation which is integral to the process $G \rightarrow n_1, n_2, \ldots$ Furthermore, this syntactic disambiguation must have occurred *before* the identification of items as content words; otherwise *été* would have been understood as 'summer'.

When asked to read the sentence again, the patient said:

'Je prends mes vacances en hiver.'
(I take my holidays in winter.)

The concept of frame allows one to draw an analogy between single word reading and sentence reading in deep dyslexia. With single word reading, the graphic input is not analysed into its components (letters or phonemes) for these to be mapped onto the output; instead, the graphic input as a whole points to the meaning of the word, and it is by using this meaning that the phonology of the word is provided; hence semantic errors. With sentence reading, the sentence is not analysed into its components (words) for these to be mapped onto the output; instead, from the sentence as a whole, using the content words as key words, some related information (a frame) is retrieved (and/or computed). From this frame, a phonological representation of some sentence is computed. Thus in the last example given above, the patient uses the key words *vacances* and *hiver* to select from his stored general knowledge the fact that holidays may be taken in winter, and says this.

Hence in deep dyslexia, (3) becomes (4):

$$(4) \quad G \rightarrow n_1, n_2 \ldots \text{ (including syntactic disambiguation)}$$
$$n_1, n_2, \ldots \rightarrow f$$
$$f \rightarrow S$$

Here S is derived not jointly from G and f as in (3) but solely from f. This is why content words are so dominant in the reading of the deep dyslexic, and why sentences which cannot be understood by recourse to stored general knowledge (e.g. 'The square is above the circle') pose such problems. If sentence understanding is restricted to frame retrieval through content words, function words are irrelevant; hence the deep dyslexic deals poorly with function words. In short, as formalized by relations (4), the understanding of a written sentence by a deep dyslexic is provided by a subset of the normal relations (3). A point worth emphasizing is that even this subset of the normal procedures includes some syntactic processing, namely, syntactic disambiguation during the identification of content words: and this form of syntactic processing is preserved in deep dyslexia, despite difficulties with other aspects of syntax (e.g. in pronouncing function words, or in understanding sentences on the basis of their syntactic structure).

3 Speed-reading and general knowledge retrieval

There are more newspaper announcements dealing with speed-reading than there are scientific research papers on the subject. Speed-reading seems so far to be generally understood in terms of eye-movement strategies; this has discouraged psycholinguistic approaches to the understanding of speed-reading. There are, nevertheless, psycholinguistic results handling relationships between these eye movements and cognitive mechanisms. According to Kouznetsov *et al.* (1976) these movements are accelerated via a feedback mechanism absent in 'normal' reading; this mechanism is driven by a cognitive procedure: the search for relevant information. The Morton (1964) hypothesis that the increase in reading speed is achieved by increased use of contextual cues, at both grammatical and semantic levels, is also supported by Marcel's results (1974). Reading rate will obviously increase if the reader reduces the number of his fixations and regressions. Since the number of fixations and regressions increases with the difficulty of the material, one determinant of reading rate must be difficulty. A direct way to assess the efficiency of reading is to correlate reading rate with the degree to which written material has been comprehended. However, since we do not know at present how to measure the 'degree of comprehension', this way of studying the efficiency of reading is not at present practicable.

The feature of speed-reading which is of importance here is that it is often considered as involving an apprehension of the meaning of print which is in some sense 'direct'. The reader builds a representation of the meaning of text without paying unnecessary attention to surface aspects of the text such as orthography or phonology. At the level of single words, one might think of this as a reliance on relations (1) and a discarding of procedure (2). Here there is an analogy with deep dyslexia, since in deep dyslexia relations (1) is at least partly intact whilst procedure (2) is abolished. At the level of sentences, speed-reading may involve a diminished emphasis upon the graphemic input and an increased emphasis upon stored general knowledge: in other words, increased use of relations (4) rather than relations (3). Once again, there is an analogy with deep dyslexia if deep dyslexics can only use relations (4) in reading sentences, as has been suggested.

Thus, whether we are considering single word reading or sentence reading, there is a similarity between deep dyslexic reading and speed reading: in both cases, surface features of written language play a less significant role in reading than is the case for the normal reader. It is the analysis of sentence reading in terms of general knowledge retrieval which allows the analogy between deep dyslexia and speed-reading to be brought out sufficiently clearly. The speed reader chooses to rely heavily upon general knowledge retrieval; the deep dyslexic has no choice but to do so.

This line of reasoning is supported by the case of deep dyslexia which we describe below, since this patient, although suffering from deep dyslexia, showed a preservation of the ability to speed-read, an ability of which he had made much use prior to the onset of his reading disorder.

4 Speed-reading and deep dyslexia: a case study

The patient, P.C., was a professor of philosophy at the university. He suffered in October 1975, at the age of 55, a right-sided hemiplegia of sudden onset with aphasia and right homonymous hemianopsia. A left carotid arteriogram showed a left parietal haematoma. At operation a left parietal infarction was found, together with a large haematoma, which was evacuated.

In October 1976, P.C. was assessed and accepted for re-education in the service of Professor Lhermitte at the Salpêtrière Hospital. Neurological examination showed:

(a)   A right-sided pyramidal syndrome, with a slight motor deficit.
(b)   Major defects in touch, vibration and position sense on the right side of the body.
(c)   A combination of alexia, agraphia, anomia and acalculia.

A CAT scan performed in September 1978 revealed a large hypodense zone in the left parietal region, reaching the occipital lobe, in continuity with the left lateral ventricle and a dilated occipital horn. The conclusion was that these appearances were typical of a porencephalic cyst as a sequel of previous infarction.

4.1 Neuropsychological assessment

This assessment, carried out on admission in October 1976, showed a picture of disturbances affecting all aspects of language:
(a)   *Speech output* was fluent, but the frequency of nominal dysphasia, and word-finding difficulties, gave rise to aborted sentences. This, and the production of semantic and phonemic paraphasias, severely restricted the patient's capacity to communicate.
(b)   *Speech comprehension* was adequate in tests requiring the patient to point out objects and to carry out simple commands, but was disturbed in the absence of context. Thus, on the oral Binoit-Pichot vocabulary test, the patient obtained an IQ of only 117, well below his formerly very high intellectual level.
(c)   *Writing* was abolished.
(d)   *Reading*: single letters could not be read aloud, but in response to spoken letters the patient could mostly point to their printed equivalents. He could only respond 'I don't know' when asked to read aloud function words or non-words. Even for single written nouns, reading aloud was often impossible. Those responses which were made were very slow, and semantic errors were frequent. Some examples are:

France   → 'Paris'
directeur   → 'gérant'
tricot   → 'chan . . . ['chandail' is a synonym for 'tricot']
          . . . un pull'

paquebot → 'bateau'
les malles → 'les bals, pas de bagages'
machine → 'mécanique'
les quais → 'les K, les K, les kiosques'
musulmans → 'Mahomet'

The patient could match printed words to pictures. He succeeded in a sentence/picture matching task, using sentences such as 'The woman is at the hairdressers' and distractor pictures involving a man at the hairdresser, a woman in the street, etc.

(e) Because of the severity of the aphasia, it was not possible to test for dyscalculia. One could, however, detect a loss of understanding of the significance of arithmetical symbols: $+ - \div$ and $\times$.

(f) There was a severe buccofacial apraxis, together with a disturbance of gestures (arbitrary and symbolic gestures were both disturbed). The patient also showed automatic-voluntary dissociation in this area of testing.

(g) Juxtaposition of details in the construction of the Figure of Rey suggested a residual constructional apraxia. Spontaneous drawing was poor and simplified.

(h) The patient showed a decrease in intellectual performance to PM 38 (75th percentile) on formal testing, although the interpretation of this result is difficult, given the extent of his difficulties with language and praxis.

It should also be added that the difficulty in comprehension of speech and print was complicated by anosognosia.

The patient claimed – although the speech therapist did not believe him – that he could still speed-read the newspapers, as rapidly as he had been able to do before his stroke.

4.2 Subsequent testing

Some improvement took place. Initial severe hemiplegia disappeared. An almost total alexia improved to a much less marked defect of oral reading. In May 1977, reading behaviour was as follows:

(a) P.C. could point to and read aloud single letters.
(b) Written non-words could still not be read aloud.
(c) Understanding of written sentences improved, but was still

very poor for reversible sentences such as 'The square is under the circle', where meaning is provided via 'under' and serial ordering of content words.

(d) The patient could give an oral abstract of a short text.

(e) The ability to write was recovered to a small extent.

Formal testing of the ability to read aloud single printed items of various syntactic categories produced the following results:

46 nouns

correct	44
no answer	1
semantic errors	1

30 adjectives, adverbs, verbs

correct	23	
no answer	6	
errors	1	(*dur* → 'doux')

25 articles, pronouns, conjunctions

correct	8	
no answer	5	
errors	12	(e.g. *les* → 'elle', *lui* → 'il', *entre* → 'contre', *ici* → 'trois lettres')

10 non-words

correct	0
omissions or errors	10

Here nouns are most successfully read, then adjectives, adverbs and verbs; function words are the most difficult words, and non-words are still more difficult (here, impossible). This syntactic ordering has been repeatedly observed in deep dyslexia (see, e.g., Chapter 2). Although all the examples of error given here involve responses which seem visually similar to the stimuli, it cannot be claimed that they are all visual errors, because the response preserves the syntactic class of the stimulus. If these responses were visual errors, we would expect the response to be less abstract than the stimulus and perhaps also would expect a bias towards nouns in the response. Neither of these tendencies is evident. We therefore consider that these errors have a genuine semantic (or syntactic) component, and that they are not straightforward visual errors. Other examples of reading error observed at the time confirm this claim. Many errors were made in attempting to read function words, and the erroneous responses themselves were function words not always visually similar to the stimuli (*immediat* → 'imminent', *clairement* → 'nettement'). Furthermore, incorrect responses to Arabic numerals were often numerically close to the stimulus, such as *13* → douze; this is a form of semantic error. Semantic errors were also made in reading sentences aloud (e.g. *David* → 'Goliath').

At this time the patient continued to claim that his previous ability to speed-read was preserved with material such as newspapers and television news. We therefore set out to investigate his claim.

4.3 Speed-reading in a deep dyslexic

(a) *Single words*. Single words were displayed on the screen of a computer terminal for 50 msec and then replaced by an alphabetic masking string. The patient was able to read aloud some of these words. Only nouns and verbs (but not their inflections) could be read. The effect of exposure duration was then studied: 20 nouns were displayed at each of four exposure durations (50 msec, 100 msec, 250 msec and 500 msec). The percentage of correct reports at each of these durations is 40, 80, 75 and 80 per cent. Thus, increasing exposure duration beyond 100 msec up to 500 msec did not improve performance. It did, however, increase the incidence of complaints from the patient. At the 500 msec duration, the patient produced long comments and complaints about the tip-of-the-tongue phenomenon; such complaints also occurred at the 250 msec duration, but not at the two shorter durations.

(b) *Sentence comprehension*. A set of 20 yes/no questions was selected. Examples are:

Is Paris the capital of Ireland?
Is Italy the capital of Rome?
Do Parisians leave Paris in August?

Each sentence was displayed briefly on the terminal screen. The answers chosen by P.C. appeared to be determined by whether or not there was some close semantic relationship between the content words of the sentence. Thus he responded 'no' to the first question above, 'yes' to the second, and 'no' to the third.

(c) *Text comprehension.* The patient says that he speed-reads the newspaper *La Croix* every day.

After short exposures to texts such as newspaper editorials (frequent both in his everyday life, and with his speech therapist), what was P.C. able to report? Written production was impossible. Oral production of a summary was in general poor but even more so with a text upon which P.C. had been drilled for hours, as compared to a speed-read text.

Here is an example of his attempts to summarize a 650-word editorial, 'Dom Helder évêque et voyageur', from *La Croix*, 2/4/78, by Pierre de Boisdeffre – reading time: 1 min 17 sec: 'Helder Camara a toujours aimé voyager pour les découvertes; il est non seulement ouvert, mais il est prêt; il est toujours ouvert sur le monde, et ça va lui permettre de découvrir quelque chose de plus . . . '. It appears that P.C. was only able to report a few of Dom Helder's characteristics (his open mindedness, his being a great traveller, etc.). Asked to give a title (the actual title had been masked), he proposed 'Portrait moral et physique d'Helder Camara' (Moral and physical portrait of Helder Camara).

Asked to sort the nouns belonging to this text out of a list of forty nouns, it was observed that the more the nouns were abstract-key-words, the better were P.C.'s scores:

List of 40 nouns			P.C. answers to the question: Did these items belong to the text?	
			yes	no
13 semantically unrelated nouns	concrete	9	0	9
	abstract	4	0	4
11 related nouns (absent from the text)	concrete	8	1	7
	abstract	3	1	2
16 nouns from the text	concrete	10	5	5
	abstract	6	4	2

P.C. rejected all unrelated items. All the data already listed for P.C. (attempts on his part to summarize, to sort out the words of a text or to give a title of his own) seem to prove that P.C. has grasped something of the text, but is not sufficient as an estimation of his comprehension.

To assess his comprehension, we experimentally checked his speed-reading, using texts from Richaudeau *et al.* (1977). A mean performance was obtained for the following text: 'Une scène de la vie parisienne' (A scene from Parisian life) from Balzac (Richaudeau, pp. 18–20). The patient's speed was 570 words per minute. Ten multiple choice questions were asked, as, for example:

Q.10   What is the frequent ambition of a petty merchant's youngest son?
(a) to take over his father's commerce
(b) to deny his humble parents
(c) to become a statesman
(d) to go in search of adventure beyond the seas.

P.C. was more accurate in answers to general ideas as above than in choosing between single items such as:

Q.3   What is the name of the newspaper cited by Balzac?
(a) The 'ami du peuple'
(b) The 'moniteur'
(c) The 'Père Duchesne'
(d) The 'Constitutionnel'

Results:

Questions		P.C. answers	
	Right	Don't know	Wrong
General ideas	5	1	0
Specific items	1	1	2

P.C.'s correct answers were 6/10 – the chance level being 2.5. This result seems to point to the patient's good comprehension of, at least, the general ideas of the text.

4.4 P.C.'s reading

This patient exhibits two types of reading behaviour. One is very slow: it is the reading of the deep dyslexic. The other is very fast: it is speed-reading. How does he switch from one reading behaviour to the other? And how can one explain the increase in comments and complaints as exposure duration is increased, and the absence of an improvement in tachistoscopic performance beyond durations of 100 msec?

When several procedures are interacting in a given system, the overall rate at which the system operates will be determined by the rate at which the slowest procedure operates. The system can be accelerated if the interactions are switched off. In deep dyslexia and also in speed-reading, the understanding of written material relies heavily upon the extraction of content words and knowledge-retrieval procedures. We suggest that these two forms of reading differ because in deep dyslexia general knowledge-retrieval procedures are interacting with the other slow and no longer reliable procedures. In speed-reading the reader has learned to switch off these interactions. When P.C. tries to read aloud or to read carefully, his performance is seriously impaired because these interactions are not only present but are malfunctioning.

When the interactions are switched off, in his speed-reading, he is no longer affected by his deep dyslexia. Thus speed reading may testify to a skilled ability to switch off the slowest procedures used for understanding print, whilst deep dyslexia involves impairments in these procedures.

5 Conclusions

Many pieces of the model of normal reading that we are trying to build up are of course still missing. The chapter is an attempt at thinking up a new piece from an old one, an attempt at generalizing from word reading to sentence reading. Analysis of the characteristics of reading in deep dyslexia provides some ideas about how a normal reader understands single printed words: in particular, the absence of the grapheme-phoneme correspondences in deep dyslexia allows one to consider their functions in normal reading.

What remains in deep dyslexia is a link between word comprehension and word utterance, so that reading aloud involves retrieval of semantic features and computation of meaning. Our attempt to generalize this 'retrieving-computing' model from single words to sentences involves concepts such as *procedure, stored general knowledge*, and *frame retrieval*. The normal system for understanding printed sentences is assumed to depend upon interactions between subsystems such as morphosyntactic procedures and frame retrieval. The rate of the system as a whole is determined by the rate of the slowest subsystems, which may be damaged in deep dyslexia (the morphosyntactic procedures being the ones damaged).

This rate can be considerably increased when subjects are trained to read mainly with frame retrieval subprocesses, i.e. when they are able to switch off the other interacting processes (speed-reading).

Such a *procedural model* is able to describe both of the forms of reading behaviour displayed by P.C. Hence our subtitle: *towards a procedural understanding of reading*.

Notes

1 Since we can read non-words aloud, there must also exist;

   (2) G → P

   Most reading models (e.g. Marshall and Newcombe, 1973; Andreewsky, 1974; Marin, Saffran and Schwartz, 1975; Coltheart, 1978) consist of (1) and (2). This describes well the reading of context-free single words.

2 An English example would be 'Did you *read* the book I *read*?'

3 An example in English:

   The *lead* was taken by a Ferrari.
   The *lead* was taken by a scrap-merchant.

References

Allport, D. A. (1977) On knowing the meaning of words we are unable to report: the effect of visual masking. In S. Dornic (ed.), *Attention and Performance*. Hillsdale, N.J.: Lawrence Erlbaum.

Andreewsky, E. (1974) Un modèle sémantique. Application à la pathologie du langage: alexie aphasique. *Traitement Automatique Informations*, 2, 3–27.

Andreewsky, E. and Seron, X. (1975) Implicit processing of grammatical rules in a classical case of agrammatism. *Cortex*, *11*, 379–90.

Andreewsky, E., Deloche, G. and Nicolas, P. (1977) Essai d'identification des processus de lecture. In *Modelisation et Maîtrise des Systèmes techniques, Economiques et Sociaux, Hommes et Techniques*, vol. 2, 147–56. Paris: AFCET.

Andreewsky, E., Kossanyi, P. and Deloche, G. (1978) Traitement cognitif des traits sémantiques dan des conditions limites de lecture. In *Psychologie et Education*. Toulouse: Université du Mirail.

Coltheart, M. (1977) Phonemic dyslexia: some comments on its interpretations and its implications for the study of normal reading. I.N.S. Meeting, Oxford, 1977.

Coltheart, M. (1978) Lexical access in simple reading tasks. In G. Underwood (ed.), *Strategies of Information Processing*. London: Academic Press.

Ellis, A. W. and Marshall, J. C. (1978) Semantic errors or statistical flukes? a note on Allport's 'On knowing the meaning of words we are unable to report'. *Quarterly Journal of Experimental Psychology, 30*, 569–75.

Fodor, J. A., Bever, T. G. and Garrett, M. F. (1974) *The Psychology of Language*. New York: McGraw-Hill.

Johnson-Laird, P. N. (1977) Procedural semantics. *Cognition, 5*, 189–214.

Kouznetsov, O. A., Korenev, A. N. and Rhomov, L. N. (1976) Speed-reading: model and learning methods. *Vopros Psychology, 4*, 90–102. (In Russian)

Lienard, J. S. (1977) *Les processus de la communication parlée. Introduction à l'analyse et à la synthèse de la parole*. Paris: Masson.

Marcel, T. (1974) The effective visual field and the use of context in fast and slow readers of two ages. *British Journal of Psychology, 65*, 4, 479–92.

Marin, O., Saffran, E. M. and Schwartz, M. F. (1975) Dissociation of language in aphasia: implications for normal functions. Paper presented at the New York Academy of Sciences Conference on origins and evolution of language and speech, 1975.

Marshall, J. C. and Newcombe, F. (1973) Patterns of paralexia: a psycholinguistic approach. *Journal of Psycholinguistic Research, 2*, 175–99.

Miller, G. (1976) Semantic relations among words. Paper presented at convocation on communication, M.I.T., June 1976.

Miller, G. (1978) Construction and selection in the mental representation of texts. In J. Costermans (ed.), *Structures cognitives et organisation du langage*. Louvain.

Minsky, M.A. (1975) Framework for representing knowledge. In P. H. Winston (ed.), *The Psychology of Computer Vision*. New York: McGraw-Hill.

Morton, J. (1964) The effects of context upon speed of reading, eye-movements and eye-voice span. *Quarterly Journal of Experimental Psychology, 16*, 340–54.

Richaudeau, F., Gauquelin, M. and Gauquelin, F. (1977) *Méthode de lecture rapide*. Paris: Retz-C.E.P.L.

Schank, R. and Nash-Webber, B. L. (eds) (1975) Theoretical issues in natural language processing. *An Interdisciplinary Workshop in Computa-*

tional Linguistics, Psychology, Linguistics and Artificial Intelligence.
Cambridge, Mass.: M.I.T.
Winograd, T. (1977) A framework for understanding discourse. *Stanford AI memo AIM – 297.*
Zurif, E. and Blumstein, S. E. (1976) Language and the brain: evidence from aphasia. Paper presented at convocation on communication, M.I.T. Cambridge, Mass., June 1976.

16 Deep dyslexia: a right-hemisphere hypothesis*

Max Coltheart

Most theoretical treatments of deep dyslexia and its neuroanatomical basis have assumed, implicitly, that the syndrome arises when some of the components of the left-hemisphere system responsible for reading have been damaged or abolished, whilst other components of this left-hemisphere system have remained intact. The reading of the deep dyslexic thus reflects the operation of a partially impaired left-hemisphere reading system.

One difficulty with this kind of view is that the syndrome of deep dyslexia involves numerous distinct reading symptoms. The deep dyslexic not only makes semantic errors; he makes visual errors, he makes derivational errors, he lacks the ability to derive phonology from print, he has particular difficulties with low-imagery words, and he also has difficulty with function words. There is no obvious relationship between these various symptoms; thus it is natural to suppose that the different symptoms are associated with different loci of damage in the left hemisphere. If these symptoms, and these loci, are independent, then it should be possible for one form of damage to occur without the others, and hence for some of the symptoms to occur without the others. As indicated in Chapter 2, all of the dyslexic patients so far described in the literature who produced semantic errors also showed phonological impairment in dealing with print, difficulties with low-imagery and function words,

* I am greatly indebted to Karalyn Patterson for her detailed criticisms of two lengthy earlier drafts of this chapter, for her suggestions as to how these might be improved, and for her patience in answering innumerable questions about her work. I thank also Alan Allport, Derek Besner, William Marslen-Wilson and Tim Shallice for valuable discussions and suggestions.

326

and visual and derivational errors. If these symptoms arise at independent neurological loci, why is it that they do not occur independently in patients? Why, for example, do we not find patients who make semantic errors but not visual errors, or patients who make semantic errors but have no impairment in dealing with phonological representations of printed words?

One way of resolving this issue is to claim that there is in fact only one basic impairment in deep dyslexia, and that all of the other symptoms of the syndrome spring from this one impairment. For example, it is sometimes argued that an inability to derive phonology from print is by itself sufficient to cause semantic errors, difficulty with function words and abstract words, and so on. Such arguments are described more fully in the chapter on phonological encoding and reading in this volume (Chapter 10); there it is suggested that no argument of this kind can deal with the full range of deep-dyslexic symptoms.

The problem, then, is that if one supposes that the deep dyslexic reads by using a left-hemisphere system from which some components have been deleted, it is difficult to avoid a dilemma: either the various symptoms of the syndrome are neurologically and functionally independent, yet do not occur independently in patients, or else the symptoms are all reflections of a single basic impairment of some particular function, yet one cannot specify what this function is.

I would not wish to suggest that this dilemma is insuperable, and that its existence is sufficient to rule out the view that the neuroanatomical system used by the deep dyslexic when he is reading is the normal left-hemisphere system minus some of its components. However, it does seem to me that the arguments put forward above raise difficulties for this view which are serious enough to suggest that one should consider looking elsewhere for a neuroanatomical interpretation of deep dyslexia.

The possibility of right hemisphere involvement in the reading of the deep dyslexic has been occasionally considered. For example, Brown (1972, p. 263) in a discussion of the semantic error, suggests that 'the phenomenon may be related to the ability of the right hemisphere to extract information from the written message in an otherwise global alexic'; and a theory of deep dyslexic reading which postulates considerable contributions from the right hemisphere was proposed by Marcel and Patterson (1979). The strongest hypothesis, namely, that the right hemisphere is *entirely* responsible for reading in the deep dyslexic, has been suggested by Saffran, Bogyo, Schwartz and Marin (Chapter 17, this volume) and by Coltheart (1977).

There are various ways in which one might attempt to develop arguments in favour of this right-hemisphere hypothesis. I will do so by first reviewing work on hemispheric asymmetries in the reading performance of people who are not deep dyslexics. There is, in fact, a considerable amount of work providing information about the reading capabilities of the right hemisphere in people whose left hemisphere is specialized for linguistic functions, though this information is scattered in nooks and crannies of the literature, and the relevant information is rather fragmentary. A review of this work allows one to develop a tentative description of the right hemisphere reading system. Once this is done, the next step is to decide whether this description of how the right hemisphere reads corresponds with a description of how the deep dyslexic reads; the closer this correspondence is, the more confidence one has in the hypothesis that the deep dyslexic reads by using his right hemisphere.

Reading by the right hemisphere

It is sometimes claimed that the right hemisphere is completely incapable of reading. If this were so, this chapter could stop here. Hence I begin with a consideration of the claim by Geschwind (1965) that the right hemisphere is 'word-blind and word-deaf'. This claim is reiterated by Benson and Geschwind (1969, p. 421). They explicitly reject the view that the right hemisphere possesses any capacity for reading; their rejection of this view is based upon results they have observed in cases of alexia without agraphia.

The classical interpretation of this syndrome, due to Déjerine and borne out by numerous post-mortem studies, is that the syndrome is due to isolation of the left angular gyrus from left and right occipital cortex. This isolation has usually occurred because of the joint presence of two different lesions: one affecting left occipital cortex (producing right hemianopia, and preventing the left angular gyrus from receiving input from the right visual hemifield) and the other affecting the splenium of the corpus callosum (which is considered to be a pathway from right occipital cortex to left angular gyrus; if this is so, a splenial lesion would prevent the left angular gyrus from receiving input from the left visual hemifield). These two lesions would isolate the left angular gyrus from the entire visual field. Visual input from the left visual hemifield to a putative right-hemisphere system for reading, however, should still occur in these patients; yet, according to Benson and Geschwind (1969), studies they have carried out on patients suffering from alexia without agraphia indicate that these patients 'not only fail to read aloud but cannot match written words with pictures or objects and fail to carry out written commands with either hand'. This implies that reading is impossible even when visual input can gain unrestricted access to the right hemisphere; so Benson and Geschwind (1969) assert that 'it can be stated with some confidence that the ability to comprehend written language is dependent upon intactness of the dominant (usually left) hemisphere in the majority of adults'. It is unfortunate that the work on reading comprehension in alexia without agraphia which they refer to has not yet been published, since substantiation of the claim that reading comprehension is absent from the right hemisphere would immediately refute any interpretation of deep dyslexia based upon contributions to reading from right-hemisphere print-comprehension mechanisms. It is also unfortunate that, in the published studies of alexia without agraphia, the ability of the patients to read has usually been assessed by asking the patients to read *aloud*; when a patient fails to do so, it is concluded that he or she 'cannot read'. Very rarely, perfunctory attempts at investigating reading *comprehension* are reported; and these in fact reveal that, in cases of alexia without agraphia, this function has *not* disappeared completely. For example, the patient described by Cohen, Salanga, Hully, Steinberg and Hardy (1976), a classical case of the syndrome, had 'complete word alexia' (for oral reading? for comprehension?) but 'was able to pick out spoken numbers from a list of numerals', suggesting that she comprehended printed numerals. An equally classical case of alexia without agraphia is described by Caplan and Hedley-White (1974). She 'could read no words'; the context suggests that the authors meant reading aloud here. However, when asked to read a number aloud, this patient would usually give a price name if the number were accompanied by a dollar or cents sign; thus she must have been able to comprehend these two signs. She could indicate that the last two letters in *catat* and the first two in *xedog* were 'wrong' or 'didn't belong'. When shown the list of words *red, hot, cold, brown, warm, pink* and *yellow*, she could not read any of them aloud, and when asked whether any of them were alike she responded 'No'. However, when asked whether there were any colours, she responded to three words, all colour words (*brown* → 'tan', *pink* → 'tan', *yellow* → 'brown'); and when asked if there were any temperatures, she responded to three words, two of them temperatures and the other the word *red* (*red* → 'warm', *cold* → 'cold', *warm* → 'hot'). A second list (*red, rose, chair, tulip, boy, daisy*) also produced no correct responses when the patient was asked to read aloud, and a 'No' to every word in response to the question 'Are there any alike?'. However, the question 'Are there any flowers?' produced the two responses *rose* → 'hyacinth' and *daisy* → 'flower'; and the question 'Are there any persons?' produced the response *boy* → 'boy'. Thus appropriate forms of testing succeeded in demonstrating that this patient *could* achieve at least some comprehension of some written words.

These two examples show that one cannot assert that reading comprehension is entirely abolished in classical cases of alexia without agraphia; therefore they are not justified in claiming that the ability to comprehend written language depends upon intactness of the speech hemisphere. Consequently, the view that there exists a right-hemisphere lexicon which can play a part in reading remains tenable. In fact, these two case studies of alexia without agraphia actually support such a view, if one accepts the orthodox interpretation that in alexia without agraphia visual input can no longer gain any access to left-hemisphere reading systems, since it follows from this view that any reading comprehension exhibited by such patients must be mediated by a right-hemisphere reading system.

There are other lines of evidence suggesting that the right hemisphere's capacity for language, even for reading, is not entirely negligible. One such line of evidence comes from studies of left hemispherectomy. The most valuable of these is the report by Smith (1966). His patient was aged forty-seven before any indication of brain pathology occurred. One year later his left hemisphere was removed. Smith reported that 'speaking, reading, writing and understanding language were present immediately after hemispherectomy', although these functions were of course all greatly impaired. Six months after the operation, when the patient was shown a printed colour word and five pens of different colours, he was able to select the pen whose colour was specified by the printed word; thus he had comprehended the meaning of this word. This is a demanding task, since it was not sufficient for the patient to understand that the printed item was a colour name; he had to understand *which* colour name it was.

When Smith's patient was studied by Zangwill (1967), it was found that 'he was on occasion able to read words, such as object or colour names' though not sentences, and 'he could print his name and copy script or designs, but could not write the names of objects spontaneously or to dictation'. This patient exhibited a considerable amount of 'automatic' or 'emotional' speech, and even some propositional speech; the degree to which he was able to speak improved gradually, but speech was present to some extent even immediately after the left hemispherectomy. On the Peabody Picture Vocabulary Test, which measures comprehension of single spoken words, the patient scored 85/112, which represents a substantial degree of speech comprehension.

Crockett and Estridge (1951) describe another case of adult left hemispherectomy. This patient 'could not read' after the operation, but the interpretation of this result is unclear, for two reasons. Firstly, the patient's pre-operative reading ability was not reported. Secondly, it is impossible to know whether by the term 'read' these authors meant 'utter aloud' or 'comprehend'. Since the patient's speech was severely limited, an inability to read words aloud would not be surprising, and would by no means indicate an inability to comprehend the printed word. Both points also apply to the case of Hillier (1954), whose fifteen-year-old left-hemispherectomized patient could read individual letters after the operation, but could not 'formulate words'. Unfortunately, it is not stated whether letter reading was perfect or merely partly preserved, nor precisely what was meant by 'formulate words'. The left-hemispherectomized patient described by Gott (1973) showed some post-operative ability to comprehend print and to utter it, but was only ten years old when the operation was performed. Only one other case of removal of the speech hemisphere has been reported (Zollinger, 1935) and no mention of reading is made in this report.

The virtue of Smith's case is that his patient's brain was mature prior to the onset of pathology. One can therefore presume that language lateralization was complete, and therefore that any linguistic capabilities exhibited by the right hemisphere of this patient should also be present in the right hemispheres of the deep dyslexics discussed in this volume, all of whom received their left-hemisphere injuries in late adolescence or adulthood. The patient described by Gott (1973), on the other hand, may not have attained a maximal degree of cerebral lateralization of language by the time of onset of pathology (eight years of age). Thus this patient's right hemisphere may have possessed linguistic capabilities superior to those enjoyed by the right hemisphere of people in whom lateralization of language is complete; if so, Gott's patient may not be an appropriate source of information about the gross linguistic capabilities of the right hemisphere of deep dyslexics.

This point is especially relevant when one is considering the implications of data obtained from commissurotomized patients. The reading, writing and spelling abilities of the right hemispheres of two of these patients, L.B. and A.A., have been described by Levy, Nebes and Sperry (1971), Zaidel (1973), Gazzaniga and Sperry (1967) and Gazzaniga and Hillyard (1971), and evidence of some capacity of the right hemisphere to comprehend print, to spell, and to write, has been obtained. However, as Levy and Trevarthen (1977, p. 106) note, both of these patients appear to have received their critical brain injury at birth. The likelihood that the two patients' language lateralization would have been abnormal because of the existence of left-hemisphere damage since birth means that one cannot safely deduce, from information about the linguistic capacities of their right hemispheres, anything about the linguistic capacities of the right hemisphere of deep dyslexics.

However, linguistic *inabilities* of the right hemisphere of split-brain patients may provide somewhat more pertinent information. Suppose one finds that split-brain patients are *unable* to perform some linguistic task using their right hemispheres in spite of the possibility that, because of an early injury to the brain, their right hemispheres may be somewhat more sophisticated at linguistic tasks than the right hemispheres of people in whom language lateralization has occurred in the normal fashion. In this case, one may argue that there is some intrinsic property of the right hemisphere which renders it incapable of performing this linguistic task, even with the advantage of biases towards the abnormal development of linguistic proficiency in the right hemisphere. One example relevant to this issue is the inability of the right hemisphere in split-brain patients to accomplish such phonological tasks as judging whether a picture has a name which rhymes with a printed word; this is discussed later.

An alternative source for this sort of evidence is the observation of patients during the course of partial recovery from an aphasia produced by left hemisphere damage. Linguistic behaviour which emerges during such partial recovery might be the product of left-hemisphere mechanisms which have recovered some temporarily lost function; alternatively, such behaviour might be produced by previously inoperative right hemisphere mechanisms. Several findings point towards the latter possibility. Neilsen (1946) found that right-hemisphere damage which was incurred during the course of recovery from an aphasia produced by left-hemisphere damage could produce an exacerbation of the aphasic symptoms. Tikofsky, Kooi and Thomas (1960) found that the prospects for recovery from aphasia were worse when there were EEG abnormalities of the right hemisphere than when there were not; left hemisphere EEG abnormalities were unrelated to prognosis. Kinsbourne (1971), using intracarotid sodium amytal, obtained direct evidence that the (very limited) speech of some aphasic patients was originating from the right hemisphere, even though their aphasia had originally been produced by left-hemisphere damage. Pettit and Noll (1972; cited in Searleman, 1977) found that aphasic subjects in a dichotic listening test with speech stimuli showed a *left*-ear advantage. Moore and Weidner (1974) found the usual right visual field advantage in tachistoscopic word recognition with a group of normal subjects, but a left visual field advantage for an aphasic group. Whilst each of these investigations was not without its individual methodological problems, all yielded evidence consistent with the view that recovery of linguistic function after aphasia is sometimes achieved by use of right hemisphere linguistic mechanisms. The results of Lesser (1974) are also relevant here, since they suggest that processing of semantic aspects of language (unlike the processing of syntax or phonology) can be impaired by damage to either hemisphere in patients with the usual left-hemisphere lateralization for speech.

It seems clear, then, that the claim that 'the right hemisphere is word-blind and word-deaf' (Geschwind, 1965) is indefensible; work on alexia without agraphia, on left hemispherectomy, and on recovery from aphasia reveals that the right hemisphere has some ability to read, and to understand speech. Thus one cannot dismiss out of hand the hypothesis that the reading performance of the deep dyslexic is mediated by a neuroanatomical system for reading which is located in the right hemisphere. This hypothesis may turn out to be wrong; but its refutation will require a detailed discussion of what is known about the right-hemisphere reading system and of how well the properties of this system correspond to the properties of the reading behaviour of the deep dyslexic. Such a discussion now follows.

The right-hemisphere reading system

The right hemisphere and the derivation of phonology from print

It has been claimed for some years, certainly since the work of Geffen, Bradshaw and Nettleton (1972), that a task which requires the derivation of a phonological from an orthographic representation is performed more quickly or more accurately when the stimulus is presented to the left hemisphere than when it is presented to the right. Any such finding however, is open to at least two interpretations. The first is that the right hemisphere can perform such phonological tasks, but is merely slower or less accurate at doing so than the left hemisphere. The second interpretation is that the right hemisphere is actually *incapable* of this kind of task; the finding that reaction times are slower with right-hemisphere presentation is taken, on this interpretation, as an indication of the time required to transfer the relevant information to the left hemisphere, and the finding that accuracy is lower with right-hemisphere presentation is taken as an indication of some information loss during inter-hemispheric transfer.

It is clearly of great importance to be able to distinguish between these two interpretations, at least for the purposes of this chapter. If the right hemisphere is merely slower or less accurate at deriving phonology from print, the inability of the deep dyslexic to perform such tasks is not obviously explicable on the right-hemisphere hypothesis, whereas it is if one can provide evidence that the right hemisphere is actually *incapable* of deriving phonology from print. Fortunately, there are experimental methods which allow one to adjudicate between these two interpretations of right-hemisphere inferiorities.

Klatzky and Atkinson (1971) presented their subjects on each trial of their experiment with a set of letters to memorize. Then a picture was presented. The subject's task was to decide whether or not the picture's name began with any of the letters in the memory set. This is a phonological task, and so it was not surprising that reaction times were slower when the picture was presented to the right hemisphere than when it was presented to the left.[1] As noted above, however, there are two possible explanations for this. The first explanation is that the right hemisphere can and does perform this phonological matching task, but it is simply slower at it than the left. The second explanation is that the right hemisphere is incapable of the task; thus when the picture is directed to the right hemisphere, it must be transferred to the left before the phonological matching can be performed. These explanations can be distinguished experimentally. If the right hemisphere is merely slower, then the more matches that are required the larger will be the right-hemisphere RT disadvantage. Consequently, the size of this disadvantage will be an increasing function of the number of items in the memory set. If the right hemisphere is not performing the task at all, then the right-hemisphere RT disadvantage is due to the time required for inter-hemisphere transfer of the picture, and this time will be the same regardless of the size of the memory set. Klatzky and Atkinson obtained the latter result, which suggests that the right hemisphere is not performing any phonological matching, even when the picture-stimulus is directed to this hemisphere.

A similar conclusion was reached by Moscovitch (1976). The task in his experiment was to decide whether or not a printed letter rhymed with a previously-presented spoken letter; this, like the task used by Klatzky and Atkinson, is a phonological matching task. The responses were made by pushing or pulling a microswitch with the index finger, and it is assumed that this response was produced from the contralateral hemisphere. Given this assumption, it follows that, if the right hemisphere is merely less efficient at this phonological task, its RT disadvantage will be less when it is producing the response (left-hand responses), since here the left hemisphere will lose some of its time advantage because of the time needed for inter-hemispheric transfer prior to response. If all the phonological matching is performed in the left hemisphere, even when the stimulus was directed to the right hemisphere, then the right-hemisphere RT disadvantage will be the same size whichever hand is responding. Since Moscovitch found a right hemisphere disadvantage of nine msec. with left-hand responding and ten msec. with right-hand responding, he concluded that 'the right hemisphere displays *no* aptitude at dealing with the task' (my italics).

When non-words in a lexical decision task are phonologically identical to English words (BRANE, SHERT), the 'No' response is slower than when they are not (BRENE, TREP) (Rubenstein, Lewis and Rubenstein, 1971; Coltheart, Davelaar, Jonasson and Besner, 1977; Patterson and Marcel, 1977; Gough and Cosky, 1977). Cohen and Freeman (1979) found that this was only true when the non-words were presented to the left hemisphere, which again suggests that the right hemisphere does not perform phonological recoding of printed stimuli. (In fact, the effect was reversed with right-hemisphere presentation; the reader is referred to Cohen and Freeman's paper for a discussion of why this might have occurred.) This result also suggests that the right hemisphere can perform lexical decisions, a suggestion discussed further at a later stage in this paper.

The three types of experiment just described used normal subjects. Levy and Trevarthen (1977) studied the phonological abilities of the right hemisphere of split-brain subjects. Although such subjects could comprehend a word or a picture directed to this hemisphere, it was impossible for them to judge whether the name of a picture presented to the right hemisphere rhymed with a previously spoken word. The left hemisphere, in contrast, could perform this phonological task.

This result would have been of much greater interest for present purposes if the stimulus presented to the right hemisphere had been a printed word, not a picture. It is frequently claimed that this experiment has been carried out with split-brain patients. According to Searleman (1977), for example, 'the right hemisphere may comprehend the meaning of the words "ache" and "lake", but it would never know that they rhyme (Levy, 1974a)'. However, the chapter by Levy referred to here by Searleman describes only the picture-rhyming experiments discussed in the previous paragraph of this chapter. According to Moscovitch (1976, footnote 8): 'The split-brain minor hemisphere can semantically decode words to derive their meaning, but it cannot phonologically recode them in order to rhyme one word with another (Levy, 1973)'. This word-rhyming experiment again eludes the reader, since there is no Levy (1973) in the reference section of Moscovitch's paper. Yet again,

Cohen and Freeman (1979) describe the results of Levy and Trevarthen (1977) thus: 'When a word was presented to the right visual field (left hemisphere), the patient could then point to a rhyming word in a list of alternatives, but when a word was presented to the left visual field (right hemisphere), performance on phonological matching was at a chance level'. This is not what Levy and Trevarthen (1977) did: they studied picture/print rhyming, and the failure of the right hemisphere is not unequivocal evidence of its inability to derive phonology from print, since an alternative explanation of the failure is an inability of the right hemisphere to access a picture's name from the picture itself. Thus, in spite of the existence of three forthright assertions that Levy has investigated the ability of the right hemisphere to judge whether two printed words rhyme, it appears that she has not in fact done so. Fortunately, however, the appropriate experiment has recently been reported by Zaidel (1978). He showed that the split-brain right hemisphere can match pictures by rhyme, match words to pictures by meaning, but is at chance on matching words to pictures by rhyme, which shows a complete inability of the right hemisphere to derive phonology from print.

One difficulty exists for the claim that the right hemisphere lacks completely the ability to convert orthography to phonology: this is Gott's left-hemispherectomy case, a girl who developed a tumour of the lateral ventricle at the age of eight. The tumour was removed, but parietal malignancy developed two years later, and her left hemisphere was removed at that age. This patient's reading, which pre-operatively was poor, was not completely abolished by the hemispherectomy. Furthermore:

> Given a list of twenty written words, 10 of which rhymed with 'son' but many of which did not have the same letters, such as sun or bun, and 10 which did not rhyme with 'son' and had some letters in common with son, such as sin or sow, she was 80 per cent correct in indicating if the word rhymed with son. Yet, the only words she could identify from the list were sun and boy. (Gott, 1973, p. 1085)

It is difficult to determine whether this is evidence for phonological recoding by the right hemisphere or not. If the target word 'son' was spoken to the patient, why should she not have spelled it as SUN,

and hence have no difficulty identifying rhymes such as *sun* or *bun*? If
the target word was presented *visually*, then even the purely visual
strategy 'Say Yes if the word ends with -ON otherwise No' (which is
the strategy used by deep dyslexics in rhyming tasks – Saffran and
Marin, 1977) would yield above-chance performance, if the list
included TON and WON and not such words as YON and NON.
Even if one accepted that this patient's right hemisphere could
perform phonological recoding, it does not follow that the right
hemisphere of a brain which had gone through a normal process of
language lateralization would be able to do so; but, if one concludes
that Gott's patient was performing the task visually, it would be
possible to maintain the stronger conclusion that even when early
brain development is abnormal (as in Gott's case and in the split-
brain patient studied by Zaidel), the right hemisphere does not
develop a phonological-recoding ability.

The data discussed in this section provide evidence that in people
whose language lateralization has been completed normally, and
perhaps even in those for whom it has not, the right hemisphere is
unable to derive phonological representations from print.

Kanji and kana

Japanese is written in a mixture of two forms of script. This dual
writing system is described elsewhere in this volume, in Chapter 3,
and will merely be summarized here. The *kana* script is a syllabary;
each symbol corresponds to a syllable, so that there is a one-to-one
(and invariant) relationship between the syllables of any spoken
word and the kana symbols used to write it down. The *kanji* script is
ideographic, like the Chinese script; a single kanji character stands
for a whole word, no matter how many syllables there are in the
spoken representation of that word. The kanji representation of a
word contains no information about precisely how that word is
pronounced, so that an unknown word written in kanji would not
only be incomprehensible, but unpronounceable; written in kana, it
could be pronounced even if it could not be understood.

Since the kana script is an ideal one if reading depends on a
phonological recoding of print prior to lexical access, whereas the
kanji script is ideographic and therefore in principle cannot permit
phonological recoding prior to access to a stored representation of

the printed word – since, putting the matter crudely, kana is designed to allow phonological reading whilst kanji demands visual reading – it is clearly of great interest to study hemispheric effects on the reading of kana and kanji, and we are fortunate that such investigations have been carried out by Japanese experimental psychologists and neuropsychologists.

The results of these experiments are straightforward. When a single kanji is presented tachistoscopically, verbal report is more accurate when presentation is to the right hemisphere than when it is to the left (Hatta, 1977a, 1977b, submitted). When the kana script is used in tachistoscopic experiments, verbal report is more accurate when presentation is to the left hemisphere than when it is to the right (Hirata and Osaka, 1967; Sasanuma, Itoh, Mori and Kobayashi, 1977; Hatta, submitted). When words written as more than one kanji are presented, a left-hemisphere advantage is found (Hatta, submitted); if nonsense words written as multiple kanji are used, a non-significant right-hemisphere advantage is found (Sasanuma *et al.*, 1977). Thus, at least when single characters are presented, the right hemisphere is better at dealing with kanji whilst the left is better at dealing with kana. One could use the Sternberg technique (as applied by Klatzky and Atkinson, 1971) or the hand-interaction technique (as developed by Moscovitch, 1976) to determine whether kanji characters are solely processed by the right hemisphere and kana by the left, or whether it is merely a matter of differential efficiency; this remains to be done. It is clear, however, that the right hemisphere is specialized for kanji and the left for kana in Japanese readers. Tzeng, Hung and Garro (1978) have obtained comparable results for the reading of Chinese characters: single characters showed a right-hemisphere advantage, whilst multiple characters showed a left-hemisphere advantage.

Sugishita, Iwata, Toyokura, Yoshioka and Yamada (1978) studied three Japanese patients suffering from sections of the splenium of the corpus callosum. Since, as discussed earlier in this chapter, it has been argued that the transmission of visual information from right occipital cortex to left hemisphere reading systems occurs via the splenium, this form of callosal section is of great theoretical interest. In these patients, verbal report of tachistoscopically-displayed kanji or kana characters representing common concrete nouns was almost perfect with left-hemisphere presentation. When the stimuli were presented to the right hemisphere, performance with kana was extremely poor; performance with kanji was much better than performance with kana. (Experiments involving picture/word and word/word matching yielded much less clear-cut results; the raw data from these studies are set out in the paper by Sugishita *et al.*, 1978). On the assumption that the spoken response in this tachistoscopic experiment was produced from the left hemisphere, these data indicate that the splenium is vital if communication is to occur between right-hemisphere kana input and left-hemisphere speech systems, whereas communication between right-hemisphere kanji input and left-hemisphere speech systems can use other callosal pathways. One interpretation of this pattern of results, considered again later in this chapter, is that the splenium is required for the transmission of purely visual information from right occipital cortex to left hemisphere; semantic information is transmitted by other pathways, but these are poorly used with kana input because the right hemisphere can derive semantic information much more effectively from kanji than from kana. The comprehension results support this proposal, but are certainly not clear-cut. Nevertheless, one can argue that the results of Sugishita *et al.* (1978) indicate that, in the right hemisphere, comprehension of kanji is superior to comprehension of kana.

Numbers

Although English is usually considered to be an alphabetically written language, ideographs are used quite frequently in printed or written English (see, e.g., Edgerton, 1941; Marshall, 1976). Mathematical signs, abbreviations, and punctuation marks are all examples of ideographic writing: but the most common examples are the Arabic numerals. If kanji characters receive privileged treatment in the right hemispheres of Japanese readers, perhaps English ideographs such as Arabic numerals are similarly privileged in the right hemispheres of English readers?

Teng and Sperry (1973) studied the performance of six commissurotomized patients in a tachistoscopic experiment with digits and letters as stimuli. Letters were dealt with better than digits in the left hemisphere; the reverse was true in the right hemisphere, and these authors concluded that 'the right hemisphere, generally speechless and less proficient in language, is nevertheless better in dealing with

digits than with letters'. Zaidel (1976) found that his three commissurotomized patients, when carrying out the Word Discrimination subtest from the Boston Diagnostic Aphasia Examination,
performed slightly better with digits than with letters when using
their right hemispheres for reading. Gazzaniga and Hillyard (1971)
found that their split-brain patient could report digits presented to
the right hemisphere. The patient achieved this by using a cross-
cueing strategy, but in order for this strategy to have been used
successfully it must have been the case that the right hemisphere
had comprehended the visually-presented digits. The young left-
hemispherectomy case studied by Gott (1973) also showed good
comprehension of digits.

It should be noted that one cannot reject this particular form of
data from split-brain patients simply on the general ground, noted
earlier, that their language lateralization is likely to be abnormal
because of their early brain injury. If abnormal lateralization
favours numbers over other linguistic entities – that is, if the right
hemisphere develops the ability to deal with numbers to a greater
extent than the ability to deal with letters or words – then this itself
suggests that there is some kind of affinity between numbers and the
right hemisphere, which is what is being argued here.

It has been suggested, during the discussion above of the work of
Sugishita *et al.* (1978), that transmission from right to left hemisphere
of information concerning kanji is at least partly possible in the
absence of an intact splenium. By analogy, this may be true of
numbers too. This may be investigated by studying the number-
naming performance of patients exhibiting alexia without agraphia,
since these patients almost always have splenial lesions. Thus the
following passage from Caplan and Hedley-White (1974, p. 258) is
of considerable significance:

> The reading of numbers is often preserved in cases of alexia
> without agraphia. In Déjerine's original case, number reading
> was normal. Symonds (1953) and Geschwind (1965) emphasize
> the sometimes striking preservation of the capability of reading
> complex numbers in patients with severe letter and word
> naming defects.

One reason why the Japanese script is of such theoretical importance is that two fundamentally different types of script, one

syllabic and the other ideographic, exist and can often serve as alternative methods of writing a single word. We should not lose sight of the fact that there are circumstances in which this is true for English too; and the best examples are the numbers, which can be written alphabetically or ideographically (or even pictographically: I II III). These two scripts may differ in fundamental ways in English. For example, Besner and Coltheart (1979) found that when subjects are asked to judge which of two numbers is numerically the greater, a Stroop-like effect of the conflicting physical sizes of the stimuli occurs with ideographic presentation but not with alphabetic presentation; that is, 1₂ was harder than 12, but ONE TWO was not harder than ONE TWO. Thus we would like to know whether number sparing in alexia without agraphia, or indeed the selective advantage of numbers in the right hemisphere, occurs because of the semantic category to which numbers belong, or to the ideographic nature of the script in which they have been written when presented to patients suffering from alexia without agraphia. This can be determined by comparing performance with ideographically and alphabetically written numbers in such patients. Fortunately, this elegant comparison can be made from data presented by Hécaen and Kremin (1976). They describe (p. 298) four alexic patients: three had no writing deficits, one a slight writing deficit. All four were better at reading aloud numbers written ideographically than numbers written alphabetically; indeed one made no errors with ideographic numbers and almost 100 per cent errors with alphabetic numbers. This implies that it is the printed form, not the semantics, which is the relevant factor in cases where number sparing is observed; the right hemisphere is relatively good at reading ideographs. A possible difficulty, however, for this idea is raised by the patient of Sasanuma and Monoi (1975): this Japanese aphasic, who had left-hemisphere damage, could comprehend printed Arabic numerals but not kanji characters.

There is surprisingly little work with normal subjects on the topic of hemispheric asymmetry in digit processing. One might argue that the findings of Dimond and Beaumont (1972) indicate a right-hemisphere advantage in digit comprehension, and Hirata and Osaka (1967) demonstrated a right-hemisphere superiority for the recall of briefly displayed Arabic digits, but virtually all of the abundant work of the past fifteen years on hemispheric effects with printed stimuli has used letters or words, not numbers. Much work with numbers is needed before one can maintain with any confidence the suggestions advanced here, that the right hemisphere inferiority usually observed in the processing of print is reduced or even reversed when the stimuli are digits and that this occurs because of the nature of the script, not the semantics of the stimuli. Worth pondering also is the finding of Brooks (1973), referred to by Bryden and Allard (1976): a left-hemisphere superiority in processing normal print accompanied by a right-hemisphere superiority in processing handwriting.

These considerations suggest that, if deep dyslexics are using their right hemispheres to read, their performance with numbers and with hand-written material might be relatively spared. This has not been systematically explored, although Patterson (1979) has observed that one of her patients is able to read John Morton's handwriting – no mean feat.

Imageability/concreteness

Some words can easily be imaged (DISASTER, FANTASY) and some not (CHARLATAN, ECONOMY); some are concrete (DISASTER, CHARLATAN) and some abstract (FANTASY, ECONOMY); these examples are taken from Richardson (1975). It is by no means clear that we need distinguish these two variables, especially since they are so highly correlated, but if we do, it appears (Marcel and Patterson, 1979) that the relevant one for our present purposes is imagery rather than concreteness. Both terms will be used here.

Ellis and Shepherd (1974) carried out a tachistoscopic experiment with normal subjects; on each trial a pair of words was presented, on opposite sides of a fixation point. One word was concrete, the other abstract, and the subject's task was to report the words he saw. Concrete words yielded an insignificant left-hemisphere advantage; abstract words a significant one. A similar experiment by Orenstein and Meighan (1976) yielded a similar interaction between hemisphere and concreteness, though this was not statistically significant (perhaps, as these authors note, because of an order-of-report artifact). Hines (1976, 1977) has also carried out similar experiments, and again observed an interaction between hemispheres and concreteness: the left-hemisphere superiority was greater for abstract words than for concrete words. A difficulty with all these experiments, addressed only by Hines (1977) but perhaps not completely adequately, is that when one is dealing with percentages as data, whether one obtains an interaction between two variables depends on what data transformation is used, and there is no way in which to make a non-arbitrary choice of transformation; even no transformation at all represents an arbitrary choice. For example, suppose concrete words yielded percentages correct of 80 per cent in the left hemisphere and 40 per cent in the right hemisphere, and abstract words yielded a percentage correct of 60 per cent in the left hemisphere. What right-hemisphere result would constitute a zero interaction? One could suggest 20 per cent (to maintain a constant 40 per cent difference between hemispheres) or 30 per cent (to maintain a constant 2:1 ratio of performance between hemispheres); and if transformations of the percentages were to be used, still other values could be taken as indicating absence of interaction.

Marcel and Patterson (1979) avoided this problem. They presented single words to the left or right of a fixation point, and followed the word with a pattern mask. The stimulus-onset asynchrony (SOA) of the mask was adjusted separately for the two visual hemifields until, with high-imageability words, the subject was equally accurate in the two hemifields. At these SOAs, low-imageability words presented to the left hemisphere were reported just as well as high imageability words; with right hemisphere presentation, low-imageability words were reported much less accurately than high-imageability words. Because concreteness and imageability were varied orthogonally, it was possible to determine that imageability was having an effect here whilst concreteness was not.

This set of tachistoscopic experiments provides evidence of a selective disability of the right hemisphere: it has difficulty in dealing with words which are low in imageability.[2] Unfortunately, this result is not unanimously obtained. Hatta (1977b), using tachistoscopic presentation of single high-frequency kanji characters, found that performance was more accurate with right hemisphere presentation and also with concrete rather than abstract kanji; but there was no trace of an interaction between hemisphere and concreteness. Saffran, Bogyo, Schwartz and Marin (see Chapter 17) presented single words or pronounceable non-words oriented vertically, to the left or right of a fixation point, with a following pattern mask. Abstract words were reported better than concrete words; performance was better with left-hemisphere presentation; but there was no interaction between hemisphere and concreteness. In a second experiment using the Marcel-Patterson method of equating performance across the hemispheres on concrete nouns by allowing SOA to vary, again no hemisphere-by-concreteness interaction was observed.

Interactions between hemispheres and imageability/concreteness have been studied by Day (1977) using reaction time rather than report accuracy. In a lexical decision experiment where the subject pressed a button if a vertically-oriented letter-string was a word and did nothing if it was not a word, the time taken to respond positively to concrete words was equivalent for left-hemisphere and right-hemisphere presentation. This implies that the right hemisphere is as capable as the left hemisphere of deciding that a concrete noun is a word. In contrast, when the stimulus was an abstract noun, mean reaction time was 35 msec. faster when the stimulus was presented to the left hemisphere than when it was presented to the right.

If the two hemispheres are equally competent at lexical decision with concrete nouns, one would expect, if control of the responding hand was primarily from the hemisphere contralateral to it, that there would be an interaction between response hand and hemifield of presentation: the left hand should be faster with left than with right visual hemifield presentation, and the reverse should be true for the right hand. This was so in Day's experiment; however, the interaction was not statistically significant, though it was in the predicted direction and was very similar in size (12 msec.) to the comparable hand-by-field interactions obtained (statistically significantly) by Moscovitch (1976). A similar interaction (also in the predicted direction but not significant) was evident in error rates: with left-hand responding, a failure to respond, i.e. a 'No' judgment, was more likely with right visual field than with left visual field presentation, and the reverse was true for right-hand responding. These two interactions, although neither is significant, do support the conclusions from the reaction-time data that the right hemisphere is as competent as the left at lexical decision with concrete nouns.

If the right hemisphere inferiority observed in lexical decisions with abstract words were due, not to a complete incapacity of the right hemisphere, but just to a relative slowness, one would expect hand-by-field interactions of the sort just described, in the response to abstract words. This did not occur: for both reaction times and errors, not only were the interactions minute (3 msec. in the case of reaction times) but both were in the opposite direction to that predicted by the view that the right hemisphere is performing the lexical decision task with the abstract words.

Thus Day's data suggest that with concrete words the two hemispheres are equally competent at lexical decision, whereas with abstract words the right hemisphere is so much inferior to the left that decisions are always made by the left hemisphere even when the stimuli are presented initially to the right hemisphere. This does not, of course, imply that the right hemisphere is incapable of deciding that an abstract noun is a word; it may simply be extremely slow at doing so.

Tzeng, Hung, Cotton and Wang (1979) carried out a lexical decision experiment exactly like Day's, except that the stimuli were pairs of Chinese characters. The subjects' task was to decide whether each character pair represented a genuine Chinese word or not. They found in this lexical decision task a left-hemisphere reaction time advantage; this advantage was greater for low-imagery than for high-imagery words, as Day found.

Day (1977) also carried out a semantic-categorization experiment to investigate the interaction of concreteness with hemisphere. On each trial of this experiment, the subject saw a centrally-presented category name, followed by a noun presented to the left or the right of centre; he pressed a button if this noun were an exemplar of the category, otherwise did nothing.

Exactly the same pattern of results emerged. When the category and its exemplar were concrete, reaction times were equivalent for the hemispheres. The hand-by-field interaction for reaction times were again in the direction predicted by the hypothesis that the hemisphere to which the concrete noun is presented is the one which performs the categorization task; the interaction was larger this time (24 msec.) but still not significant. The error-rate interaction of hand-by-field was also in the direction predicted by this hypothesis, but also not significant.

When the category and its exemplar were abstract, reaction times were 36 msec. faster with left-hemisphere presentation, and neither reaction times nor error rates yielded interactions of the kind implying any right-hemisphere involvement in decision-making (in any case, these interactions were not only statistically insignificant, but very small).

Bradshaw and Gates (1978) studied the effects of hemisphere of presentation and abstractness/concreteness on naming latency. Their Figure 5 suggests larger effects of abstractness in the right than in the left hemisphere on naming latency but the relevant interactions were not significant. However, abstract words showed a larger left-hemisphere advantage than concrete words in terms of number of naming *errors* made. Thus some evidence in support of Day's conclusions was obtained.

These studies of the effects of imageability/concreteness on hemispheric asymmetry provide a substantial amount of evidence that for words high in imageability or concreteness the two cerebral hemispheres differ little or not at all in the ability to perform such tasks as lexical decision, semantic classification, or tachistoscopic identification; in contrast abstract words or those rated low on imageability are dealt with much better by the left hemisphere than by the right. Whether the right hemisphere can deal with such words at all remains to be discovered. (It also remains to be discovered why the interaction between hemispheres and imageability has failed to appear in some studies.)

Lexical decision

As has just been discussed, the results of Day (1977) suggest that the right hemisphere is as competent as the left at lexical decision provided that words are high in imageability or concreteness.

There is confirmatory neuropsychological evidence: the patient of Caplan and Hedley-White (1974) who, it can be argued, was reading with the right hemisphere, could not only judge that *catat* and *xedog* were non-words, but could point to the letters *-at* and *xe-* indicating that these letters were 'wrong'.

There have been several other studies of hemispheric effects in lexical decision tasks. In two experiments, Cohen and Freeman (1979) found no differences between the two visual hemifields in the mean reaction time of the Yes response. Leiber (1976) found that Yes responses were slower in the left visual hemifield, and that this hemispheric effect was larger for five-letter than for four-letter words; the latency of No responses did not differ between hemifields.

Bradshaw, Gates and Nettleton (1977) found a left-hemisphere superiority in Yes latency, and in No latency, only for male, right-handed subjects. Bradshaw and Gates (1978) found a left-hemisphere superiority in Yes latency, except for female subjects in the first half of the experiment. The results of these studies are of limited interest, since in none of them is information provided about the imageability values of the words used, and as discussed above this appears to determine whether or not a left hemisphere advantage in lexical decision will occur. However, the interaction of hemisphere of presentation with handedness and sex noted by Bradshaw *et al.* (1977) deserves attention; Day (1977) noted that six of his subjects showed a right-hemisphere advantage for abstract nouns, and of these subjects five were women, and both Bradshaw *et al.* (1977) and Bradshaw and Gates (1978) demonstrated reduced left-hemisphere advantages for women in the lexical decision task.

Semantic errors

There are two fragments of information which suggest that, when the right-hemisphere reading system is dealing with a word, it is liable to make a semantic error, i.e. to confuse this word with another, semantically related, word.

Firstly, the patient with alexia without agraphia studied by Caplan *et al.* (1974) and discussed earlier in this chapter was induced to make such responses as *red* → 'warm', *daisy* → 'flower' and *yellow* → 'brown' when attempting to select and read aloud words of a specific semantic category from a semantically heterogeneous list of printed words. As discussed above, it can be inferred that this patient must have been using a right-hemisphere reading system, in view of her syndrome and her lesion sites.

The patient studied by Gott (1973) must have been using her right hemisphere to read, since her left hemisphere had been removed. Table 1 of Gott's paper lists twenty words which the patient was asked to read aloud. Nine responses were made; five were correct, and the other four were the semantic errors *egg* → 'eat', *cup* → 'coffee, tea', *book* → 'poem', and *cake* → 'yum yum'. It is true that this patient suffered cerebral damage at a very early age (a tumour was discovered when she was eight), and so would be unlikely to have normal cerebral lateralization of language; but, while one could argue that this explains the existence of some reading capacity in the right hemisphere, it does not explain why semantic errors should be one aspect of this capacity.

A related characteristic of this patient was that, when a number was pointed to and she was asked to name it 'the only way she could do so was to begin with one and count until she reached the desired number'. The same behaviour is observed in the deep dyslexic; when asked to read aloud the printed name of a day of the week, the patient may begin 'Monday, Tuesday . . .' and proceed until the correct day is reached (Saffran, personal communication; Patterson, personal communication). Brown (1972, p. 260), discussing the deep dyslexic's attempts at naming letters, notes that 'series speech is ordinarily used as an aid in evoking the desired letter name'. (It should be mentioned here that Patterson's patients do not employ the series stratagem for *letters*.) In Gott's hemispherectomy case, the patient could signal with her fingers the correct number, even though, if asked to name it aloud, she needed to fall back on the counting stratagem. Such a dissociation between comprehension and pronunciation is a major characteristic of deep dyslexia. These points are relevant to a discussion of semantic errors and the right hemisphere because the fact that a number engages the counting strategy in the first place means that the patient recognizes it as a number, even though she cannot pronounce it; if prevented from using the counting strategy and forced to make a vocal response, she would therefore presumably have produced some number or other, and, unless she guessed correctly, this response would be a semantic error.

The observations described here in connection with the possibility of a proneness of the right hemisphere reading system to semantic errors may not be especially compelling, but they do describe circumstances in which the right hemisphere has established the superordinate semantic category to which a printed word belongs without deciding which exemplar of the category the word actually is, and also circumstances in which the word chosen by the right hemisphere is an associate of, or shares some semantic features with, the word displayed. Thus one could hardly dismiss such observations as irrelevant to a discussion of the characteristics of a right-hemisphere reading system and their relationship to deep dyslexia.

Résumé

This section began by arguing that one cannot reject outright the view that the right hemisphere can read. The question is not whether or not this can happen; the question instead is what are the characteristics of the reading system located in the right hemisphere? Clinical and experimental investigations provide some hints as to what these characteristics might be:

1 It can be claimed with some confidence that the right hemisphere appears to be entirely unable to convert a printed representation into a phonological representation. This appears to be the case both for pre-lexical phonological recoding (e.g. the results of Cohen and Freeman, 1979) and for post-lexical phonological recoding (e.g. the results of Klatzky and Atkinson, 1971), especially since the task employed by Zaidel (1978), on which the right hemisphere failed completely, could have been performed using either kind of phonological recoding.

2 In Japanese readers, the right hemisphere is better at processing kanji characters than kana characters; the left hemisphere shows the reverse specialization.

3 The right hemisphere has a special affinity for numbers; it seems likely that it occurs only when the numbers are written as Arabic numerals, and that therefore it is not a semantic effect, but an effect due to form of orthography.

4 The right hemisphere reading system has selective difficulty in processing words which are abstract or of low imageability; though this finding is not unanimous, it is found that the hemispheres are equally proficient if a word is concrete or highly imageable, whereas the right hemisphere is worse than the left with words which are low in imageability or abstract.

5 There is sparse but intriguing evidence that, when reading relies on a right-hemisphere system, a susceptibility to semantic errors occurs.

Deep dyslexia as right-hemisphere reading

Preliminary considerations

Numerous findings, not only those concerning phonology and mentioned earlier in this chapter, suggest that of all linguistic capabilities it is speech which is least well represented in the right hemisphere. Even when speech appears to be originating from the right hemisphere of an aphasic patient whose now damaged left-hemisphere had been specialized for speech, this right-hemisphere speech is extremely impoverished (Kinsbourne, 1971) and certainly far worse than the speech of deep dyslexics, even those who display the characteristics of Broca's aphasia. I begin, therefore, with the assumption that when a deep dyslexic pronounces print, his speech is produced by the left hemisphere. This assumption is testable; if it turns out to be false, then the right-hemisphere hypothesis developed below will require some modifications, but these would not be major ones. Of course, if it turns out that the deep dyslexic's oral reading responses *are* generated by his right hemisphere, this would in itself provide compelling reasons for believing that his reading comprehension also depends upon the right hemisphere, i.e. reasons for accepting a right-hemisphere hypothesis for deep dyslexia.

A second preliminary point which needs to be made here concerns the locus of speech *comprehension* in the deep dyslexic. At least some deep dyslexics make semantic errors when writing to dictation (see, e.g., Marshall and Newcombe, 1966; Saffran, Schwartz and Marin, 1976). If the hypothesis advanced in this chapter concerning how a deep dyslexic reads were to be extended to writing, it might be necessary to claim that the deep dyslexic who makes semantic errors in writing to dictation is comprehending speech with his right hemisphere whilst generating written output from his left hemisphere. Since not much is yet known about semantic errors in writing to dictation, this issue will not be explored further here.

A third preliminary point which seems worth mentioning has to do with the extent and locus of the left hemisphere lesion in deep dyslexia. Tomographic scans are available for five deep dyslexic patients; all five scans are reproduced in this volume; and all five show extremely extensive left-hemisphere lesions. The sheer size of these lesions may predispose one towards arguing that reading comprehension must depend upon the right hemisphere in these patients, since the damage to the left hemisphere, especially to regions of that hemisphere normally associated with linguistic functions, is so extensive. A proponent of the right-hemisphere hypothesis, however, needs to be wary in advancing this argument, if at the same time the view is being taken that the deep dyslexic's spoken output is originating from the left hemisphere. If the left-hemisphere damage is so extensive as to make reading by the left hemisphere seem an unlikely prospect, why is speech by the left hemisphere not also unlikely? This is not a devastating difficulty, since the right-hemisphere hypothesis is not committed to the assumption that it is the left hemisphere which controls speech when the deep dyslexic reads aloud; but it is clearly an issue which needs to be kept in mind.

Because deep dyslexia can occur even when speech is only mildly impaired, and certainly not impaired in ways which correspond to the reading impairment (e.g., Low, 1931; Shallice and Warrington, 1975; Yamadori, 1975; Sasanuma, 1974; and patient W.S. of Saffran *et al.*, referred to in Chapter 2), it is difficult to claim that deep dyslexia is produced by some general impairment internal to left-hemisphere linguistic systems (e.g. destruction of left-hemisphere lexical entries for abstract words or for function words). The particular version of the right-hemisphere hypothesis advanced here instead suggests that what is lost in deep dyslexia is access from print to the left-hemisphere lexicon, i.e. orthographic access to this lexicon. When the deep dyslexic is asked to read a word aloud, then his problem, put very crudely, is this: orthographic input to a right hemisphere linguistic system is possible, but speech output is not; speech output from a left hemisphere linguistic system is possible, but orthographic input is not. If so, the task of reading aloud will require (a) orthographic input to a right-hemisphere reading system, followed by (b) transfer from the right hemisphere to the left of information which can be used (c) to select from amongst the phonological forms of words stored in the left hemisphere that form which corresponds to the word being looked at.

One can produce reasonable arguments concerning the nature of the information used for this interhemispheric communication. The information cannot be phonological, since, as argued earlier, the right hemisphere lacks the ability to derive phonology from print. It cannot be orthographic since, *ex hypothesi*, the left hemisphere of the deep dyslexic lacks the ability to be accessed orthographically. Two remaining possibilities are that the information is semantic, or that it takes the form of an image. The latter cannot be the only explanation because one common error in deep dyslexia is to read one function word as another, completely unrelated, function word, and no imaginal representation could be linking two such words. Other reasons for rejecting an account of deep dyslexic errors in terms of imaginal mediation are given elsewhere in this volume (Chapter 6). It may be that an imaginal code is used sometimes, and a semantic code used sometimes, for interhemispheric communication; but the assumption will be made here that only one form of code is used, and it follows that this code is semantic, if an imaginal code can sometimes be ruled out.

The argument, then, is that when a deep dyslexic reads aloud, he does so by firstly accessing (correctly or incorrectly) an entry in a right-hemisphere lexicon. From this entry, he retrieves a semantic representation and transmits this representation to the left-hemisphere, where it is used to access an entry in the left-hemisphere lexicon. Once a left-hemisphere entry is identified, phonological information can be retrieved and, finally, articulated.

This view runs into difficulties[3] when one considers alexia without agraphia (pure alexia). Many of the patients suffering from this syndrome have intact right hemispheres, with splenial and left-occipital lesions. Their reading performance is far worse than that of deep dyslexics. Why is this so if the right hemisphere is intact? It seems necessary for a proponent of the right-hemisphere hypothesis to suppose that the pathway for communicating between the right-hemisphere reading system and the left-hemisphere speech-output system relies to a considerable extent on the splenium; thus, the crucial interhemispheric intercommunication is unimpaired in deep dyslexia, but impaired in pure alexia because of the splenial lesion.

However, although a splenial lesion has severe consequences for reading English, its consequences for Japanese are much less severe, as far as kanji is concerned. The patients studied by Sugishita *et al.* (1978), who had splenial sections, could nevertheless read kanji quite well in the left visual field; reading of kana in this field was much more impaired. This implies that in these Japanese patients there is a non-splenial callosal pathway, which can be used for kanji far more successfully than it can for kana.

If such a non-splenial pathway existed in English readers, then the right hemisphere reading system could communicate with the left hemisphere speech-output system even when there is a splenial section. Consequently, the reading deficit in pure alexia should not be severe; yet it is.

We are left with what looks like a direct contradiction. Data from Japanese patients suggest the existence of a useful non-splenial pathway from the right-hemisphere reading system to the left-hemisphere speech-output system; data from English patients with pure alexia suggest that there is no such pathway. In fact there is no contradiction here. If this non-splenial pathway is specifically related to ideographic printed symbols it will allow the Japanese reader to read ideographic symbols (kanji) presented in the left visual field even when he has a splenial lesion, and it will allow the English patient suffering from pure alexia to read ideographic symbols (e.g. numerals) even when he cannot read alphabetically-printed words. Number sparing is, of course, a distinctive feature of pure alexia, as noted earlier in this chapter.

One can therefore maintain the view that the splenium is important for interhemispheric transmission of semantic representations of alphabetically-printed words, and hence that the superior reading of deep dyslexics in comparison with pure alexics is due to the intactness of the splenium in deep dyslexia.

If the deep dyslexic can use only a right-hemisphere reading system for dealing with print, then one can infer what deep dyslexic reading must be like from those characteristics of the right hemisphere reading system revealed by studies of non-dyslexic subjects or patients and described earlier in this chapter. The deep dyslexic's inability to derive phonology from print (pre-lexically or post-lexically) is a consequence, it can be argued, of the *independently* demonstrable inability of the right hemisphere to perform such phonological tasks. The fact that, if a Japanese reader suffers from deep dyslexia, he will also always show a relative sparing of kanji over kana is likewise a consequence of the selective ability of the right hemisphere to process kanji. The deep dyslexic is better with concrete/high-imagery words than abstract/low-imagery words, as is the right hemisphere; and both the deep dyslexic and right hemisphere are prone to make semantic errors.

It seems fair to claim that the arguments advanced so far in this chapter make a reasonable *prima facie* case for the hypothesis that the deep dyslexic's reading is mediated by a right-hemisphere reading system. Considerably more detailed arguments would be required, however, to make this case really compelling. Furthermore, some of the major characteristics of deep dyslexia have not been mentioned yet in this chapter, the reason being that there are no results from work with non-dyslexic patients or normal subjects which are relevant to these characteristics. One could claim that, since the deep dyslexic makes visual errors and has difficulty with function words, these problems must characterize the right hemisphere reading system too, and such claims could be investigated with normal subjects; but this has not yet been done. Hence, there is no *independent* evidence for such an interpretation of the deep dyslexic's visual errors and function-word difficulties.

In the remainder of the chapter, I will consider how a right-hemisphere hypothesis might deal with some of the characteristics of deep dyslexia not discussed so far. These considerations will be more speculative and tentative than any advanced earlier in this chapter, since studies of other kinds of readers which could yield useful supporting evidence simply have not been carried out. The particular symptoms to be dealt with in the remainder of the chapter are semantic errors, function-word difficulties, syntactic analysis, the abstractness/imageability effect, visual errors, and derivational errors.

Semantic errors

It was suggested in Chapter 3 that one can distinguish at least two categories of semantic error: associative errors and shared-feature errors. Associative errors are those which are like word-association responses: examples are *next* → 'exit', *merry* → 'Christmas', *income* → 'tax', *sad* → 'sack', *pale* → 'ale' and *ideal* → 'milk'. The relationship of stimulus to response in such examples is not one of sharing a subset of semantic features. Shared-feature errors are those in which stimulus and response *do* share a subset of semantic features: *draw* → 'paint', *est* → 'nord', *found* → 'lost', *tulip* → 'crocus', and *sepulchre* → 'tomb'.

How might these shared-feature semantic errors be explained, in the context of a right-hemisphere hypothesis? There are several possible avenues to be pursued. Firstly, the lexical entry for a word in the right hemisphere might lack some semantic features, so that what is available for transmission to the left hemisphere is an incomplete semantic representation. Secondly, it might instead be argued that, even if the right hemisphere lexical entry is semantically complete, not all the semantic information is despatched to the left hemisphere. Thirdly, it might be argued that complete semantic information is dispatched, but some semantic information is lost en route – similar arguments are made to explain the right-ear advantage in dichotic listening. There are too many theoretical alternatives here, and it is fortunate that powerful constraints upon the alternatives are provided by some results obtained by Patterson (1978). She showed that a patient who produces a response such as *Thermos* → 'flask' will not only tend to give such semantic-error responses a low confidence rating (in contrast to visual errors, where the patient is often confident that his response is correct), but when later asked which of the spoken words 'Thermos' and 'flask' corresponds to the printed word *thermos* will often be able correctly to choose 'thermos'.

This suggests that, although the patient responded 'flask' when trying to read *thermos* the semantic information reaching the left hemisphere is closer to a characterization of *thermos* than of *flask*. The patient accepts the match between the semantic representation of *thermos* (sent from the right hemisphere) and the semantic representation of *flask* (obtained from the left-hemisphere lexical entry for *flask*) since there is a reasonable correspondence between the two representations; but the correspondence is not perfect, and the appreciation of this is what makes the patient lack some confidence in the correctness of his response. When his attention is drawn to the left-hemisphere entry for *thermos* as well as that for *flask*, which is what happens in the forced-choice task, he can determine that the semantic information coming from the right hemisphere matches *thermos* even more closely than it matches *flask*, and hence can correct his original semantic error.

Shallice and Warrington (1975, p. 198) originally proposed that semantic errors occur either when stimulus and response are semantically very similar (e.g. *pencil* → 'biro') or are both abstract (e.g. *fiction* → 'acting'). In fact, many semantic errors do not fit either of these patterns. However, Patterson (1978) provides evidence that those semantic errors which *do* fit one or other pattern are the errors which are not likely to be corrected in the forced-choice task.

The difficulty in correcting errors where stimulus and response are approximately synonymous is obviously consistent with the argument being advanced here; in the limit, where stimulus and response are exact synonyms, the semantic information transmitted from print via the right hemisphere to the left hemisphere is equally consistent with both left-hemisphere lexical entries, so the forced-choice response can only be a guess.

The difficulty in correcting errors with abstract words is attributed to the impoverishment of semantic information in the right-hemisphere lexical entries of abstract words. This is discussed at more length shortly; if abstract words have impoverished semantic representations in the right hemisphere, semantic errors which cannot be corrected in the forced choice test will arise because inadequate semantic information reaches the left hemisphere.

It is argued, then, that shared-feature semantic errors arise because, when the patient is searching the left-hemisphere lexicon for an entry whose semantic representation matches that which has been sent from the right hemisphere, he is willing to accept imperfect matches. The more specific (the lower in the semantic hierarchy) the mismatching feature is, the more willing the patient is to overlook the mismatch; hence the finding that semantic error responses tend to differ from the stimuli at a highly specific semantic level whilst preserving generic semantic information.

Since associative semantic errors lack shared semantic features, they cannot be interpreted in terms of feature loss or semantic ambiguity. Instead, it will be proposed that they reflect the existence of an associative network within the right-hemisphere lexicon. This network may have functional significance for reading, since, when a lexical entry is accessed, the entries of words which are now contextually likely are primed so that they are temporarily more accessible. Hence several lexical entries are excited even though only a single word is presented. An incorrect choice from the set of associatively related candidate entries would produce an associative semantic error. This is a familiar approach to theorizing about the genesis of semantic errors. Since normal readers do not make associative semantic errors, there must be a procedure available to the normal reader, but not to the deep dyslexic, which prevents associative semantic errors. This procedure is usually considered to involve the use of some non-lexical stimulus record which is matched against each lexical candidate until the correct one is identified. The nature of this non-lexical record is problematical. It is tempting to suppose that the record uses a phonological code, because the demonstrable inability of the deep dyslexic to derive phonology from print would explain his susceptibility to associative semantic errors. However, as Chapter 10 indicates, there is little or no evidence that normal skilled readers need to use phonological recoding at all. On the other hand, if the non-lexical stimulus record uses a visual code, then one must postulate that the deep dyslexic is deficient in the formation of visual codes; and there is no independent evidence for such a deficit. Theoretical resolution is needed here; even without this, it is suggested that associative semantic errors occur in deep dyslexia because a set of associatively related candidate words become available in the right hemisphere lexicon in response to the presentation of a single word, and an incorrect choice from this set is sometimes made; this incorrect choice is then transmitted to the left hemisphere and eventually uttered.

Function words

When a deep dyslexic is asked to read a printed function word aloud, a common form of response is an omission – no response is made at all. One might explain this by supposing that one characteristic of the right hemisphere lexicon, as yet not studied directly because the appropriate experiments have not been done with normal readers, is that many function words are simply absent from that lexicon. This might be one aspect of the generally poor syntactic ability of the right hemisphere.

However, one cannot adopt this approach to the deep dyslexic's difficulties with function words; the results of Patterson (1979) refute any such approach. She gave her two patients a list of sixty function words to read aloud. One patient produced 38 per cent correct responses, the other 8 per cent. When the sixty functions were randomly intermingled with sixty similar pronounceable non-words, and the patients asked to classify these 120 items as words or non-words, they performed almost perfectly: 97.5 per cent and 98.3 per cent correct responses respectively. Thus one cannot claim that the right hemisphere lacks lexical entries for function words; if it did, almost perfect performance on a lexical decision task with function words could not occur.

Furthermore, since one common form of response to a function word is another, completely unrelated, function word (e.g. *up* → 'and'), it is sometimes the case that the deep dyslexic not only knows that a function word is a word; he knows that it is a *function* word. He simply does not know *which* function word. This stage, evident in the reading of deep dyslexics, also arises in the writing of aphasic patients, as is revealed by the introspections of an aphasic studied by Head (1926, p. 254): discussing spontaneous writing, the patient said: 'I always have to spell out every word, even the little ones; I have to say "of" – I know it's a preposition, but then I have to think is it "to" or "of" or "from". Prepositions are always a bother to me.'

The occurrence of function-word substitutions in reading aloud shows that sometimes the effective semantic representation of the word consists of a single feature, 'function-word'; but this is not always the case. Appendix 2 includes a breakdown of the kinds of responses deep dyslexics produce with printed function words; sometimes the response is a semantically related function word (*usually* → 'sometimes') and sometimes even a semantically related content word (*she* → 'woman'). Here semantic features of function words more specific than the generic feature 'function word' are linking stimulus to response. Thus one cannot claim that all the right hemisphere knows about function words is that they are function words.

Another reason for rejecting such a claim is that the deep dyslexic can sometimes *understand* printed function words:

> although the patient cannot read prepositions aloud, he had no difficulty in correctly selecting pictures on the basis of descriptions containing prepositions. Given, for example, the sentence 'The cup is under the table', he could point to the correct picture of a pair with a cup under and on a table. (Marshall and Newcombe, 1966, p. 175)

Similar observations have been reported by Marin, Saffran and Schwartz (1975):

> a majority of the errors with pronouns involved the substitution of other pronouns. These substitutions were typically unrelated to the target in number, gender or case, but it was possible to demonstrate that at least some of this information was available to the patients by having them indicate to whom the word referred. Thus, in a typical instance, the patient read 'me' as 'him' while pointing to himself.

Chapter 13 describes some systematic explorations of a deep dyslexic's ability to comprehend printed function words. In that chapter, Morton and Patterson argue that function words carry both semantic and syntactic information, and that the patient could appreciate semantic aspects of function words but not syntactic aspects. He could, for example, choose which of two function words goes with a third when the distinction depended upon gender, number, frequency or spatial location, but not when it depended on part of speech (this/thus/that) or case (he/him/her).

These results suggest that the deep dyslexic's behaviour when he attempts to read function words is influenced by two factors: lack of syntactic information about a function word, plus the generation of semantic errors due to the necessity for interhemispheric communication using a semantic representation, as discussed above in the section on semantic errors. If the right hemisphere has difficulties in appreciating syntactic distinctions such as that between *he* and *him*, information allowing such distinctions will be difficult to transmit to the left hemisphere, and hence function-word errors where stimulus and response differ only syntactically will arise: *me* → 'I', *us* → 'we'.

Semantic aspects of function words, such as their gender, are appreciated by the right hemisphere and can be transmitted to the left, but not all of this information is necessarily used when a response is being selected. The patient is willing to tolerate some degree of mismatch between the semantic representation arriving from the right hemisphere and the semantic representation obtained from the left-hemisphere lexical entry for the word he chooses as his response. The more specific the non-matching semantic information is, the more willing the patient is to tolerate the mismatch: hence errors such as *often* → 'sometimes' or *usually* → 'sometimes', where stimulus and response differ semantically only at a highly specific level, or errors such as *where* → 'whither', where stimulus and response are actually synonyms.

Sometimes the only semantic feature of the stimulus used in selecting a response is the most generic feature 'function word'. My impression is that, when this occurs, it is usually with the kind of function word whose function is almost entirely syntactic and which has little or no semantic representation: conjunctions, articles, some prepositions and some adverbs, for example. If this is so, one might argue that with such words the only semantic information the right hemisphere has for the purposes of communication with the left is the semantic feature 'function word'. On this view, semantically rich function words such as personal pronouns, spatial prepositions, or adverbs of time should rarely produce error responses consisting of completely unrelated function words, whereas such responses should be relatively common with semantically sparse function words such as articles, conjunctions, or abstract prepositions and adverbs. There certainly are some counter-examples to this view (*you* → 'why', *in* → 'he', *between* → 'sometimes') but they appear to be rare. More detailed analysis of a corpus of responses to function words will allow this view to be assessed adequately.

What is being suggested concerning the deep dyslexic's difficulties with function words, then, is that they arise from three sources. Firstly, some function words have very sparse semantic representations; interhemispheric communication using a semantic code will not be able to deal satisfactorily with such words. In such cases, sometimes all that can be communicated is that a word is a function word, and perhaps it is even sometimes the case that no semantic information at all can be communicated – hence the high rate of omission responses to function words. Secondly, for function words which have a richer semantic representation, more adequate inter-hemispheric communication is possible, and semantic errors arise for the same reason as with content words. Thirdly, purely syntactic aspects of function words (case, for example) are poorly appreciated by the right hemisphere and thus cannot be reliably communicated to the left.

Syntactic analysis by deep dyslexics

It was shown by Andreewsky and Seron (1975) that a deep dyslexic who could not read aloud conjunctions, prepositions, adverbs, or pronouns, and who read inflected verbs without producing their inflections, was nevertheless able correctly to assign part of speech to the words in a printed sentence. They showed this by using sentences such as *Le car ralentit car le moteur chauffe*. The first *car*, here meaning 'bus', was uttered by the patient, whilst the second, here meaning 'because', was not. This must mean that the patient identified the first *car* as a content word and the second as a function word. Since the two words are orthographically identical, this differential assignment of part of speech could only occur if the syntactic structure of the sentence was understood. This was confirmed by using pseudo-sentences such as *Le train ralentit mer le moteur chauffe*. The word *mer* presented in isolation could be read aloud with ease, since it is a common concrete noun; in the sentence context, it could not be read, presumably because it was assigned the syntactic category 'function word'.

An analogous result was reported by Marin, Saffran and Schwartz (1975). They showed that a word which might be a verb or a noun is more likely to be read aloud when its accompanying context specifies that it is a noun. For example, the underlined word in *The fly buzzed in my ear* was more likely to be read aloud correctly than the underlined word in *The bird will fly away*.

Morton and Patterson (Chapter 13) have explored the deep dyslexic's abilities at syntactic analysis by asking a patient to judge whether printed sentences are grammatical or not: the ungrammatical sentences used personal pronouns having the wrong case (e.g. *Me gave it to him*). The patient made some errors, but performed above chance, even though this patient was at chance in deciding which of *he* and *him* goes with *her*, i.e. at performing this triad task on the basis of case of personal pronouns. His ability to appreciate the case of personal pronouns in a sentence context but not when they are presented in isolation suggests that the sentence context assists processing of individual words; perhaps this is why the patient of Andreewsky and Seron (1975) refused to begin reading a sentence aloud until the entire sentence had been shown to him.

These examples indicate that the deep dyslexic has some, perhaps a considerable, ability to analyse a sentence syntactically, at least implicitly. If deep dyslexics read with their right hemisphere, then it will be necessary to credit the right hemisphere with at least this level of syntactic ability. The finding that a patient utters the first *car* but not the second in *Le car ralentit car le moteur chauffe* might be explained as follows. Since *car* has two quite different meanings, it has two distinct lexical entries in the right hemisphere. At some stage, a decision must be taken as to which of these entries is to be the source of the semantic information to be transferred to the left hemisphere. The right hemisphere is capable of using sentence context to determine that, for the first *car*, information must be retrieved from the noun entry whilst for the second it must be retrieved from the conjunction entry. In the pseudo-sentence *Le train ralentit mer le moteur chauffe*, this decision process rejects the noun entry for *mer* since the syntactic context makes it impossible for the fourth word in the sentence to be a noun.

When a single word whose meaning and part of speech is ambiguous is presented without context, both lexical entries are accessed, and the choice is made in terms of a bias towards content words, and, amongst content words, towards nouns. Hence the French patient treats *est* as 'East' not 'is'; and hence *nice* → 'place in the South of France' (Marshall and Newcombe, 1966).

The abstractness/imageability effect

The deep dyslexic makes numerous errors and omissions when attempting to read abstract words. This is consistent with the claim that deep dyslexics use the right hemisphere to read, if we accept the (not entirely unequivocal) evidence for selective impairment of the right hemisphere for abstract words, demonstrated in experiments with normal subjects. The term 'selective impairment' is a vague one, however. It could be taken to mean that lexical entries for some abstract words are simply not present in the right hemisphere. Alternatively, it could be that such entries are present, but are selectively impoverished or inaccessible. The experiments carried out with normal subjects do not allow us to distinguish between these different ways in which the right hemisphere impairment with abstract words could be characterized.

A similar question was raised above in connection with function words; the resolution of this issue was provided by Patterson (1979) who showed that her two patients were virtually perfect at lexical decision with function words and so argued that their difficulties with such words cannot be due to absence of lexical entries. She has also investigated (Patterson, 1979) the performance of her patients in lexical decision tasks with abstract words, and therefore has collected evidence which allows clarification of the basis of the deep dyslexic's difficulties with abstract words.

One of these experiments involved 150 abstract words and 149 non-words (all non-words being pronounceable and differing by one letter from an abstract word, e.g. *sufframe, origilate*). The instruction to the patient was 'go through the list of mixed words and non-words; if it is a word try to say it; if it is not a word, say No'. Patient D.E. missed 40 of the 150 words. This implies that the entries for these abstract words are absent from the right-hemisphere lexicon of this patient. However, of the remaining 110 words, D.E. was unable to read 78 of them aloud, or even to produce an erroneous reading response; his response to these was 'Yes, but can't say it'. If the abstract-word lexical entries which are present in his right-hemisphere lexicon are intact, this high rate of 'omission' responses is inexplicable. One is forced to conclude that, for those abstract words which are actually present in the right-hemisphere lexicon, the lexical entries are often impoverished: whatever semantic information is present in these impoverished entries is insufficient for the interhemispheric semantic communication upon which oral reading depends. Thus the pattern of results displayed by D.E. when performing lexical decision with abstract words suggests that some abstract words are not represented as lexical entries in the right hemisphere, whilst others possess lexical entries but suffer because these entries contain impoverished semantic information or no semantic information at all. For these latter words, lexical decision Yes responses can be made because lexical access occurs; but the words cannot be uttered because the semantic representations required for transmission to the left hemisphere are absent or inadequate. This is consistent with the fact that, of D.E.'s 13 paralexic reading responses to the 150 abstract words, only one was a clear semantic error, and it was of the associative type, a class of error attributed here to intrahemispheric associations, not interhemispheric communication; this error was *ideal* → 'milk'.

The performance of Patterson's second patient on lexical decision with abstract words was considerably better. This is not surprising, as Patterson notes, because the first patient, D.E., suffered his cerebral injury at the age of sixteen, claims that he rarely read before his accident, and had left school at fifteen, whilst the second patient, P.W., is a former civil servant who suffered a stroke at the age of fifty-seven. This second patient responded No only to six of the 150 abstract words; but again the patient often indicated that a word was a word without being able to utter it; this occurred with 47 words. Semantic errors did occur, implying that semantic representations of some of the abstract words became available.

The performance of P.W. in classifying items as words or nonwords was within normal limits, implying that his right-hemisphere lexicon is not selectively deficient in lexical entries for abstract words (unlike the right hemisphere of D.E.), but the high rate of 'omission' responses suggests a selective deficiency of the semantic information contained in these entries. This semantic deficit is thus evident in both patients. The lexical deficit additionally evident in D.E. may not be specific to abstract words. A possibility considered by Patterson (1979) is that the missed words were never known to this patient, and so were never present even in the left-hemisphere lexicon; it could also have been a word-frequency rather than an abstractness effect. Thus it is unclear whether we should conclude that abstract words selectively lack right-hemisphere lexical entries; but it will be concluded here that semantic representations of abstract words are selectively impaired in the right hemisphere lexicon. Semantic errors to abstract words (*procrastinate* → 'late') indicate some comprehension; however, the most direct way of investigating this is to study the comprehension of printed abstract by these patients. If they show substantial comprehension of abstract words which they can classify as words but cannot utter, the hypothesis of a selective semantic deficit will have to be rejected.

Visual errors

Shallice and Warrington (1975) suggested that the abstractness effect and the visual error may be related, noting that when a deep dyslexic makes a visual error his response is usually much less abstract than the stimulus: raters judged that in 73 per cent of visual errors, the response was more concrete than the stimulus. A related, but different, claim is that abstract words are more likely than concrete words to generate visual errors. An analysis of data kindly provided by N. Kapur, consisting of the responses of his patient (Kapur and Perl, 1978) to the 650 words of the list drawn up by Brown and Ure (1969), showed that the mean concreteness of the words producing visual errors was 4.31, and of the words producing semantic errors 5.26, a significant difference (median split $\chi^2 = 5.22$, p<.05). Thus there is some evidence that abstract words are particularly likely to generate visual errors.

Shallice and Warrington (1975) proposed the following explanations of visual errors:

> A visual error would . . . result when a more abstract semantic unit cannot be adequately stimulated by the maximally

activated graphemic unit. A more concrete semantic unit which is excited by a less activated graphemic unit would then become the most strongly excited and dominant semantic unit. Visual error responses are indeed more concrete than the stimulus as would be predicted.

Essentially this view will be adopted here, except that it will be suggested that patients are capable of exerting some strategic control over the process of activation of 'semantic units' by 'graphemic units' (to use Shallice and Warrington's terms). It will be argued (and for very similar arguments see Patterson, 1978) that this occurs because, on those occasions where the abstract word a deep dyslexic is looking at lacks a lexical entry in his right-hemisphere lexicon, and hence is effectively a non-word, the patient uses a strategy which might be called 'approximate visual access' in his effort to pronounce a word. This strategy consists of finding, amongst those lexical entries which *are* present in the right hemisphere, that entry which is orthographically maximally similar to the word being viewed. If no very similar entry is found, the patient does not respond, i.e. produces an omission error.

There seems no doubt that deep dyslexics can and do use this strategy when they are attempting to pronounce genuine non-words. For example, Low (1931, p. 565) reported the results of presenting 60 nonsense syllables to his patient, and asking him to read them aloud. The patient produced a response to 19 of these. Amongst the responses were *sto* → 'story', *fal* → 'fat', *ser* → 'serve', *tla* → 'atlas', *cor* → 'corrupt', *jun* → 'jump', *lom* → 'lemon'. Goldstein (1948) reported that his patient was as good as, if not better than, normals at uttering mutilated words, such as *hsptl* → 'hospital', *starcase* → 'staircase', *gradn* → 'garden'. Patterson and Marcel (1977) presented their patients with pronounceable non-words, some of which were phonologically identical to English words. One patient correctly read three (*toun* → 'town', *flore* → 'floor' and *wurk* → 'work'); the other none. Amongst their incorrect responses were *dake* → 'drake', *sprade* → 'spade', *rud* → 'naughty', and *glem* → 'jewel'.

All of these examples demonstrate that a deep dyslexic can, and is sometimes willing to, proceed from a printed non-word to the lexical entry of a word whose spelling approximates that of the non-word. He will rarely, if ever, produce a non-word as his spoken response. If asked to pronounce a non-word, he will either remain silent, or else will access the lexical entry of a word visually similar to the non-word, and say that word as his response (or even make a semantic error, as in *rud* → 'naughty' and *glem* → 'jewel').

This was shown most directly by Saffran and Marin (1977) who presented their subject with 60 non-words, all phonologically identical to English words; they were to be read aloud. The fewer letters the non-word had in common with the word whose pronunciation it shared, the less likely the subject was to say the latter word. Thus no response was made to *koppee, kowtch, foan* or *mewzik*, whereas responses such as *poynt* → 'point', *nife* → 'knife', *paynt* → 'paint' and *bootes* → 'shoes' were made.

Now, the response *paynt* → 'paint' is not regarded as a visual error here; but if *paynt* were really a word, and the patient believed it to be the word *paint*, then his response would be classified as a visual error. If the word *origin* is not present in the lexicon used by the deep dyslexic, then he will treat it as a non-word, and so may carry out the kind of approximate visual access he uses to produce 'paint' from *paynt*; hence *origin* → 'organ'. Because some abstract words are absent from the right hemisphere lexicon, a visual error will take the form of responding to an abstract word (effectively a non-word) with a visually similar less abstract word, as Shallice and Warrington (1975) pointed out; and for the same reason abstract words will be particularly likely to evoke visual errors, which appears to be the case, as noted above.

It seems evident from the work of Patterson and Marcel (1977), Saffran and Marin (1977) and Patterson (1978) that the deep dyslexic, although reluctant to attempt to pronounce a non-word, can be persuaded to make this attempt, especially if the non-word is visually very similar to some real word. This is analogous to the situation where only real words are used, but some are abstract and hence absent from the patient's right-hemisphere lexicon; since in these situations the patient expects *all* the stimuli to be words, this expectation might have the effect of inducing him to use the approximate visual access strategy which he is usually reluctant to attempt. Thus instead of an omission in response to an abstract word, he produces a visual error, if he finds an entry with a sufficient degree of visual similarity.

Here it is instructive to return to the work of Patterson (1979) involving lexical decision with abstract words. It was argued that for patient D.E. a substantial proportion of the words used in this work were not represented as lexical entries in his right-hemisphere lexicon. It might be expected that on some occasions when confronted with such a word, D.E. might have used the strategy of approximate visual access in order to try to utter it. But if so, since uttering a real word was counted as a Yes response, even if the word uttered was not the word being inspected, the use of this strategy would have had disastrous consequences for lexical decision performance. In the limit, if D.E. behaved like this with every letter-string for which he lacked a lexical entry, he would produce a false positive for every non-word. He did not do so; he made only 20 false positive responses to the 149 non-words. Putting the problem another way: D.E. always responds 'sandals' to *scandal*. If he does this by using approximate visual access, why would he not always respond 'sandals' to *smandal* also? But if so, how could he perform adequately in a lexical decision task involving abstract words such as *scandal* and non-words visually similar to these, such as *smandal*? Yet D.E. did achieve respectable performance here ($d' = 1.74$).

Detailed inspection of the data of this experiment provides a possible answer. Of D.E.'s twenty false positive responses in the lexical decision task, five were words very similar visually to the non-words which evoked them, and fifteen were 'Yes, but I can't say it' responses. Suppose that D.E. were using the approximate visual access strategy, but only accepting approximate access when visual similarity was sufficiently high. Because every non-word was derived from an abstract word by changing a single letter, it should often have been the case that the lexical entry accessed from a non-word by this strategy would be the entry for an abstract word, and the semantic impoverishment of such entries would prevent effective communication to the left hemisphere. This would produce a 'Yes, but . . .' response to non-words. When interhemispheric communication *was* possible, this would produce a visual error (or conceivably a visual then semantic error, hence perhaps *evel* → 'devil' which D.E. produced).

Consequently, in this situation D.E. was using a criterion for approximate visual access which resulted in accessing a visually similar lexical entry for 20 of 149 non-words: a rather conservative criterion, no doubt because about 50 per cent of the letter-strings seen were non-words and lexical decisions were required. This strategy would have to operate with words too, on those occasions where the word presented lacked a lexical entry; and some of D.E.'s incorrect readings with words were visual errors.

There is further evidence that D.E. was using such a strategy. In reading situations where all the items are words, 'D.E.'s reading yields paralexic errors and omissions in roughly equal proportions'. However, in the lexical decision task with 299 items, 149 of them non-words, D.E. produced in response to the words only 13 paralexic responses, compared to 40 omissions of one kind (responding 'No') and 78 omissions of another kind (responding 'Yes', then indicating that he could not pronounce the word). This would occur if the presence of non-words and the necessity to perform lexical decision had induced D.E. to adopt an unusually stringent criterion for approximate visual access; normally, when only words are presented to him, he uses a loose criterion, which reduces omissions but increases visual errors.

The puzzle involving *scandal*, *smandal* and 'sandals' – how can a high rate of visual errors co-exist with good lexical decision performance, if visual errors are produced by approximate visual access? – is thus dealt with by denying that these two effects do co-exist. A high rate of visual errors occurs in situations where D.E.'s criterion for approximate visual access is lax; good lexical decision performance occurs when he adopts a stringent criterion. A direct test of this would be to present the 150 words used in this lexical decision task for oral reading with no non-words present; the rate of visual errors should now increase greatly and the rate of omissions decrease.

It was suggested above that P.W. differs from D.E. in that P.W.'s right hemisphere lexicon is well stocked with lexical entries for abstract words (even though some of these may be semantically deficient). Thus the situation in which immediate lexical access fails through lack of the appropriate lexical entry, and the approximate visual access strategy would therefore become relevant, will be rare for P.W. Since this strategy produces visual errors it would be expected that P.W. should make relatively few visual errors, and this is so (Patterson, 1978). It would also be expected that the presence of non-words should not perturb P.W.'s reading strategies in the way it perturbed D.E.'s, since P.W. doesnot often need approximate visual access, the use of which causes difficulty in these lexical decision experiments. This could explain why, unusually, P.W. made more visual errors than D.E. in these experiments.

In terms of the right-hemisphere hypothesis, then, it is argued that visual errors arise when a printed word lacks a lexical entry and the patient adopts the approximate visual access strategy; the association between abstractness and visual error occurs because lack of a right-hemisphere lexical entry is more likely to occur when a word is abstract than when it is concrete. This account makes the strong prediction that a word to which a visual error is made will not be comprehended correctly; this contrasts with function-word errors, where an incorrect response can occur with correct comprehension.

Patterson (1978) has shown that when patients rate their confidence in their responses, semantic errors are given lower ratings than visual or derivational errors. The low confidence associated with semantic errors was attributed, earlier in this chapter, to the patient's usually being aware that the semantic representation of the word he has selected as his response does not match exactly the semantic representation of the stimulus as delivered from the right hemisphere. The high confidence associated with visual errors must thus be taken as indicating that patients tend not to be aware that the orthographic representation of the word whose right-hemisphere lexical entry has been accessed does not match exactly the orthographic representation of the word being displayed to the patient. If this lack of awareness occurs because the relevant events are going on in the right hemisphere, then one might expect a patient to be unaware of the associative type of semantic error, if, as argued, this arises in the right hemisphere. Comparisons of the two types of semantic error in terms of confidence ratings and forced-choice testing would be of interest here.

The deep dyslexic is worse at reading aloud adjectives and verbs than at reading aloud nouns. If this effect is partly or wholly due to differential representation of these syntactic classes in the right hemisphere, then, according to the arguments advanced here, adjectives and verbs should generate visual errors more than nouns do. Marshall and Newcombe (1966) report exactly this. This effect, however, could be due to differences in concreteness between the three syntactic categories. The effect of part of speech on oral reading is not due to a confounding with concreteness (Shallice and Warrington, 1975).

This discussion of visual errors has depended heavily on the observation that such errors tend to occur to abstract words and that the response tends to be more concrete than the stimulus; but these are only tendencies. Visual errors *do* occur to highly concrete words, and the error response *can* be more abstract than the stimulus. One can still argue that on such occasions the stimulus, although not belonging to any class of words with respect to which the right hemisphere has been demonstrated to be deficient, is still absent from or inaccessible in the right-hemisphere lexicon; but too frequent a recourse to this argument would clearly be dubious.

An alternative possibility is that orthographic access to the left hemisphere, assumed throughout this chapter to be completely abolished in deep dyslexia, may merely be impaired. An impaired orthographic-access system could produce visual errors (though not semantic or function-word errors, nor derivational errors if they are not merely visual errors). This cannot be the *sole* explanation of visual errors, since it does not explain their association with abstractness; but it may explain *some* visual errors (e.g. those unrelated to abstractness), and so this variant of the right-hemisphere hypothesis may need to be pursued in the future.

Derivational errors

The problem here is not devising a plausible theoretical account of this form of error, but of finding some way of adjudicating between a number of possible accounts. A response such as *had* → 'have' could be (a) an associative semantic error, since this response to this stimulus occurs in word-association norms; (b) a shared-feature semantic error, since *had* and *have* possess common semantic features; (c) a visual error; or (d) a genuinely distinct category of error, the derivational error, in which stimulus and response possess the same root morpheme but different inflectional morphemes. Patterson (1978) has argued that derivational errors cannot be semantic errors because they differ with respect to the confidence ratings assigned them by patients, and also because the two types of error yield different results in her forced-choice task. She has also argued that derivational errors are not visual errors either, since these two error types also yield somewhat different patterns of results. Her arguments will be accepted here, and the view taken that errors which preserve the root morpheme of the stimulus word whilst differing from it in inflectional or derivational morpheme(s) are a distinct category of error and require an explanation independently of the explanation of a semantic or visual error.

Once again, tests involving lexical decision and comprehension provide much valuable evidence. Marin, Saffran and Schwartz (1975) studied comprehension and pronunciation of singular and plural nouns in their patients. These patients were scarcely above chance at giving the correct number of a noun in their oral reading, even when they produced the correct root morpheme. Nevertheless, they could often indicate whether the noun was singular or plural by holding up one or two fingers, even when their oral reading incorporated an incorrect specification of number. However, Patterson (see Chapter 14) found that her patients performed at or near chance when asked to cross out the wrong word in such sentences as *Prince Charles will one day (ruler/rule) the country*, the bracketed pair of words consisting of a word and its derivational error response. It may turn out that the patient's ability to comprehend inflected forms depends on whether the inflections convey semantic information or purely syntactic information: the words *bee* and *bees* differ semantically, whilst the words *she* and *her* differ only syntactically; this kind of possibility was suggested by Morton and Patterson (see Chapter 13) to account for their results on comprehension of function words. Alternatively, it may be that inflections can be comprehended when attached to nouns but not when attached to parts of speech more difficult for the patients. More work on the deep dyslexic's comprehension of inflected forms is needed before such possibilities can be assessed. The situation is complicated further still by the existence of a theoretical dispute concerning how inflected forms are read by normal readers. There are two views: the 'independence' (Mackay, 1978) or 'single-unit' (Manelis and Tharp, 1977) view, according to which the various derivational forms of a root morpheme each has its own independent lexical entry, and an alternative view according to which only root morphemes have lexical entries, so that lexical access requires morphological decomposition, and linguistic production requires morphological composition (Murrell and Morton, 1974; Taft and Forster, 1975; Mackay, 1978). This issue, and relevant data from deep dyslexia, is considered in more detail by Patterson in Chapter 14.

One difficulty with the concept of morphological decomposition is that, while it is easy to see how some early system could strip the inflectional morphemes from such words as *walked* or *socks*, it is very difficult to see how the root morpheme *go* could be retrieved from *went*, and also to see how a system could remove the terminal -*s* from *socks* without removing it from *trousers*. It has sometimes been suggested (Low, 1931; Marin, Saffran and Schwartz, 1975) that derivational errors are much less likely to occur with nouns or verbs whose derivational structure is irregular; and Marin *et al.* found that patients who tended to omit the terminal -*s* from plural nouns in reading aloud did not do so to regular plurals which have no singular nominal form (e.g. *trousers, clothes, news, suds*). Further studies of these effects would provide more insight into the nature of the derivational error; some such studies are described by Patterson in Chapter 14.

As far as the implications of derivational errors for the right-hemisphere hypothesis are concerned, one can draw attention to the work of Zurif and Sait (1970), Heeschen and Jurgens (1977) and Lesser (1974), all of whom concluded that the right hemisphere lacked syntactic abilities. It is thus consistent with the right-hemisphere hypothesis that the deep dyslexic should have particular trouble with inflections; but this consistency may merely be a consequence of the fact that we still know very little about the basis of derivational errors, and even less about precisely which syntactic abilities the right hemisphere lacks.

Summary and conclusions

It is proposed here that deep dyslexia is the result of a lesion which abolishes access from orthography to the left-hemisphere lexicon. It is assumed that the spoken responses of these patients are generated from the left hemisphere. Thus reading aloud will require orthographic access to a right-hemisphere lexicon, interhemispheric transmission of information (which, it is argued, is semantic information) and the use of this information to access an entry in the left-hemisphere lexicon: from this entry a pronunciation is retrieved and articulated.

Sometimes the patient will tolerate a small degree of difference between the semantic representation dispatched from the right hemisphere and the semantic representation in the left-hemisphere lexical entry of the word he chooses as a response. This tolerance produces feature-loss semantic errors and also function-word substitution errors. The more specific a semantic feature is, the more willing a patient is to tolerate a mismatch of that feature.

Associative semantic errors are attributed to the generation of an associatively related set of candidate words in the right-hemisphere lexicon (this occurring because of the associative organization of that lexicon), followed by an incorrect choice from this set, and then interhemispheric transmission of the semantic representation of that incorrect choice.

Difficulties with function words arise for at least two reasons. The right hemisphere is poor at appreciating purely syntactic properties of words and many function words serve a largely syntactic function, having little semantic characterization: hence there are difficulties in interhemispheric communications concerning function words. When such communication is possible, with semantically rich function words, then shared-feature semantic errors can occur.

Lexical entries for abstract words in the right-hemisphere lexicon are sometimes semantically impoverished. This in itself can generate semantic errors; when the impoverishment is so severe that it prevents any interhemispheric transfer of semantic information, such words cannot be uttered nor can shared-feature semantic errors occur in response to these words. Nevertheless, it will still be possible for the deep dyslexic to classify these words as words. There may also be *lexical* impoverishment, abstract words selectively lacking lexical entries in the right hemisphere; the extent to which this is so may depend on the pre-morbid educational level of the patient. When a word has no lexical entry, the patient must treat the word as a non-word, and hence either fail to respond to it (an omission) or else, using the strategy of approximate visual access, produce a visual error.

Derivational errors – responding 'rule' to *ruler* and being unable to decide which of these two words fits correctly into a sentence context – may reflect the inability of the right hemisphere to deal with inflected forms, although much more work needs to be done on the deep dyslexic's comprehension of various syntactic forms before anything secure can be said about derivational errors.

This chapter has been devoted to efforts at interpreting, within the framework of a right-hemisphere hypothesis, the body of data which has so far been collected from deep-dyslexic patients. If the interpretations provided by this hypothesis are judged to be satisfactory, then one can next proceed by deriving predictions from the hypothesis concerning what should happen in experimental situations which have not yet been investigated. The hypothesis has been stated in enough detail to generate a great many predictions; one obvious line to take is to look at visual hemifield effects in the reading of the deep dyslexic. Not all patients can be used to test such predictions, since some have right visual hemifield defects; but some do not. In such patients, it is an obvious expectation that there will be left visual field advantages in reading tasks. Preliminary investigations along these lines are reported by Saffran, Bogyo, Schwartz and Marin in the following chapter; and indeed the results of their tachistoscopic experiments provide evidence that when deep dyslexics carry out reading tasks they do so more accurately with stimuli in the left visual hemifield than with those in the right hemifield, as is predicted by the right-hemisphere hypothesis.

Notes

1 Since in intact subjects a stimulus present in one hemisphere will also reach the other, it is perhaps more precise to discuss laterality experiments in terms of visual hemifields or ears, rather than cerebral hemispheres. However, this requires continual translation between 'left' and 'right' for the reader. In the interests of ease of exposition, I will write 'presented to the right hemisphere' as a short form of 'presented in the left visual hemifield, hence initially reaching the right hemisphere and subsequently via commissural transfer reaching the left hemisphere'.

2 This may be related to the finding of Seamon and Gazzaniga (1973): in their task imagery instructions produced a right-hemisphere superiority in performance, whilst verbal instructions produced a left-hemisphere superiority.

3 These problems were pointed out to me by K. Patterson.

References

Andreewsky, E. and Seron, X. (1975) Implicit processing of grammatical rules in a case of agrammatism. *Cortex, 11,* 379–90.

Benson, D. F. and Geschwind, N. (1969) The alexias. In P. J. Vinken and G. W. Bruyn (eds), *Handbook of Clinical Neurology,* vol. 4. Amsterdam: North Holland.

Besner, D. and Coltheart, M. (1979) Ideographic and alphabetic processing in skilled reading of English. *Neuropsychologia, 17,* 467–72.

Bradshaw, J. L. and Gates, E. A. (1978) Visual field differences in verbal tasks: effects of task familiarity and sex of subject. *Brain and Language, 5,* 166–87.

Bradshaw, J. L., Gates, A. and Nettleton, N. C. (1977) Hemispheric involvement in lexical decisions: handedness and a possible sex difference. *Neuropsychologia, 15,* 277–86.

Brooks, L. R. (1973) Treating verbal stimuli in a novel manner. In M. P. Bryden and F. Allard, *op. cit.*

Brown, J. S. (1972) *Aphasia, Apraxia, Agnosia.* Springfield, Ohio: Thomas.

Brown, W. P. and Ure, D. M. J. (1969) Five rated characteristics of 650 word association stimuli. *British Journal of Psychology, 60,* 223–50.

Bryden, M. P. and Allard, F. (1976) Visual hemifield differences depend on typeface. *Brain and language, 3,* 191–206.

Caplan, L. and Hedley-White, T. (1974) Cueing and memory dysfunction in alexia without agraphia. *Brain, 97,* 251–62.

Cohen, D., Salanga, V., Hully, W., Steinberg, M. and Hardy, R. (1976) Alexia without agraphia. *Neurology, 26,* 455–9.

Cohen, G. and Freeman, R. (1979) Individual differences in reading strategies in relation to handedness and cerebral asymmetry. In J. Requin (ed.), *Attention and Performance,* VII. Hillsdale, N.J.: Lawrence Erlbaum.

Coltheart, M. (1977) Phonemic dyslexia: some comments on its interpretation and its implications for the study of normal reading. Paper presented at International Neuropsychology Society Meeting, Oxford.

Coltheart, M., Davelaar, E., Jonasson, J. T. and Besner, D. (1977) Access to the internal lexicon. In S. Dornic (ed.), *Attention and Performance,* VI. Hillsdale, N.J.: Lawrence Erlbaum.

Crockett, H. G. and Estridge, N. M. (1951) Cerebral hemispherectomy: a clinical, surgical and pathologic study of four cases. *Bulletin of the Los Angeles Neurological Society, 16,* 71–87.

Day, J. (1977) Right-hemisphere language processing in normal right-handers. *Journal of Experimental Psychology: Human Perception and Performance, 3,* 518–28.

Dimond, S. J. and Beaumont, J. G. (1972) A right-hemisphere basis for calculation in the human brain. *Psychonomic Science, 26,* 137–8.

Edgerton, W. F. (1941) Ideograms in English writing. *Language, 17,* 148–50.

Ellis, H. D. and Shepherd, J. W. (1974) Recognition of abstract and concrete words presented in left and right visual fields. *Journal of Experimental Psychology, 103,* 1035–6.

Gazzaniga, M. S. and Hillyard, S. A. (1971) Language and speech capacity of the right hemisphere. *Neuropsychologia, 9,* 273–80.

Gazzaniga, M. S. and Sperry, R. W. (1967) Language after section of the cerebral commissures. *Brain, 90,* 131–48.

Geffen, G., Bradshaw, J. L. and Nettleton, N. C. (1972) Hemispheric asymmetry: verbal and spatial encoding of visual stimuli. *Journal of Experimental Psychology, 93,* 25–31.

Geschwind, N. (1965) Disconnection syndromes in animals and man. *Brain, 88*, 327–94 and 585–644.

Goldstein, K. (1948) *Language and Language Disturbances*. New York: Grune & Stratton.

Gott, P. S. (1973) Language after dominant hemispherectomy. *Journal of Neurology, Neurosurgery and Psychiatry, 36*, 1082–8.

Gough, P. B. and Cosky, M. L. (1977) One second of reading again. In J. N. Castellan, D. B. Pisoni and G. P. Potts (eds), *Cognitive Theory*, vol. 2. Hillsdale, N.J.: Lawrence Erlbaum.

Hatta, T. (1977a) Recognition of Japanese kanji in the left and right visual fields. *Neuropsychologia, 15*, 685–8.

Hatta, T. (1977b) Lateral recognition of abstract and concrete kanji in Japanese. *Perceptual and Motor Skills, 45*, 731–4.

Hatta, T. (submitted) Recognition of Japanese kanji and hirakana in the left and right visual fields.

Head, H. (1926) *Aphasia and Kindred Disorders of Speech*. Cambridge University Press.

Hécaen, H. and Kremin, H. (1976) Neurolinguistic research on reading disorders resulting from left hemisphere lesions: aphasic and 'pure' alexia. In H. Whitaker and H. A. Whitaker (eds), *Studies in Neurolinguistics*, vol. 2. New York: Academic Press.

Heeschen, C. and Jurgens, R. (1977) Pragmatic, semantic and syntactic factors influencing ear differences in dichotic listening. *Cortex, 13*, 74–84.

Hillier, W. (1954) Total left cerebral hemispherectomy for malignant glioma. *Neurology, 4*, 718–21.

Hines, D. (1976) Recognition of verbs, abstract nouns and concrete nouns from the left and right visual half fields. *Neuropsychologia, 14*, 211–16.

Hines, D. (1977) Differences in tachistoscopic recognition between abstract and concrete words as a function of visual half-field and frequency. *Cortex, 13*, 66–73.

Hirata, K. and Osaka, R. (1967) Tachistoscopic recognition of Japanese letter materials in left and right visual fields. *Psychologia, 10*, 7–18.

Kapur, N. and Perl, N. T. (1978) Recognition reading in paralexia. *Cortex, 14*, 439–43.

Kinsbourne, M. (1971) The minor cerebral hemisphere as a source of aphasic speech. *Archives of Neurology, 25*, 302–6.

Klatzky, R. L. and Atkinson, R. C. (1971) Specialization of the cerebral hemispheres in scanning for information in short-term memory. *Perception and Psychophysics, 10*, 335–8.

Leiber, L. (1976) Lexical decision in the right and left cerebral hemispheres. *Brain and Language, 3*, 443–50.

Lesser, R. (1974) Verbal comprehension in aphasia: an English version of three Italian tests. *Cortex, 10*, 247–63.

Levy, J., Nebes, R. D. and Sperry, R. W. (1971) Expressive language in the surgically separated minor hemisphere. *Cortex, 8*, 49–58.

Levy, J. and Trevarthen, C. (1977) Perceptual, semantic and phonetic aspects of elementary language processes in split-brain patients. *Brain*, *100*, 105–18.

Low, A. A. (1931) A case of agrammatism in the English language. *Archives of Neurology and Psychiatry*, *25*, 555–97.

Mackay, D. G. (1978) Derivational rules and the internal lexicon. *Journal of Verbal Learning and Verbal Behaviour*, *17*, 61–71.

Manelis, L. and Tharp, D. A. (1977) The processing of affixed words. *Memory and Cognition*, *5*, 690–5.

Marcel, A. J. and Patterson, K. (1979) Word recognition and production: reciprocity in clinical and normal research. In J. Requin (ed.), *Attention and Performance*, VII. Hillsdale, N.J.: Lawrence Erlbaum.

Marin, O. S. M., Saffran, E. M. and Schwartz, M. F. (1975) Dissociations of language in aphasia: implications for normal function. *Annals of the New York Academy of Science*, *280*, 868–84.

Marshall, J. C. (1976) Neuropsychological aspects of orthographic representation. In R. J. Wales and E. Walker (eds), *New Approaches to Language Mechanisms*. Amsterdam: North Holland.

Marshall, J. C. and Newcombe, F. (1966) Syntactic and semantic errors in paralexia. *Neuropsychologia*, *4*, 169–76.

Moore, W. H. and Weidner, W. E. (1974) Bilateral tachistoscopic word perception in aphasic and normal subjects. *Perceptual and Motor Skills*, *38*, 1003–11.

Moscovitch, M. (1976) On the representation of language in the right hemisphere of right-handed people. *Brain and Language*, *3*, 47–71.

Murrell, G. A. and Morton, J. (1974) Word recognition and morphemic structure. *Journal of Experimental Psychology*, *102*, 963–8.

Neilsen, J. (1946) *Agnosia, Apraxia, Aphasia: Their Value in Cerebral Localization*. New York: Hoeber.

Orenstein, H. B. and Meighan, W. B. (1976) Recognition of bilaterally presented words varying in concreteness and frequency: lateral dominance or sequential processing? *Bulletin of the Psychonomic Society*, *7*, 179–80.

Patterson, K. (1978) Phonemic dyslexia: errors of meaning and the meaning of errors. *Quarterly Journal of Experimental Psychology*, *30*, 587–601.

Patterson, K. (1979) What is right with 'deep' dyslexic patients? *Brain and Language*, *8*, 111–29.

Patterson, K. and Marcel, A. J. (1977) Aphasia, dyslexia and the phonological coding of printed words. *Quarterly Journal of Experimental Psychology*, *29*, 307–18.

Pettit, J. M. and Noll, J. D. (1972) Cerebral dominance and the process of language recovery in aphasia. Presented at American Speech and Hearing Association, San Francisco. In A. Searleman, A review of right hemisphere linguistic capabilities. *Psychological Bulletin*, *84*, 503–28.

Richardson, J. T. E. (1975) The effect of word imageability in acquired dyslexia. *Neuropsychologia*, *13*, 281–8.

Rubenstein, H., Lewis, S. S. and Rubenstein, M. A. (1971) Evidence for phonemic recoding in visual word recognition. *Journal of Verbal Learning and Verbal Behaviour, 10,* 647–57.

Saffran, E. M. and Marin, O. S. M. (1977) Reading without phonology: evidence from aphasia. *Quarterly Journal of Experimental Psychology, 29,* 515–25.

Saffran, E. M., Marin, O. S. M. and Schwartz, M. F. (1976) Semantic mechanisms in paralexia. *Brain and Language, 3,* 255–65.

Sasanuma, S. (1974) Kanji vs. kana processing in alexia with transient agraphia: a case report. *Cortex, 10,* 89–97.

Sasanuma, S., Itoh, M., Mori, K. and Kobayashi, Y. (1977) Tachistoscopic recognition of kana and kanji words. *Neuropsychologia, 15,* 547–53.

Sasanuma, S. and Monoi, H. (1975) The syndrome of Gogi (wordmeaning) aphasia: selective impairment of kanji processing. *Neurology, 25,* 627–32.

Seamon, J. G. and Gazzaniga, M. S. (1973) Coding strategies and cerebral laterality effects. *Cognitive Psychology, 5,* 249–56.

Searleman, A. (1977) A review of right hemisphere linguistic capabilities. *Psychological Bulletin, 84,* 503–28.

Shallice, T. and Warrington, E. K. (1975) Word recognition in a phonemic dyslexic patient. *Quarterly Journal of Experimental Psychology, 27,* 187–99.

Smith, A. (1966) Speech and other functions after left (dominant) hemispherectomy. *Journal of Neurology, Neurosurgery and Psychiatry, 29,* 467–71.

Sugishita, M., Iwata, M., Toyokura, Y., Yoshioka, M. and Yamada, R. (1978) Reading of ideograms and phonograms in Japanese patients after partial commissurotomy. *Neuropsychologia, 16,* 417–26.

Taft, M. and Forster, K. I. (1975) Lexical storage and retrieval of prefixed words. *Journal of Verbal Learning and Verbal Behaviour, 14,* 638–47.

Teng, E. L. and Sperry, R. W. (1973) Interhemispheric interaction during simultaneous bilateral presentation of letters and digits in commissurotomized patients. *Neuropsychologia, 11,* 131–40.

Tikofsky, R. S., Kooi, K. A. and Thomas, M. H. (1960) Electroencephalographic findings and recovery from aphasia. *Neurology, 10,* 154–6.

Tzeng, O. J. L., Hung, D. L., Cotton, W. and Wang, W. S.-Y. (1979) Visual lateralization effects in reading in Chinese characters. Unpublished manuscript.

Tzeng, O. J. L., Hung, D. L. and Garro, L. (1978) Reading the Chinese characters: an information processing view. *Journal of Chinese Linguistics, 6,* 287–305.

Yamadori, A. (1975) Ideogram reading in alexia. *Brain, 98,* 231–8.

Zaidel, E. (1973) Linguistic competence and related functions in the right hemisphere of man following cerebral commissurotomy and hemispherectomy. Doctoral dissertation, California Institute of Technology.

Zaidel, E. (1976) Auditory vocabulary of the right hemisphere following brain bisection or hemidecortication. *Cortex, 12,* 191–211.

Zaidel, E. (1978) Lexical organization in the right hemisphere. In P. Buser and A. Rougeul-Buser (eds), *Cerebral Correlates of Conscious Experience.* Amsterdam: Elsevier.

Zangwill, O. (1967) Speech and the minor hemisphere. *Acta Neurologica Psychiatrica, 67,* 1013–20.

Zollinger, R. (1935) Removal of left cerebral hemisphere: report of a case. *Archives of Neurology and Psychiatry, 34,* 1055–62.

Zurif, E. B. and Sait, P. E. (1970) The role of syntax in dichotic listening. *Neuropsychologia, 8,* 239–44.

17 Does deep dyslexia reflect right-hemisphere reading?

Eleanor M. Saffran, Lola C. Bogyo,
Myrna F. Schwartz and Oscar S. M. Marin

In another chapter in this volume, Coltheart (Chapter 16) argues the case for right-hemisphere mediation of reading in deep dyslexia. We have adopted a similar view, which we have begun to test experimentally. Coltheart presents the arguments for right-hemisphere reading in detail, and we will not elaborate them again here. Following a brief rationale of the right-hemisphere hypothesis, we turn to some experimental approaches to the question.

The right-hemisphere hypothesis

It is generally accepted that reading in deep dyslexia depends on a means of access to lexical information that is mediated by an orthographic rather than a phonological code (e.g. Saffran and Marin, 1977). This orthographic-lexical pathway is the sole reading mechanism available to the deep dyslexic. Unable to translate print directly into sound, the patient can read a word aloud only by accessing a lexical entry that specifies its pronunciation; when there is no lexical entry for a letter-string (as in the case of nonsense words), the deep dyslexic is unable to read it aloud (Patterson and Marcel, 1977; Saffran and Marin, 1977).

Given that oral reading performance in deep dyslexia depends on lexical information, how do we account for the differences in performance across word categories? Why should concrete (or imageable) words be easier to read than abstract words, nouns

This research has been supported by N.I.H. grant NS 13992 to
E. Saffran and N.I.M.H. pre-doctoral fellowship MH07316 to L. Bogyo.

easier than verbs, and function words be by far the most difficult (Marshall and Newcombe, 1966; Shallice and Warrington, 1975; Richardson, 1975; Schwartz, Saffran and Marin, 1977)?

One possible explanation is that the word class effects reflect the more general language disturbance that accompanies the reading deficit in deep dyslexia. If there is lexical impairment, which there generally is in aphasia, the lexical deficit should be reflected in the reading performance of patients who read via lexical mediation. The nature of the aphasic impairment should therefore account for the pattern of reading performance in deep dyslexia.

This parallelism does, in fact, hold in most of the published cases of deep dyslexia. Almost all of the patients would be classified as agrammatic, and there is a strong similarity between language output in agrammatism and oral reading in deep dyslexia. Agrammatic speech consists mostly of concrete nouns (Goodglass, Hyde and Blumstein, 1969), contains relatively few verb forms (Myerson and Goodglass, 1972; Saffran, Schwartz and Marin, 1979) and is notably lacking in functors. These considerations led to our earlier view that the reading deficit in deep dyslexia was the product of two underlying disturbances: (1) a syntactic disorder, which compromises 'syntactically-related' lexical items (which we took to include abstract words), as well as the morphemes and rules of the grammar; and (2) loss of the ability to use spelling-sound correspondence rules, which, if functional, would allow the agrammatic reader to bypass his deficient lexicon when reading aloud (Marin, Saffran and Schwartz, 1976).

The problem with this approach is that it fails to account for the occasional deep dyslexic who is *not* agrammatic. There are at least two non-agrammatics (more, if we consider earlier cases that were not as thoroughly tested) who satisfy the definition of deep dyslexia as proposed elsewhere in this volume by Shallice and Warrington: their own patient K.F. (Shallice and Warrington, 1975) and our patient W.S. (Schwartz, Saffran and Marin, 1977). W.S. produces well formed though simply structured and somewhat anomic speech; in reading, however, he is agrammatic, paralexic (his error corpus includes the remarkable example, package → 'pack-old') and unable to apply grapheme-phoneme correspondence rules.[1] The disparity between the agrammatism in reading and the relative well-formedness of the spontaneous speech in such patients forces us to reconsider this 'aphasic' hypothesis for deep dyslexia.

In at least this non-agrammatic subset of deep dyslexics, it appears that graphemic input lacks complete access to the set of language capacities that are available in the auditory-vocal mode. How can we account for this modality difference? One possibility is that semantically-mediated reading is necessarily 'agrammatic'; perhaps the lexical route does not provide access to words (like functors) that do not have isolable (i.e. non-contextually dependent) meanings. Another possibility is that such patients are utilizing two different language systems, one (agrammatic) for reading, and another (not agrammatic) for speaking. (It should be noted that these alternatives are not mutually exclusive.) We have chosen to test a form of the second hypothesis – more specifically, that the language system that deep dyslexics use for reading is that of the intact right hemisphere.

The argument for right hemisphere reading in deep dyslexia rests primarily on the similarities between right hemisphere language abilities and the reading performance of deep dyslexics. Since this evidence is reviewed by Coltheart elsewhere in this volume (Chapter 16), it will be summarized only briefly here.

1   The strongest evidence for language capacity in the minor hemisphere is that there is some form of lexical representation. The right hemisphere seems to be able to comprehend single words, whether spoken or written, reasonably well (see Zaidel, 1976).
2   The phonological capacities of the minor hemisphere are less well developed. In particular, the right hemisphere seems to be unable to match objects on the basis of the phonological properties of their names (e.g. 'key' and 'bee'), although it can recognize the relation between objects and names (Levy and Trevarthen, 1977; Zaidel, in press). There is no evidence that the right hemisphere can translate graphemic input directly into a phonological code (Zaidel, in press), although, as Coltheart (Chapter 16) points out, stringent tests for this capacity have not yet been performed.
3   When tested auditorily, the right hemisphere's syntactic abilities are poorly developed relative to its capacity for lexical representation (Zaidel, 1978). As yet, there have been no comparable tests of syntactic comprehension using written stimuli.
4   Finally, split-field studies of normal subjects have indicated

that the right hemisphere lexicon is biased toward imageable words (see Coltheart, Chapter 16, for a summary of these experiments). There is also evidence that the isolated right hemisphere has some difficulty reading verbs, at least when they are presented in the gerundive (-ing) form (Zaidel, in press).

On these grounds, we would expect a right-hemisphere reader to display most of the salient features of deep dyslexia: grapheme-phoneme impairment, a bias toward imageable words, and difficulty with the syntactic aspects of written language. While there is little evidence that specifically predicts semantic errors in oral reading (although the errors of Gott's hemispherectomy patient, discussed in Coltheart's chapter, were of this sort), a right-hemisphere theory could easily accommodate this feature of deep dyslexia (as in Coltheart, Chapter 16, and below).

The right-hemisphere hypothesis is therefore consistent with the available data on right-hemisphere language. It also has the virtue of accounting for the uniformity of the reading pattern in a group of patients whose language impairments may, in other respects, be quite different: whatever the source of their expressive speech, all would be relying on the same right hemisphere mechanisms for reading. As Coltheart points out, the right hemisphere hypothesis receives additional support from neurological data; all of the tomographic scans presently available for deep dyslexics show very extensive lesions involving most of what is generally considered the language cortex of the left hemisphere (e.g. Penfield and Roberts, 1959). Thus it would be surprising if reading (or indeed any other language function) is subserved entirely by the left hemisphere in these patients. Evidence for right-hemisphere involvement comes in fact from the dichotic listening performances of deep dyslexics tested in our laboratory; all four patients showed a strong left-ear advantage, three of them a total suppression of the right-ear stimulus in a digit recognition task.

Testing the right-hemisphere hypothesis

Our efforts to test the hypothesis that deep dyslexia reflects right-hemisphere reading have taken two major directions. First, we have attempted to determine directly, by means of split-field experiments in deep dyslexic patients, which of the two hemispheres is responsible for reading. Second, we have conducted experiments in normal readers to determine whether the characteristics of right-hemisphere reading are consistent with the pattern of performance in deep dyslexia. These studies are still in progress, and this paper constitutes a preliminary report of this work.

Some general methodological comments are in order here. Throughout these studies we have used the technique of split-field presentation to restrict the initial reception of the stimulus to one hemisphere or the other. However, there is no sure way (short of callosal section) to constrain the subsequent processing of the graphemic information to the hemisphere that receives it. Information can pass freely to the other hemisphere via the corpus callosum, and we do not have a way to 'tag' that information (as the biochemist can do) with the imprint of one hemispheric processor or the other. Thus it is difficult to determine the extent to which the two hemispheres have contributed to the performance of a particular cognitive task. In most instances,[2] the experimenter can only infer from differences arising from the field of presentation (differences which are usually small) that one hemisphere has some advantage over the other in performing the task. Too often, the results of split-field studies have been given a much stronger interpretation (for example, on the basis of a right visual field superiority, that the right hemisphere is incapable of reading).

Split-field experiments in deep dyslexics

The difficulties inherent in the split-field method are multiplied when the subjects have hemispheric lesions. Of necessity, stimulus presentation must be brief; otherwise, eye movements would allow stimulation in both visual fields. But should the damaged hemisphere perform poorly in the split-field task, it could be as a result of perceptual limitations that might not apply under more adequate reading conditions. Thus it would not necessarily follow, from a tachistoscopic demonstration of left visual field (right hemisphere) superiority for word recognition in deep dyslexics, that these patients are normally relying on right hemisphere mechanisms for reading.

To give the results more generality, it is necessary to control for any lesion-related perceptual deficits that might occur under conditions of rapid presentation. Previous split-field studies of patients with unilateral lesions have not utilized such controls (Shai, Goodglass and Barton, 1972; Moore and Weidner, 1974). Indeed, it is even difficult to conceptualize what an adequate control procedure should be. Ideally, if the experiment involves word recognition, one would like to equate the two visual fields for the perceptibility of the letter-strings *per se*. However, we know from the word superiority effect (Reicher, 1969) that words can be identified at lower exposures than strings of unrelated letters. This effect can be observed in deep dyslexics, as well as in normal subjects (Saffran and McClelland, unpublished data). Thus, what might seem to be the best control for word recognition – the ability to process strings of unrelated letters – turns out to be quite unsuitable. Furthermore, we do not know, *a priori*, at what stage in the processing of graphemic information the damaged left hemisphere might be disrupted; it is conceivable that the deficit extends to the level of letter identification itself.

The first objective, then, was to find an adequate control task, and to do this we subjected one of our deep dyslexics, V.S. (for a case report, see Saffran and Marin, 1977), to a series of exploratory studies.

Pilot study: V.S.

The following conditions applied in the pilot study and, with minor exceptions, in all succeeding experiments. After determination (using standard perimetry) that the patient was free of visual field defects, the two hemifields were tested tachistoscopically in dot-counting and letter-recognition tasks at low (10 msec.) exposures. This was done to assure that there were no gross perceptual deficits in either visual field. The materials for the experimental and control tasks were letter-strings (white, upper case) which were arrayed vertically on a black background 1.5° from fixation. The fixation point was a white dot on a black background which was exposed for two seconds prior to stimulus presentation. The stimulus was immediately followed by a 200 msec. mask, made of white letter fragments on a black field; the mask was used in the hope that it might help to restrict at least the early stages of processing to the hemisphere that initially received the input. In the pilot study, the use of a two-field tachistoscope necessitated exposure of the mask, along with the fixation point, prior to stimulus presentation as well.

The goal was to equate the two visual fields for the ability to process graphemic input similar in complexity to the stimuli to be used in the experimental task, which would involve lexical decision on four-letter strings. Several paradigms proved to be too difficult for both visual fields, but equal and better-than-chance performance was finally achieved in these two tasks: the forced-choice recognition of pronounceable letter-strings (e.g. BAME, where the distractors were BAFE, RAME, BIME and BAMN); and the determination of identity (e.g. RRRR) vs. non-identity (e.g. RFRR) in four-letter strings. The latter task (henceforth referred to as the 'identity task') was adopted as the control procedure for further experiments.

V.S. was also given several lexical decision tasks at this time. The stimuli in the first task, which has served as the basic experimental paradigm in subsequent studies with dyslexic subjects, consisted of 40 four-letter concrete nouns and 40 pronounceable pseudo-words (generated by changing a single letter in a real word). Each item was presented twice, once to each visual field, at an exposure of 150 msec. (the level determined by performance on the control tasks). The instructions were to say 'Yes' when the stimulus was a word, 'No' when it was not. The results (Table 17.1) were striking. Lexical decision performance was very good when the stimulus was

TABLE 17.1 *V.S.: Lexical decision in the two hemifields*

	Words	Per cent correct Pseudo-words	Mean per cent correct
LVF	87.5	65.0	76.3
RVF	25.0	80.0	52.5

projected to the right hemisphere; with right visual field (RVF) stimuli, however, there was a strong tendency to say 'No', whether the stimulus was a word or not. A significant left visual field (LVF) superiority was again obtained in a lexical decision task in which the four-letter words came from several different lexical categories[3] (Table 17.2), and also in another lexical decision task in which shorter (two- and three-letter) stimuli were used (Table 17.3). In

TABLE 17.2 *V.S.: Lexical decision across word categories*

	Per cent correct						Mean per cent correct
	Concrete nouns	Abstract nouns	Function words	Proper names	All words	Pseudo-words	
LVF	66.7	75.0	79.2	62.5	70.8	44.8	57.8
RVF	33.3	50.0	37.5	29.2	37.5	61.5	49.5

TABLE 17.3 *V.S.: Lexical decision on two- and three-letter words*

	Per cent correct		Mean per cent correct
	Words	Psuedo-words	
LVF	96.7	83.3	90.0
RVF	70.0	76.7	73.3

contrast, the RVF performed as well as the LVF in another lexical decision task in which the non-word strings consisted of unrelated letters (e.g. RLBE) rather than the orthographically regular pseudo-words used in the other experiments; this task differed from the other three in that lexical information was not necessary for distinguishing words from non-word strings.

The results of the pilot study in V.S. therefore provided consistent and rather strong support for right-hemisphere involvement in at least this deep dyslexic's reading.

Split-field lexical decision in three deep dyslexics

With these results and a control task in hand, we proceeded to test two other deep dyslexics, as well as V.S., in the lexical decision task with four-letter concrete words. Since this and all subsequent studies were performed on a four-field tachistoscope, we were able to dispense with the pre-stimulus pattern mask that had been used in the pilot experiments. Otherwise, the conditions were as described above.

Like V.S., the other patients (B.L. and H.T.)[4] are agrammatic as well as dyslexic. Neither showed evidence of visual field deficits on standard perimetry, and both performed well on lateralized dot-counting and letter recognition tasks at low (10 msec.) exposures.

To equate the two visual fields, all three patients were given the control task involving identity judgments on four-letter strings. Exposure times were adjusted until performance in both fields ranged between 75 to 85 per cent correct, with a discrepancy between them of at most five per cent. Since there were no differences between the two hemifields in B.L. and H.T., both fields were subsequently run at the same exposures. In V.S., performance was matched at 90 msec. for the LVF and at 100 msec. for the RVF.

After some practice in lexical decision, the patients were given the experimental task. As in the pilot study, 40 four-letter concrete nouns and 40 pseudo-words were presented twice, once to each visual field. The results, presented separately for each subject, are summarized in Table 17.4. V.S. and B.L. both show a slight LVF superiority. In H.T. both hemifields performed poorly, with a small difference in favor of the RVF. The combined results from the three patients fail to show a significant LVF superiority (across items, t=1.30, df=79, p=0.10).

TABLE 17.4 *Lexical decision in three deep dyslexics*

		Per cent correct		Mean per cent correct
		Words	Pseudo-words	
V.S.	LVF	87.5	90.0	88.8
	RVF	75.0	80.0	77.5
B.L.	LVF	70.0	85.0	77.5
	RVF	57.5	82.5	70.0
H.T.	LVF	40.0	87.5	63.8
	RVF	45.0	95.0	70.0
		Mean per cent correct LVF		76.7
		RVF		72.5

While the results do not disprove the right-hemisphere hypothesis, neither do they offer convincing support. It was particularly surprising to find such a small LVF advantage in V.S., who had consistently shown large effects in the pilot studies. We wondered whether the change in performance could be attributed to more efficient transfer of information from the left hemisphere to the right, or whether the left hemisphere itself had become more able to deal with graphemic stimuli.

To explore these questions, and, in general, to find more adequate ways of determining which hemisphere is actually performing the lexical decision task, we turned to paradigms which involve some degree of bilateral stimulation.

Split-field studies with bilateral stimulation

When two words are presented simultaneously, one in each visual field, they may compete for the use of a set of limited-capacity processing mechanisms that are necessary for word recognition. If some or all of these mechanisms are concentrated in one hemisphere, the stimulus that projects directly to that hemisphere should have privileged access to the specialized processing mechanisms; the stimulus that projects to the other hemisphere will have to cross the callosum, suffering information loss in transfer and in delay. In such cases, it is to be expected that a visual field advantage obtained under unilateral conditions (the effect of transfer) will be increased by bilateral presentation (the effect of competition). It has, in fact, been found that bilateral presentation significantly increases the RVF superiority for word recognition in normal subjects[5] (McKeever, 1970). This effect has been shown to be independent of order of report tendencies that might be expected to favor verbal stimuli presented to the RVF (McKeever, 1970; Rosen, Curcio, MacKavey and Herbert, 1975).

If the competition argument is correct, it should be possible to use bilateral stimulation to help constrain processing to the hemisphere that initially receives the information (see Hines, 1975, for a similar argument). With this goal in mind, we have begun to use bilateral presentation paradigms with our deep dyslexics; if these patients are indeed relying on their minor hemispheres in reading, we should expect to find an enhanced LVF superiority on lexical decision tasks under conditions of bilateral presentation.

This is, in fact, what we found. Initially, there were serious difficulties in matching the two visual fields on a bilateral control task. (These failures to match the fields under bilateral stimulation conditions, due to the continued poor performance in the RVF across a range of exposure durations, are of interest in their own right and will be discussed below.) Eventually, a paradigm was found in which, for each patient, a match was achieved between the two fields. The control stimuli used in the unilateral experiment appeared in one hemifield and a single letter appeared simultaneously in the other. The task was to report the identity judgment (i.e. whether the four letters in the string were all the same) and then to identify the single letter. To encourage letter encoding, as opposed to visual matching, the single-letter stimuli were presented in upper case and the recognition set (a card containing the whole alphabet) in lower case. Exposures were adjusted until the two visual fields performed equivalently on the identity task; differences on letter recognition were ignored. These exposure levels would then be used in a lexical decision task of similar design, that is, with a single letter appearing in the other visual field.

To equate the two visual fields on control task performance, it was necessary, in two of the patients (V.S. and B.L.), to extend the range of possible exposure times by eliminating the post-stimulus pattern mask. Without the mask, B.L.'s visual fields were matched at 30 msec. In V.S., equal performance was achieved when RVF strings were exposed for 40 msec., as opposed to 20 msec. in the LVF. H.T.'s visual fields were matched, at 150 msec., *with* the post-stimulus mask.

Consequently, the lexical decision task, with a single letter appearing simultaneously in the other visual field, was run under somewhat different conditions in the three subjects: for H.T., all stimuli were exposed for 150 msec., followed by the pattern mask; for B.L., stimuli were exposed for 30 msec., but without the mask; and V.S. was run without the mask, with exposures set at 20 msec. when the lexical decision string was in the LVF, and at 40 msec. when it was in the RVF. The competing letter stimulus was exposed simultaneously and for the same duration as the lexical decision string; in V.S.'s case, the letters therefore appeared longer in the LVF (40 msec.) than in the RVF (20 msec.). The lexical decision stimuli were the same as those used in the earlier study with unilateral presentation.

The results of this study are summarized in Table 17.5. In all three patients, performance was better when the lexical decision string appeared in the LVF; this effect is significant in the combined data from the three patients (t=2.31; df=79; p<0.01). When these results are compared with those of unilateral experiment (Figure 17.1), two of the subjects (H.T. and B.L.) show a greater LVF advantage under bilateral conditions. This is the effect predicted by the competition hypothesis, on the assumption that lexical decision is performed by the right hemisphere. There is little effect in V.S., who shows a negligible shift in the opposite direction. Overall, the magnitude of the LVF advantage in the bilateral condition does not differ significantly from that obtained in the unilateral condition (t=1.14, df=79, p<.2).

TABLE 17.5 *Lexical decision and letter recognition in deep dyslexics under bilateral conditions*

		Per cent correct		Mean per cent correct	Per cent letters correct	
		Words	Pseudo-words		Control task	Experimental task
V.S.	LVF	75.0	87.5	81.3	71.1	77.5
	RVF	60.0	85.0	72.5	7.7	7.5
B.L.	LVF	72.5	90.0	81.3	94.2	78.8
	RVF	57.5	77.5	67.5	53.8	48.8
H.T.	LVF	55.0	70.0	62.5	75.0	83.8
	RVF	35.0	72.5	53.8	93.8	51.3
Mean per cent correct	LVF			75.0	80.1	80.0
	RVF			64.6	51.8	35.9

Thus, the results of the bilateral experiment point to right-hemisphere involvement in the reading performance of these deep dyslexic patients. Given that the two visual fields were matched on the control task, it is unlikely that the LVF advantage obtained in the lexical decision task is the result of general perceptual or processing deficits in the damaged left hemisphere.

It is of interest, however, that the effects of bilateral presentation were not uniform across patients. In particular, V.S. failed to show the predicted enhancement of LVF superiority with bilateral stimulation. In the next section, we would like to consider the possibility that these differences in lexical decision performance reflect differences in the degree to which the patients' damaged left hemispheres are able to process letter information. If the left hemisphere is sufficiently impaired, performance of the identity judgment (control task) on RVF stimuli may shift to the right hemisphere. If we control for this effect (by increasing RVF exposures, as we did in V.S.), there may be no further differences arising from field of presentation in the lexical decision task. We turn now to evidence that favors this interpretation.

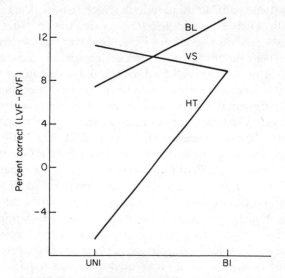

FIGURE 17.1 Differences in lexical decision performance in the two visual fields under unilateral (UNI) and bilateral (BI) conditions in three deep dyslexics

Information transfer at different stages of processing?

In our first attempts at using a bilateral paradigm to lateralize word recognition in deep dyslexics, the manipulation proved almost too effective. One patient (V.S.) was given a lexical decision task in which a word or pseudo-word was presented to one visual field and a string of unrelated letters (e.g. LRNE) to the other; the instructions were to say 'Yes' whenever a word appeared in either visual field. Responses to RVF stimuli were unfailingly negative. The control (letter-string identity) task of the unilateral experiment was then given to both V.S. and B.L. under these same bilateral conditions (i.e. with a string of letters, all different, in the other visual field); the task was to say 'Yes' whenever a string of identical letters appeared in either field. In both subjects, RVF responses were again over-whelmingly negative. These effects were difficult to interpret, how-ever. In the absence of a control for fixation,[6] it was possible that the patients were consistently fixating to the left. Alternatively, there might have been a strong attentional bias in that direction.

In an effort to encourage processing of the contents of both visual fields, we turned to a bilateral paradigm which requires the report of both stimuli. This is the single-letter competition paradigm dis-cussed in the previous section. First, the two hemifields were equated for performance on the letter-string identity task, with a single letter in the other visual field. But in only one subject (H.T.) was it possible to achieve equal visual field performance under the standard experimental conditions. V.S. and B.L. consistently failed to detect identical strings in the RVF; both, and especially V.S., also had difficulty identifying single letters in the RVF (see Table 17.5). The discrepancy between the two visual fields on the identity task persisted even when RVF stimuli were 30 msec. longer than LVF stimuli (RVF = 150 msec.; LVF = 120 msec.). To determine whether this difficulty might reflect sensory extinction on the side of the lesion, the identity task was given again, this time without the requirement to report the letter in the contralateral field. The identity judgment on RVF stimuli was performed adequately under the no-report condition. Thus, it seemed to be the requirement to encode and to remember the letter in the LVF that was interfering with processing of the letter strings in the RVF.

These data support the notion that the patients differ in the degree to which the damaged left hemisphere is able to process letter information presented to the RVF. H.T.'s left hemisphere seemed more capable in this respect than B.L.'s or V.S.'s. Unlike the other patients, H.T. had no difficulty performing the identity judgment for RVF stimuli under bilateral conditions; he also had no difficulty identifying single letters in the RVF in the control task (less difficulty, in fact, than in the LVF; Table 17.5). In his case, the RVF stimulus was at a disadvantage only in the bilateral lexical decision task, where performance on both lexical decision and letter recognition was poorer in the RVF. In contrast, B.L. and V.S. had difficulty with both the identity judgment and letter recognition in the bilateral control task (Table 17.5).[7] This would suggest that, in these two patients, the competing stimulus in the LVF interferes with the processing of *letter* information in the RVF. The implication is that the left-hemisphere deficit in B.L. and V.S. occurs at an earlier stage than lexical decision, and that the right hemisphere plays some role in the analysis of letter information received by the left. The role of the right hemisphere must be particularly important in V.S.,[8] who showed the bilateral competition effect so dramatically. However, having controlled for the competition effect at a relatively early stage of processing (i.e. having matched the two-fields on the control task), we should not expect to find any further effect in the lexical decision task. We do not, in V.S.; and in the case of B.L. the effect is intermediate.

Clearly, more experiments with these patients, and, importantly, with left hemisphere lesioned but non-dyslexic controls,[9] will have to be done before we can draw any firm conclusions from these studies. Thus far, however, the results would seem to indicate that the processing of graphemic information in deep dyslexia involves, to a varying but significant degree, the intact right hemisphere.

Word category effects in the right hemisphere of normal subjects

If the reading performance of the deep dyslexic reflects the language capacities of the right hemisphere, we might expect to find the same word category effects in the reading performance of the normal right hemisphere that we see in deep dyslexia; that is, the right hemisphere should be better able to read concrete (or imageable) words than abstract words, and it should be particularly deficient in reading functors. The abstract-concrete effect has been reported in a number of split-field experiments with normal subjects (Ellis and Shepherd, 1974; Hines, 1976, 1977; Day, 1977; Marcel and Patterson, 1978), but these laterality studies have not yet been extended to function words.

We therefore performed a study in which we examined laterality differences across several lexical categories in normal subjects. The categories were concrete (high-imagery) nouns, abstract (low-imagery) nouns, function words, and proper names (this being a class of relatively low frequency words that deep dyslexics are able to read surprisingly well; Saffran, Schwartz and Marin, 1976). The response was written report. To discourage guessing, which might be influenced by orthographic factors that differ across categories, a set of pronounceable pseudo-words was also included. There were 24 four-letter words from each of the four lexical categories (these are listed in the Appendix) and 48 pseudo-words. The abstract and concrete nouns, matched for frequency, were selected (with a few exceptions) from Paivio, Yuille and Madigan (1968). Presentation conditions (vertical, white letters on a black field, post-stimulus pattern mask) were as described for the unilateral experiments in dyslexics; the only difference was the distance of the stimuli from fixation (1.3° as opposed to 1.5°). Exposures were set individually for each of the 13 subjects, all of whom were right-handers with no family history of sinistrality.

The results are summarized in Figure 17.2. Overall performance was significantly better in the RVF, but except for proper names, there are no interactions between word category and visual field. The predicted effects – that abstract nouns and functors would show a larger RVF advantage than concrete nouns – were not obtained. It is particularly noteworthy that with the exception of proper names, real word stimuli produced as large a RVF advantage as pseudo-words. This would suggest that the right hemisphere had as little to do with the processing of words as it did with non-word stimuli, and, possibly, that all types of letter-strings presented to the LVF were transferred to the left hemisphere for analysis. It may be that the requirement to report pronounceable non-words, a task that the right hemisphere is probably unable to perform, had the effect of shifting all higher level processing to the left hemisphere. But this would not account for the rather different performance with proper names, an effect for which we have no adequate explanation.

The most surprising result of this study was the failure to replicate the abstract-concrete effect reported by other investigators. We decided to address this problem specifically in a separate experiment. A new set of words was used (Appendix, List B); these were four- and five-letter nouns, matched for frequency, and selected on

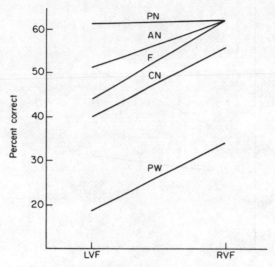

FIGURE 17.2 Split-field performance across lexical categories in normal subjects. PN = proper names; AN = abstract nouns; F = functors; CN = concrete nouns; PW = pseudo-words

the basis of subjective criteria of very high and very low image-ability. Twelve right-handed subjects served in this experiment, which was performed under the same conditions as the previous study, with two exceptions: for each subject, the two hemifields were matched for equal performance on a set of high-imageability nouns; and, to be congruent with other studies in the literature, the response mode was oral rather than written report.

As is evident in Figure 17.3, we again failed to obtain the abstract-concrete effect; if anything, the visual field asymmetry is greater with concrete words (although this effect is not significant). On the basis of our experience, then, the imageability effect does not appear to be a robust one. But while observation of the deep dyslexic pattern of category-dependent reading in the normal right hemisphere would certainly lend support to a right hemisphere theory of deep dyslexia, the failure to observe this pattern is by no means critical for the hypothesis. It may be that *when* the right hemisphere reads, it reads like a deep dyslexic; but it may not necessarily read – not in all of us, and not under all experimental conditions.

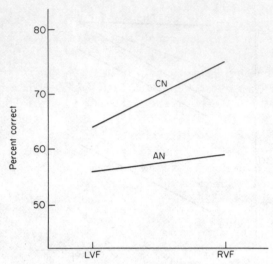

FIGURE 17.3 Split-field performance on concrete (CN) and abstract (AN) nouns in normal subjects

Toward a right-hemisphere model for deep dyslexia

Our efforts to test the right hemisphere hypothesis do not, as yet, permit any firm conclusions. While the split-field studies of deep dyslexics are clearly supportive, further experiments are necessary to rule out alternative explanations. It is unlikely, however, in view of the difficulties discussed earlier in this paper, that the split-field paradigm will ever provide an unequivocal answer to the question. Converging evidence, particularly from studies of the isolated right hemisphere, will be essential.

Having tangled with the difficulties of subjecting the right hemi-sphere theory to empirical test, we think we have earned the right to indulge in some speculation. In the rest of this chapter, we would like to consider how a right-hemisphere model might account for the salient features of deep dyslexia. We take a somewhat different approach than Coltheart, who has also addressed this question (Chapter 16).

The thrust of our argument is that reading in deep dyslexia is mediated by a right-hemisphere language mechanism that is geared to the *comprehension* of language and not its production (for evidence on this characterization of right hemisphere language abilities, see Marin, Schwartz and Saffran, 1979). The characteristics of reading performance in deep dyslexia derive, in part, from the fact that the sole pathway from print to sound depends on language comprehension; they also reflect the special character of the right hemisphere language mechanism, which deals primarily with lexical (particularly referential) aspects of meaning, and has little capacity for the syntactic aspects of language comprehension (evidence on this point is cited earlier in this chapter and also in Coltheart, Chapter 16).

We assume that word recognition in deep dyslexia is mediated entirely by the right-hemisphere language system, which lacks the capacity for phonemic recoding of orthographic information. Words are recognized by matching the input to a set of stored orthographic entries (called 'visual logogens' or 'visual word forms' by other authors in this volume). As indicated by the deep dyslexics' failure to recognize many real words as words (Patterson, in press),[10] the store of orthographic entries would seem to be incomplete; relative to the normal left-hemisphere, entries for abstract (i.e. nonreferential) words, particularly those of low frequency, are somewhat lacking. The right hemisphere orthographic entries have no direct access to phonological codes that might be used for pronunciation (i.e. 'output logogens'; see Morton and Patterson, Chapter 4, and Schwartz, Saffran and Marin, Chapter 12); their output is exclusively to the right-hemisphere semantic system.

The result of activating a right-hemisphere orthographic entry is the elaboration of a semantic representation for the input. This process may involve widespread activity in the right-hemisphere semantic network (as, for example, in lexical activation effects in normal subjects; see, e.g. Meyer and Schvaneveldt, 1971). An output device that interfaces with this system will therefore be faced with a selection problem: what piece of this semantic representation should it encode? It is understandable that the verbal response will sometimes be off-target (i.e. that a semantic error will be produced), even if the word has been adequately understood. In some cases, particularly in the more fluent patients, the response will consist of a semantically appropriate phrase or sentence, rather than a single word.

Except for semantic errors, reading performance is fairly adequate for concrete nouns. There are two problems, however, with abstract words: they are less likely to be represented in the right hemisphere;

and it is more difficult to derive an oral response for an abstract word via a semantic representation. While the core meaning of a reference term is relatively fixed (a rose *is* a rose), the meaning of an abstract word depends to a large extent on the linguistic context in which it is embedded (e.g. the *phase* of the moon, the *phase* of development, and so on). An isolated abstract word may not generate enough semantic information to specify an oral response.

There are similar problems with function words. Although the right hemisphere may have orthographic entries for these high frequency words (as indicated by the lexical decision performance of deep dyslexics; see Patterson, in press, and data for V.S., above), it will have difficulty, given its syntactic deficiency, specifying their meanings. Furthermore, the contextual dependency that charac- terizes abstract nouns also applies (if anything, more so) to functors. If we take agrammatic aphasia as the model for a syntactically impoverished language comprehender (with the features of agram- matic comprehension as described in Saffran, Schwartz and Marin, 1980), we would expect the right hemisphere to be able to extract from grammatical morphemes only their most direct semantic implications (e.g. the gender of pronouns and the type of spatial relation signified by locative prepositions); but it should not be able to comprehend grammatical morphemes that serve a purely syntactic function (e.g. case marking prepositions). We would predict, then, that the deep dyslexic will have more success reading aloud those grammatical words that can be represented semantically than those that serve a purely syntactic function.[11] This prediction is borne out in our own corpus: 90 per cent of the correct reading responses to functors are spatial prepositions or pronouns; these are also the functors that give rise to the highest proportion of meaning-related errors (e.g. *her* → 'she').

Thus, whatever its own deficiencies (e.g. whether it is agrammatic or not), an output mechanism that interfaces with the right- hemisphere language comprehender (whether it is also in the right hemisphere, or not) will have certain difficulties. It is charged, in the oral reading task, with recovering a specification for the target word from an elaborated semantic representation. In the case of refer- ential words, this representation is likely to be a rich one; in addition to the core meaning (e.g. rose), related information will be available (e.g. flower). Hence, the likelihood of semantic errors. In the case of abstract nouns and function words, the semantic representation is likely to be too vague to specify an output, and there may be no response at all. This is precisely the performance that is seen in deep dyslexia.[12]

We have not specified the laterality of the output system that interfaces with the right hemisphere comprehension mechanism. It may reside in the left hemisphere, as Coltheart (Chapter 16) suggests, in which case semantic information would have to be transmitted across the callosum for encoding; or, in some cases, the right hemisphere itself may have the capacity to produce speech. Perhaps patients differ in this respect. In any case, the laterality of the output mechanism is not, on this view, a critical feature of a right hemisphere model for deep dyslexia.

The result of this theorizing is that we are very far from our point of departure when we, at least, took up the study of deep dyslexia. We hoped to learn something about normal reading. Now we believe that the patients are telling us more about the nature of right-hemisphere language capacity, and about language mechanisms in general.

Appendix

A   Stimuli for the first experiment with normal subjects

Concrete nouns	Abstract nouns	Function words	Proper names
frog	mode	more	Paul
oats	soul	does	Jack
golf	sane	from	Bert
toad	life	your	Chad
desk	ease	both	Hans
hoof	fact	were	Matt
page	cult	ours	Kent
soil	pact	them	Jane
lime	mood	must	Mack
seed	tact	then	Walt
path	myth	that	Phil
face	mind	what	Hugh
corn	oath	been	Saul
crag	goal	some	John
wife	fate	with	Beth
door	gall	most	Joan
drum	feat	they	Pete
rust	past	this	Joel
moth	sake	when	Lynn

colt	plea	than	Fred
jail	hint	here	Carl
harp	hour	whom	Anne
chin	hope	till	Jill
cane	noun	such	Kate

B   Stimuli for the second experiment with normal subjects

Concrete nouns		*Abstract nouns*	
star	wagon	fact	event
dish	cloud	fate	truth
army	clock	duty	fault
lake	table	life	power
pipe	cabin	sake	glory
jail	tiger	goal	pride
claw	penny	mode	folly
toad	porch	feat	mercy
wine	scarf	debt	poise
pole	robin	term	proof
sand	mouth	task	sense
bulb	skull	role	creed
cave	grass	mood	peace
moth	chalk	plea	phase
cane	whale	oath	fraud
fern	bride	pang	skill
horn	straw	fame	theme
door	candy	loss	basis
tent	broom	tale	error
oven	shelf	unit	scope
gate	apple	mind	habit
flute	puppy	merit	logic
camel	skirt	topic	faith
armor	towel	prose	rumor

Notes

1 This disability, which was total when we first saw W.S. two years ago, has been partially remediated. W.S. is now able to 'sound out' the first syllable of a word with some success, in most instances using the most common pronunciation of the vowel. He also shows a limited ability to read simple nonsense words by analogy (he read 'vad', for example, by first saying 'dad' and then 'v-ad'). W.S.'s progress with phonics is greater than we have seen in other deep dyslexics, and may perhaps be attributed to his relative immaturity at the time of the lesion (he was 11, and in the first stages of puberty), and possibly to the fact that he is receiving intensive phonics instruction in school. However, W.S.'s limited command of

phonics has not, thus far, proved to be of much assistance in reading. He still shows the essential characteristics of deep dyslexia, including a substantial proportion of semantic errors in reading aloud.

2 Given a number of assumptions, some reaction time methods do allow the experimenter to infer that beyond some level of processing (usually unspecifiable) the task has been carried out entirely by one hemisphere or the other (see Coltheart, Chapter 16, for a discussion of these techniques).

3 The words in this task were the same as those used in the study with normal subjects which is reported later in this chapter.

4 Other data on H.T. and B.L. can be found in Marin, Saffran and Schwartz (1976) and in Schwartz, Saffran and Marin (1977). Two other deep dyslexics failed to qualify for this study; one (W.S.) had a visual field defect, and the other (J.R.) performed poorly on free-field tests of lexical decision.

5 In order to produce this effect (rather than a reversal to LVF superiority) it is necessary to minimize left-to-right scanning habits in readers of European languages. This is accomplished by presenting the stimulus array vertically and/or for very short durations (Mackavey, Curcio and Rosen, 1975).

6 We have avoided the use of a fixation control task (such as report of a central digit) because it imposes an additional verbal load on the subject and may have other complicating effects (Moscovitch and Klein, 1977).

7 Letter recognition in the two fields under bilateral stimulation in V.S. must be compared under conditions where RVF and LVF exposures were identical, which is not the case for the data in Table 17.5. When the identity task was run under these conditions, RVF letter recognition performance was still very poor.

8 We still lack an adequate explanation for the substantial changes in V.S.'s performance over the course of these studies. From the first pilot experiment to the bilateral series, there has been a trend towards increasing similarity in the lexical decision performance of the two visual fields. The devastating effect of a competing stimulus to the right hemisphere on performance in the control task would seem to suggest that the change does not reflect improved performance in the left hemisphere. More likely, it is the result of an increased tendency to transfer RVF information to the right, perhaps because this strategy became progressively more efficient, or perhaps because the left hemisphere became less able to deal with the letter information. There was independent evidence (the onset of weakness in the right hand, which had not been evident before) to suggest a change in the status of V.S.'s left hemisphere during the course of these experiments.

9 Control studies are in progress as this chapter goes to press. The results from the first two control patients (aphasics, with left hemisphere lesions, who are not deep dyslexics) are indicative of a normal RVF superiority.

10 One of Patterson's patients (P.W.) performed normally on lexical decision tasks with abstract words; the other (D.E.) did not. We have recently performed a similar study with our own patients, who also varied in their performance with abstract words.

11 In the case of agrammatic deep dyslexics, the problem with functors is compounded by the agrammatism of the language production mechanism, which might be unable to encode the grammatical morpheme even if presented with a complete semantic/syntactic specification.

12 We have not tried to account for visual errors. We agree with the approach taken by Morton and Patterson (Chapter 4) and by Coltheart (Chapter 16), which does not involve any commitment to the laterality of the reading mechanism in deep dyslexia.

References

Day, J. (1977) Right-hemisphere language processing in normal right-handers. *Journal of Experimental Psychology: Human Perception and Performance, 3*, 518–28.

Ellis, H. D. and Shepherd, J. W. (1974) Recognition of abstract and concrete words presented in left and right visual fields. *Journal of Experimental Psychology, 103*, 1035–6.

Goodglass, H., Hyde, M. R. and Blumstein, S. (1969) Frequency, picturability, and availability of nouns in aphasia. *Cortex, 2*, 74–89.

Hines, D. (1975) Independent functioning of the two cerebral hemispheres for recognizing bilaterally presented tachistoscopic visual half-field stimuli. *Cortex, 11*, 132–43.

Hines, D. (1976) Recognition of verbs, abstract nouns and concrete nouns from the left and right visual half-fields. *Neuropsychologia, 14*, 211–16.

Hines, D. (1977) Differences in tachistoscopic recognition between abstract and concrete words as a function of visual half-field and frequency. *Cortex, 13*, 66–73.

Levy, J. and Trevarthen, C. (1977) Perceptual, semantic and phonetic aspects of elementary language processes in split-field patients. *Brain, 100*, 105–18.

Mackavey, W., Curcio, F. and Rosen, J. (1975) Tachistoscopic word recognition performance under conditions of simultaneous bilateral presentation. *Neuropsychologia, 13*, 27–33.

Marcel, T. and Patterson, K. (1978) Word recognition and production: reciprocity in clinical and normal studies. In J. Requin (ed.), *Attention and Performance*, VII. Hillsdale, N.J.: Lawrence Erlbaum.

Marin, O. S. M., Saffran, E. M. and Schwartz, M. F. (1976) Dissociations of language in aphasia: implications for normal function. *Annals of the New York Academy of Sciences, 280*, 868–84.

Marin, O. S. M., Schwartz, M. F. and Saffran, E. M. (1979) Origins and distribution of language. In M. Gazzaniga (ed.), *Handbook of Behavioral Neurology*. New York: Plenum Press.

Marshall, J. C. and Newcombe, F. (1966) Syntactic and semantic errors in paralexia. *Neuropsychologia, 4,* 169–76.

Meyer, D. E. and Schvaneveldt, R. W. (1971) Facilitation in recognizing pairs of words: Evidence of a dependence between retrieval operations. *Journal of Experimental Psychology, 90,* 227–34.

McKeever, W. F. (1970) Bilateral word recognition: effects of unilateral and bilateral presentation, asynchrony of bilateral presentation, and forced order of report. *Quarterly Journal of Experimental Psychology, 23,* 410–16.

Moore, W. H. and Weidner, W. E. (1974) Bilateral tachistoscopic word perception in aphasic and normal subjects. *Perceptual and Motor Skills, 39,* 1003–11.

Moscovitch, M. and Klein, D. (1977) Material specific interference effects and their relation to functional hemispheric asymmetries. Paper presented to the International Neuropsychology Society, Santa Fe, New Mexico, February, 1977.

Myerson, R. and Goodglass, H. (1972) Transformational grammars of three agrammatic patients. *Language and Speech, 15,* 40–50.

Paivio, A., Yuille, J. C. and Madigan, S. A. (1968) Concreteness, imagery and meaningfulness values of 925 nouns. *Journal of Experimental Psychology, Monograph Supplement, 76* (1).

Patterson, K. E. (1978) Phonemic dyslexia: Errors of meaning and the meaning of errors. *Quarterly Journal of Experimental Psychology, 30,* 587–607.

Patterson, K. E. and Marcel, A. J. (1977) Aphasia, dyslexia and the phonological coding of written words. *Quarterly Journal of Experimental Psychology, 29,* 307–18.

Penfield, W. and Roberts, L. (1959) *Speech and Brain-Mechanisms.* Princeton, N.J.: Princeton University Press.

Reicher, G. M. (1969) Perceptual recognition as a function of meaning-fulness of stimulus material. *Journal of Experimental Psychology, 81,* 275–80.

Richardson, J. T. E. (1975) The effect of word imageability in acquired dyslexia. *Neuropsychologia, 13,* 281–8.

Rosen, J. J., Curcio, R., Mackavey, W. and Herbert, J. (1975) Superior recall of letters in the right visual field with bilateral presentation and partial report. *Cortex, 11,* 144–51.

Saffran, E. M. and Marin, O. S. M. (1977) Reading without phonology: evidence from aphasia. *Quarterly Journal of Experimental Psychology, 29,* 515–25.

Saffran, E. M., Schwartz, M. F. and Marin, O. S. M. (1980) Evidence mechanisms in paralexia. *Brain and Language, 3,* 255–65.

Saffran, E. M., Schwartz, M. F. and Marin, O. S. M. (1979) Evidence from aphasia: isolating the components of a production model. In B. Butterworth (ed.), *Language Production.* London: Academic Press.

Schwartz, M. F., Saffran, E. M. and Marin, O. S. M. (1977) An analysis of agrammatic reading in aphasia. Paper presented to the

International Neuropsychology Society, Santa Fe, New Mexico, February, 1977.

Shai, A., Goodglass, H. and Barton, M. (1972) Recognition of tachisto-scopically presented verbal and non-verbal material after unilateral cerebral damage. *Neuropsychologia, 10,* 185–92.

Shallice, T. and Warrington, E. K. (1975) Word recognition in a phonemic dyslexic patient. *Quarterly Journal of Experimental Psychology, 27,* 187–99.

Zaidel, E. (1976) Auditory vocabulary of the right hemisphere following brain bisection or hemidecortication. *Cortex, 12,* 191–211.

Zaidel, E. (1978) Auditory language comprehension in the right hemisphere following cerebral commissurotomy and hemispherectomy: a comparison with child language and aphasia. In A. Caramazza and E. Zurif (eds), *The Acquisition and Breakdown of Language: Parallels and Divergencies.* Baltimore: Johns Hopkins University Press.

Zaidel, E. (in press) Lexical organization in the right hemisphere. In P. Buser and A. Rougeul-Buser (eds), *Cerebral Correlates of Conscious Experience.* Amsterdam: Elsevier.

Appendix 1
CAT scans of five deep dyslexic patients

with comments by O. S. M. Marin

Anatomical distribution of cerebral lesions in deep dyslexias as demonstrated by computerized tomograms

We were able to gather head computed tomograms in five of our cases of deep dyslexic patients (H.T. and V.S. from the Baltimore group; D.E. and P.W. from the Cambridge group; and patient P.D., described by Kapur and Perl, 1978). Computed tomograms were studied with particular attention given to the identification of the classical areas of speech. In this we followed the radiological anatomical criteria used by other authors in pursuing the same aim (Naeser and Hayward, 1978). All the computerized tomograms were performed during the chronic stable phase of the stroke, in some cases years after it. Figure 1 is a composite picture showing the most representative C.T. picture of each case; Figure 2 is a composite diagram of the areas of cortical damage of the five patients drawn upon the classical picture from Dejerine's *Semiology of the Nervous System* (1926). Figure 3 is a composite diagram of the subcortical extent of the lesions in five patients drawn upon a horizontal section of the brain; another classical picture from Dejerine's *Semiology*. The anatomical distribution of the areas of damage merit the following general comments:

1   The cortical damage is in all cases quite extensive, and, in some intuitive way, out of proportion to the overall degree of language impairment observed in the patients. Lesions in all cases involved the left hemisphere (all patients were right-handed).

2   Classical Broca's area was involved in all cases but in two (V.S., P.W.) the damage was probably partial. The inferior pre-central involvement was minimal in V.S., relatively extensive in P.D., and only moderate in the rest.

3   Superior temporal cortical damage was clearly present in only one case (V.S.) but in all cases there were superior temporal sub-cortical areas of damage.

4   The posterior aspects of the superior temporal gyrus was mostly isolated and damaged in only one case (P.W.), with relative sparing in all the other cases.

5   Supramarginal gyrus involvement was present in all cases, with complete destruction in four cases, and only very anterior damage in one (H.T.).
6   Angular gyrus was partially involved in three cases but with significant damage in only one of these (P.W.).
7   Superior and middle parietal involvement was present in four cases. with sparing in one case (H.T.).
8   Subcortical damage was extensive in all cases, affecting, in all of them, the subcortical fronto-central white matter, and often reaching the ventricular frontal horns. Insular cortical and subcortical damage was present in all cases, and in at least one (D.E.) the damage involved the left thalamus.

Oscar S. M. Marin, M.D.

References

Kapur, N. and Perl, N. T. (1978) Recognition reading in paralexia. *Cortex, 14,* 439–43.
Naeser, M. A. and Hayward, R. W. (1978) Lesions localization in aphasia with cranial computed tomography and the Boston Diagnostic Aphasic Exam. *Neurology, 28,* 545–51.
Dejerine, J. (1926) *Sémiologie des Affections du Système Nerveux.* Paris: Masson et Cie.

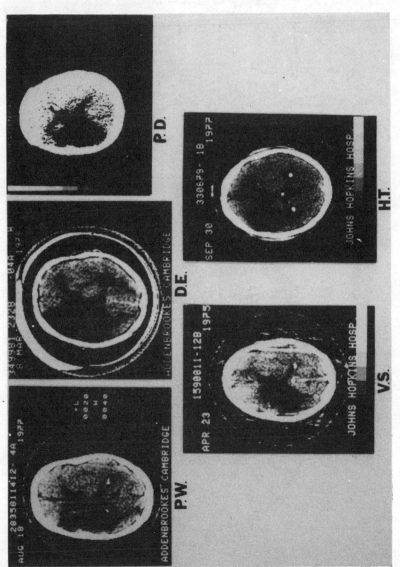

FIGURE 1 This is a composite of the most representative area of damage as shown by the head computerized tomography of five cases of deep dyslexias

409

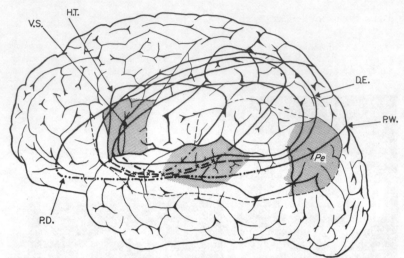

FIGURE 2 Composite diagram of the cortical involvement of five cases of deep dyslexias drawn on the classical diagram by Dejerine

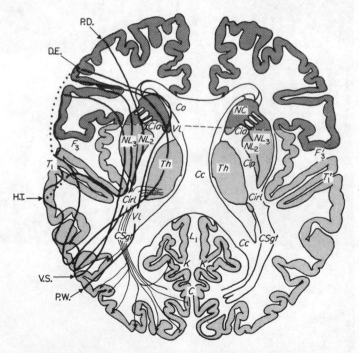

FIGURE 3 Composite of the subcortical damage in five cases of deep dyslexias drawn on the horizontal section of the brain from Dejerine

K.F.: Post-mortem findings

K.F. died in 1973 as a result of a head injury sustained in the course of an epileptic seizure. This injury resulted in a second lesion in addition to the older one sustained in 1957. Only the older lesion is relevant for interpreting his performance in psychological experiments. (It should be noted that the reading corpus was obtained in 1969 prior to the operation described in Warrington, Logue and Pratt, 1971.)

The post-mortem findings of Dr W. G. Mair concerning the old lesion site are:

An extensive lesion involved the inferior parietal lobule and the temporo-occipital region of the left cerebral hemisphere. This lesion in which the cortex and white matter were gliosed and hard, extended 4 cm antero-posteriorly and 4 cm vertically. There was a loss of tissue from the inferior part of the parietal lobe and from the occipito-temporal region; from the posterior part of the parietal lobe to within 3 cm of the occipital pole. The lesion involved much of the optic radiations on the left side. The trigone and the occipital horn of the left lateral ventricle were greatly dilated. Throughout the left cerebral hemisphere there was less white matter than in the right cerebral hemisphere.

Tim Shallice
Elizabeth Warrington

Reference

Warrington, E. K., Logue, V. and Pratt, R. T. C. (1971) The anatomical localisation of selective impairment of short-term memory. *Neuropsychologia*, *9*, 377–87.

Appendix 2
Error corpora from four deep dyslexic patients D.E., P.W., P.D. and K.F.

This Appendix contains collections of reading responses from four deep dyslexic patients: P.D. (Kapur and Perl, 1978), D.E. and P.W. (Patterson and Marcel, 1977; see also Chapters 13 and 14) and K.F. (Shallice and Warrington, 1975). The data for P.D. consist of his responses to each of the 650 words of the Brown and Ure (1969) list; these data were collected on 8 August 1977. The data for D.E. and P.W. consist of their incorrect responses to a collection of words drawn from a variety of sources; all of the incorrect responses they have made in testing sessions up to the time of writing are included. The data for K.F. come from two sources: his reading of all the AA words from this list of Thorndike and Lorge (1944) – 977 words in all – and his reading of the 650 words from the Brown and Ure (1969) list. For all four patients, these words were presented singly, without time pressure, and the patients were asked to read each single word aloud.

Reading responses of P.D. Data kindly provided by Narinder Kapur

One-word correct responses (Brown and Ure list, 1969)

action, afraid, alert, altar, ambulance, angel, angry, applaud, army, art, ask, attack, autumn, baby, bag, bake, bandage, barracks, bath, battle, beating, beautiful, beauty, bed, bible, bird, bitter, black, bleed, blue, bomb, book, box, boy, boy friend, breast, brother, bully, butter, butterfly, cabbage, camera, candy, career, carpet, caution, cemetery, census, cheese, child, church, clay, clean, client, coarse, cold, colour, command, conduct, conscience, cook, cooking, cork, corpse, corridor, courage, cow, curtains, cut, daddy, dance, danger, dark, daughter, dead, dear, dentist, deputy, description, dirt, divorce, doctor, dog, door, dream, dress, drink, dwarf, eagle, earth, eating, engine, estate, evil, expensive, fairy, false, farm, farmhouse, father, female, fiction, fire, flower, flush, foster, free, frog, fur, gamble, garage, ginger, girl, girl friend, glass, gossip, gray, habit, hammer, hand, happy, hat, hate, hay, head, healthy, heart, history, home, homosexual, horse, hospital, house, humour, industry, ink, insult, island, ivory, jelly, jerk, jolly, journey, joy, jump, key, king, kiss, kissing, kneel, lake, lamp, laugh, lawyer, lick, lie, light, lighthouse, limp, lion, long, loud, love, malice, man, memory, milk, money, monkey, month, moon, mother, music, name, narrow, nasty, needle, new, nipple, notice, office, old, paddock, painting, paper, part, parting, peace, perfume, person, phone, pirate, plant, plum, poetry, police, priest, prosper, punch, race, red, religion, rich, ring, rug, sad, salt, salute, scandal, scent, school, scissors, scrub, shadow, sheep, shut, shy, sick, sin, sleep, slow, small, smell, smooth, sniff, soft, soldier, son, spider, spit, sponge, spring, square, stammer, star, state, stomach, stork, story, street, stupid, sweet, swim, table, tame, tattoo, taxi, thief, thirsty, tickle, time, tired, tobacco, toilet, torture, train, treasure, trumpet, trunk, uncle, valentine, vehicle, village, virgin, voyage, walk, war, water, weak, whiskey, whistle, white, windmill, window, wine, woman, women, work, working, world, writer, yellow, youth, zero.

Omissions (Brown and Ure list, 1969)

absorption, accent, accordance, acorn, agency, agility, alone, antelope, anxiety, applause, apprehension, aquarium, argon, bad, baronet, beat, beef, behind, big, bite, blossom, bodice, bowl, branch, bread, bring, broad, bury, bust, capacity, caress, caring for, carrot, carry, caught, centre, chair, change, choice, choose, choosing, chore, climb, clumsy, column, comfort, comparison, compete, contents, context, corrupt, cottage, coward, crutch, damage, dancer, darn, debate, decade, deceive, deep, defeat, defect, definition, depressed, despise, detail, dimension, direct, dirty, dismal, distribution, dump, enter, erosion, errand, esteem, excel, faith, faithless, fall, family, famous, fasten, fearing, fight, finger, forbid, frame, friendly, fringe, froth, future, garment, give, glacier, glisten, go, good, green, grief, grime, grudge, hard, heavy, hinder, hoist, hostage, hungry, inferior, intercourse, iodine, kerosene, kindness, lantern, leisure, levity, loveliness, maintenance, make, mallet, mane, manner, masturbate, measurement, medley, melody, menace, mental, misfortune, modification, mural, museum, mutton, nation, nature, nectar, nice, nitrogen, obtain, occurrence, odd, offend, opinion, option, orgasm, pamphlet, patriotism, pencil, penis, perch, phase, pinch, pity, plenty, power, prairie, pray, preach, prick, pride, priority, proud, pure, purpose, qualm, quarrel, quarrelling, quart, quick, quota, radiator, rally, ram, ratio, rattle, revolt, riddle, ridicule, rip, rotation, rough, rude, rustle, sap, scar, screen, seen, sequel, should, sickness, silly, slap, slime, smash, sneak, sneer, social, socialism, soothe, sour, sphere, spill, splash, sprinkle, squeak, squeeze, stalk, statue, steady, steeple, stem, stern, stool, stove, strict, stumble, success, suicide, supplicate, swear, swift, swing, tangle, tease, tempt, theory, threat, timid, travel, tree, trouble, try, unjust, upset, vagina, valour, vanity, veneer, vigorous, violation, virtue, vision, vulgar, wagon, warmth, whine, wicked, wild, wink, wish, wishing, woo, wound, wretch, wrinkle, wrinkles.

Errors (Brown and Ure list, 1969)

abusing	→ 'abused'	indignation	→ 'digestion'
anger	→ 'angry'	injure	→ 'injury'
ascend	→ 'ascension'	insane	→ 'insanity'
baker	→ 'bakery'	insomnia	→ 'obsomnia'
barber	→ 'barbers'	instep	→ 'footstep'
beggar	→ 'beg'	justice	→ 'judge'
bowel		kitchen	→ 'not house but,
movement	→ 'bowels'		don't know'
brave	→ 'courage'	kite	→ 'Yacht, no, air'
bride	→ 'girl'	legend	→ 'deed'
bright	→ 'brightness'	little	→ 'please'
chapter	→ 'chaplain'	lose	→ 'slow'
citizen	→ 'cizinet'	luck	→ 'lucky'
city	→ 'town'	marry	→ 'married'
class	→ 'classes'	mature	→ 'mate'
clothing	→ 'clothes'	mitten	→ 'mittens'
comedy	→ 'comedian'	modest	→ 'modesty'
cripple	→ 'crippled'	moment	→ 'memory'
cry	→ 'crying'	motor	→ 'car'
cushion	→ 'seat you know'	mountain	→ 'mountains'
custom	→ 'custody'	movies	→ 'pictures'
death	→ 'dead again, don't	muddy	→ 'mud'
	know'	navigation	→ 'navigator'
decent	→ 'ascension . . . up'	normal	→ 'formal'
die	→ 'dead'	ocean	→ 'sea'
disgust	→ 'disgusted'	orchestra	→ 'orchester'
eldest	→ 'elderly'	party	→ 'parties'
elevator	→ 'lift'	passage	→ 'travel'
employ	→ 'employment'	patent	→ 'patient'
excuse	→ 'excuses'	penalty	→ 'guilty'
fail	→ 'failed'	ploughing	→ 'plough'
fear	→ 'afraid'	pond	→ 'pool'
foolish	→ 'stupid'	puppy	→ 'pup'
foot	→ 'feet'	quiet	→ 'silent'
friend	→ 'pal'	removal	→ 'moving'
fruit	→ 'cream'	river	→ 'swim'
fuss	→ 'fussy'	salad	→ 'salad-cream'
grease	→ 'greasy'	scold	→ 'cold'
guilty	→ 'jail'	seat	→ 'seats'
hatred	→ 'hateful'	secret	→ 'silent'
health	→ 'healthy'	secure	→ 'security'
hide	→ 'hidden'	seed	→ 'plant'
high	→ 'heights'	ship	→ 'slip'
hug	→ 'rug'	short	→ 'walk'
hunger	→ 'hungry'	shove	→ 'shovel'
income	→ 'tax'	sing	→ 'singing'

sister	→ 'sisters'		*taxes*	→ 'tax'
sleeping	→ 'sleepy'		*temper*	→ 'tempered'
smoking	→ 'smoke'		*thermometer*	→ 'thermostat'
speak	→ 'speech'		*thigh*	→ 'high'
stolen	→ 'steal'		*think*	→ 'thinking'
stripes	→ 'strip'		*thirst*	→ 'thirsty'
strong	→ 'strength'		*truth*	→ 'true'
suck	→ 'sucker'		*wait*	→ 'sit'
sweat	→ 'sweaty'		*wealth*	→ 'wealthy'
tackle	→ 'tacks'		*worry*	→ 'worried'

Reading errors of P.W. and D.E.
Karalyn Patterson

Comments on error corpora

1   As discussed or mentioned in several of the chapters in this book (e.g. 2 and 14), the algorithm for classifying errors is less than perfect. In particular, some paralexic errors meet the criteria for more than one category. For example, *bit* → 'bite' could be visual, derivational, or visual and/or semantic. One of the reasons for including the corpora in the book is to allow the reader to make his own judgements about these classifications.
2   When the same stimulus word appears more than once in a patient's corpus, it was presented for reading on separate occasions and evoked different paralexic responses. This may be slightly misleading as an indication of variability of reading performance, since a stimulus word which evoked the same response on different occasions is listed only once. In other words, the corpora should be used as a description of error types rather than to infer characteristics such as consistency of reading responses.
3   As indicated by Shallice and Warrington (Chapter 5), various deep dyslexic patients differ in their proportions of the various types of error. But it must be emphasised that probability of a given error type is partly a function of the type of stimulus word. To take an extreme example, patient P.W.'s corpus contains a great many function word paralexias; but this reflects the fact that he has been extensively tested on reading function words and not necessarily that he is especially prone to this type of error. The caution is the same as in (2) above: these lists should be treated as individual examples of error types rather than as comprehensive pictures of a patient's reading behaviour.
4   The occasional response in patient P.W.'s corpus is presented with the initial syllable set off in parentheses, e.g. *oblivion* → '(in)finity'. As is typical in Broca's aphasia, P.W.'s articulation shows problems with initial unstressed syllables; none the less it is usually easy to understand what word he is intending to produce. The '(in)finity' format is merely an attempt to give a more accurate picture of what he says.

Corpus of paralexic errors for P.W.

Semantic paralexias

block	→	'boulder'	*bough*	→	'branch'
thermos	→	'flask'	*bead*	→	'bauble'
directing	→	'straight'	*drove*	→	'car'
archer	→	'arrow'	*office*	→	'business'
fence	→	'wire'	*carnation*	→	'narcissus'
dial	→	'sun'	*team*	→	'football'
capsule	→	'tablets'	*turtle*	→	'crocodile'
probing	→	'digging'	*shame*	→	'wrong'
confining	→	'hospital'	*spirit*	→	'whisky'
amphibian	→	'tiddlers'	*gift*	→	'present'
hit	→	'bat'	*style*	→	'dress'
soil	→	'grass'	*amount*	→	'figures'
stock	→	'trust'	*agony*	→	'anguish'
pair	→	'two'	*amount*	→	'money'
most	→	'big'	*amount*	→	'sums'
she	→	'girls'	*answer*	→	'query'
her	→	'girl'	*beauty*	→	'love'
inch	→	'rule'	*danger*	→	'accident'
guide	→	'sightseeing'	*danger*	→	'urgent'
arrest	→	'caught'	*decree*	→	'judge'
competitor	→	'event'	*disaster*	→	'accident'
contain	→	'amount'	*edition*	→	'journal'
decay	→	'rubbish'	*event*	→	'athletics'
desire	→	'sweet'	*fact*	→	'truth'
direct	→	'straight'	*grown*	→	'harvest'
earnest	→	'genuine'	*hint*	→	'nudge'
employ	→	'working'	*lecture*	→	'talking'
extend	→	'outside'	*merry*	→	'happy'
fortune	→	'riches'	*occasion*	→	'event'
glorious	→	'valour'	*occasion*	→	'incident'
resist	→	'rebuff'	*phase*	→	'moon'
upset	→	'quarrel'	*position*	→	'place'
goddess	→	'girl'	*reality*	→	'fact'
reflection	→	'mirror'	*reason*	→	'right'
investigation	→	'query'	*revolt*	→	'rebel'
admiral	→	'colonel'	*savage*	→	'killing'
evidence	→	'police'	*savage*	→	'terrible'
product	→	'amount'	*savage*	→	'cannibals'
oxygen	→	'air'	*scene*	→	'drama'
contribution	→	'helping'	*unit*	→	'one'
inhabitant	→	'people'	*artist*	→	'picture'
fault	→	'wrong'	*emergency*	→	'accident'
limb	→	'hip'	*jury*	→	'judge'
rope	→	'hanging'	*deed*	→	'solicitors'

cost	→ 'money'	conscience	→ 'honesty'
demon	→ 'Satan'	sepulchre	→ 'tomb'
bush	→ 'tree'	diseased	→ 'dead'
pouring	→ 'raining'	beguile	→ 'bedevilled'
coach	→ 'bus'	stage	→ 'coach'
elk	→ 'yak'	pulling	→ 'come'
delight	→ 'pleasure'	negative	→ 'minus'
assaulting	→ 'hurting'	classes	→ 'school'
destruction	→ 'disaster'	shoulder	→ 'arms'
coast	→ 'seashore'	small	→ 'little'
hoisting	→ 'pulling'	poster	→ 'sign'
bereavement	→ 'burial'	pilot	→ 'air'
canine	→ 'dog'	glasses	→ 'eyes'
confining	→ 'measles'	cemetery	→ 'burial'
gable	→ 'eaves'	student	→ 'thinking'
amphibian	→ 'zoo'	spectacles	→ 'binoculars'
cascade	→ 'purge'	directions	→ 'forward'
genealogist	→ 'babies'	excavations	→ 'shovel'
concentric	→ 'compass'	furlong	→ 'miles'
cornice	→ 'curtains'	tandem	→ 'cycle'
fettered	→ 'tying'	brass	→ 'band'
university	→ 'boys'	prize	→ 'present'
parting	→ 'away'	clothes	→ 'dress'
paddock	→ 'horses'	guilty	→ 'judge'
mutton	→ 'meat'	shadow	→ 'ghost'
malice	→ 'nasty'	true	→ 'sure'
shadow	→ 'dark'	sty	→ 'pig'
nephew	→ 'cousin'	curse	→ 'swearing'
product	→ 'factory'	responsive	→ 'question'
bring	→ 'towards'	able	→ 'navy'
melody	→ 'music'	keen	→ 'zeal'
vision	→ 'view'	guessed	→ 'query'
alimony	→ 'judge'	belief	→ 'real'
oblivion	→ '(in)finity'	cite	→ 'judge'
rescind	→ 'negative'	stanza	→ 'piano'
attractive	→ 'beautiful'	lessen	→ 'minimal'
applaud	→ 'clap'	condemn	→ 'prison'
soloist	→ 'piano'	aid	→ 'helping'
procrastinate	→ 'late'	pause	→ 'wait'
disposal	→ 'dustbin'	dash	→ 'streak'
satirical	→ 'scaustic'	hit	→ 'kick'
somnambulist	→ 'sleeping'	age	→ 'old'
postage	→ 'stamps'	originate	→ 'new'
nourished	→ 'warm'		

Derivational paralexias

tackling	→ 'tackle'	hovering	→ 'hover'
assaulting	→ 'assaulted'	angling	→ 'angler'

transportation	→ 'transport'		*mercantile*	→ 'merchant'
excavation	→ '(ex)cavation'		*think*	→ 'thinking'
height	→ 'high'		*tyrannical*	→ 'tyrant'
ride	→ 'rider'		*classification*	→ 'classes'
arched	→ 'arch'		*heroic*	→ 'heroine'
calculate	→ 'calculation'		*heroine*	→ 'hero'
classify	→ 'class'		*fictitious*	→ 'fiction'
delight	→ 'delightful'		*typing*	→ 'type'
gratefully	→ 'grateful'		*projection*	→ 'projector'
swear	→ 'swearing'		*hurting*	→ 'hurt'
upper	→ 'up'		*territory*	→ 'territorial'
beauty	→ 'beautiful'		*beautiful*	→ 'beauty'
danger	→ 'dangerous'		*bedevilled*	→ 'devils'
edition	→ 'editor'		*sparkle*	→ 'sparkling'
grown	→ 'growing'		*drink*	→ 'drinking'
kingdom	→ 'king'		*graduate*	→ 'graduation'
lovely	→ 'love'		*success*	→ 'successful'
lovely	→ 'loving'		*courageous*	→ 'courage'
marriage	→ 'married'		*occupied*	→ 'occupational'
murder	→ 'murdered'		*cowardly*	→ 'coward'
reality	→ 'real'		*blood*	→ 'bloody'
slavery	→ 'slaving'		*hardly*	→ 'hard'
warmth	→ 'warm'		*solemnity*	→ 'solemn'
management	→ 'manager'		*pacifism*	→ 'pacifist'
death	→ 'dead'		*foolish*	→ 'fool'
wash	→ 'washing'		*unreality*	→ 'unreal'
pour	→ 'pouring'		*abdication*	→ 'abdicate'
speak	→ 'speech'		*cowardice*	→ 'coward'
freedom	→ 'free'		*knowledge*	→ 'knowledgeable'
length	→ 'long'		*abhor*	→ '(ab)horrent'
youth	→ 'young'		*banned*	→ 'ban'
fail	→ 'failed'		*nearer*	→ 'near'
series	→ 'serial'		*rejected*	→ 'rejection'
bat	→ 'batting'		*patience*	→ 'patient'
twist	→ 'twisted'		*burn*	→ 'burned'
wailing	→ 'wail'		*dive*	→ 'diver'
appraising	→ 'appraisal'		*worth*	→ 'worthy'
graduated	→ 'graduation'			

Visual paralexias

tying	→ 'typing'		*was*	→ 'wait'
bush	→ 'brush'		*edge*	→ 'wedge'
picking	→ 'pickles'		*indeed*	→ 'deed'
goggles	→ 'gaggle'		*organize*	→ 'organ'
tumble	→ 'rumbling'		*overcome*	→ 'over'
signal	→ 'single'		*decree*	→ 'degree'
gable	→ 'gage'		*gain*	→ 'grain'
hassock	→ 'hammock'		*narrow*	→ 'marrow'

charter	→ 'garters'	*bibliography*	→ 'bible'
loose	→ 'noose'	*stitching*	→ 'sitting'
break	→ 'breakfast'	*political*	→ 'police'
bead	→ 'bread'	*crab*	→ 'crag'
crouch	→ 'crush'	*forge*	→ 'ford'
moment	→ 'money'	*appliance*	→ 'applying'
grief	→ 'greed'	*raise*	→ 'rise'
orate	→ 'over'	*banality*	→ 'ban'
embossed	→ 'boss'	*lack*	→ 'slack'
sulky	→ 'surly'	*said*	→ 'and'
canary	→ 'carry'	*appraise*	→ 'arise'
smoulder	→ 'boulders'	*innate*	→ 'inn'
terrestrial	→ 'territory'	*drag*	→ 'rag'
campaign	→ 'camping'	*own*	→ 'owing'

Visual and/or semantic paralexias

fragment	→ 'segment'	*judicature*	→ 'jury'
appraising	→ 'assessing'	*question*	→ 'query'
flavour	→ 'savouring'	*once*	→ 'one'
incident	→ 'accident'	*mystic*	→ '(my)sterious'
newspaper	→ 'papers'	*jibe*	→ 'jab'
cone	→ 'cornet'	*least*	→ 'less'
trouble	→ 'terrible'	*sell*	→ 'sale'
jolly	→ 'joy'	*debtor*	→ 'debit'
peacock	→ 'cockerel'	*leader*	→ 'head'
hovering	→ 'hovercraft'	*grown*	→ 'grown-up'
submerge	→ 'submarine'	*raise*	→ 'rise'
preliminary	→ 'primary'	*cause*	→ 'because'

Visual then semantic paralexias

brought	→ 'buying'	*then*	→ 'chick'
copious	→ 'carbon'	*there*	→ 'she'
since	→ 'yours'	*when*	→ 'chick'
their	→ 'earl'		

Function-word paralexias

(a) SUBSTITUTION OF OTHER FUNCTION WORD

where	→ 'because'	*both*	→ 'perhaps'
off	→ 'of'	*his*	→ 'yours'
had	→ 'of'	*for*	→ 'of'
was	→ 'with'	*on*	→ 'of'
where	→ 'whither'	*under*	→ 'in'
to	→ 'which'	*to*	→ 'it'
my	→ 'me'	*not*	→ 'no'
his	→ 'in'	*just*	→ 'it'
of	→ 'if'	*by*	→ 'of'
the	→ 'is'	*or*	→ 'with'

we	→ 'I'		*about*	→ 'out'
down	→ 'under'		*again*	→ 'because'
not	→ 'no'		*all*	→ 'or'
most	→ 'sometimes'		*almost*	→ 'sometimes'
while	→ 'sometimes'		*although*	→ 'from'
and	→ 'of'		*am*	→ 'it'
your	→ 'yours'		*am*	→ 'one'
something	→ 'sometimes'		*am*	→ 'me'
ever	→ 'over'		*any*	→ 'all'
are	→ 'with'		*any*	→ 'many'
such	→ 'whither'		*are*	→ 'or'
you	→ 'yours'		*as*	→ 'is'
for	→ 'or'		*at*	→ 'what'
from	→ 'with'		*away*	→ 'always'
generally	→ 'sometimes'		*away*	→ 'outside'
had	→ 'and'		*been*	→ 'because'
had	→ 'must'		*before*	→ 'because'
had	→ 'it'		*beside*	→ 'because'
has	→ 'because'		*beside*	→ 'inside'
has	→ 'is'		*between*	→ 'sometimes'
has	→ 'and'		*between*	→ 'because'
her	→ 'she'		*between*	→ 'whether'
here	→ 'she'		*both*	→ 'with'
hers	→ 'she'		*but*	→ 'if'
him	→ 'his'		*by*	→ 'away'
his	→ 'is'		*did*	→ 'is'
if	→ 'yet'		*does*	→ 'for'
if	→ 'it'		*does*	→ 'is'
is	→ 'why'		*each*	→ 'which'
it	→ 'is'		*either*	→ 'near'
its	→ 'too'		*every*	→ 'always'
instead	→ 'because'		*every*	→ 'because'
just	→ 'which'		*nor*	→ 'and'
many	→ 'yours'		*nor*	→ 'or'
may	→ 'my'		*now*	→ 'no'
me	→ 'I'		*now*	→ 'soon'
might	→ 'yet'		*of*	→ 'off'
mine	→ 'my'		*often*	→ 'sometimes'
more	→ 'sometimes'		*on*	→ 'one'
more	→ 'or'		*or*	→ 'by'
much	→ 'some'		*our*	→ 'when'
neither	→ 'no'		*out*	→ 'under'
never	→ 'no'		*quite*	→ 'perhaps'
was	→ 'is'		*seldom*	→ 'sometimes'
where	→ 'she'		*should*	→ 'she'
who	→ 'when'		*soon*	→ 'some'
why	→ 'me'		*some*	→ 'many'
your	→ 'always'		*some*	→ 'so'

the	→ 'and'		*us*	→ 'we'
there	→ 'she'		*us*	→ 'is'
therefore	→ 'because'		*usually*	→ 'sometimes'
these	→ 'he'		*usually*	→ 'very'
they	→ 'the'		*very*	→ 'yours'
this	→ 'is'		*what*	→ 'why'
though	→ 'through'		*while*	→ 'yours'
to	→ 'we'		*who*	→ 'why'
to	→ 'of'		*yet*	→ 'if'
until	→ 'near'			

(b) SUBSTITUTION OF CONTENT WORD

across	→ 'cross'		*more*	→ 'little'
again	→ 'gain'		*most*	→ 'big'
any	→ 'sure'		*must*	→ 'musk'
around	→ 'round'		*near*	→ 'ear'
at	→ 'hat'		*near*	→ 'night'
beneath	→ 'downstairs'		*none*	→ 'negative'
both	→ 'buying'		*quite*	→ 'question'
did	→ 'pip'		*rather*	→ 'rats'
do	→ 'doll'		*several*	→ 'seven'
down	→ 'downstairs'		*that*	→ 'hat'
each	→ 'way'		*them*	→ 'ham'
either	→ 'eiderdown'		*then*	→ 'hen'
few	→ 'little'		*those*	→ 'hose'
he	→ 'man'		*through*	→ 'rough'
he	→ 'heel'		*was*	→ 'wait'
her	→ 'girl'		*were*	→ 'way'
if	→ 'query'		*what*	→ 'hat'
it	→ 'hit'		*yet*	→ 'yak'
last	→ 'late'		*you*	→ 'truly'

? Paralexias

more	→ 'little'		*wail*	→ 'mine'
piece	→ 'little'		*thinking*	→ 'helpful'
shape	→ 'rule'		*opportunity*	→ 'event'
particular	→ 'amount'		*apart*	→ 'amount'
hint	→ 'nub'		*plot*	→ 'stroll'
hint	→ 'new'		*descend*	→ 'inside'
picking	→ 'stitching'		*else*	→ 'little'
nape	→ 'nub'		*difference*	→ 'minimal'
encumbered	→ 'broken'		*drab*	→ 'nub'
recent	→ 'first'		*admonish*	→ 'ban (sem?)'
systematic	→ 'political'		*sake*	→ 'away'
susceptible	→ 'judge'			

Circumlocutions*

aunt	→	'uncle and cousin, no'
triviality	→	'little, silly, serious no'
craft	→	'sawing, no, clever'
curse	→	'naughty boy, swearing'
chemical	→	'medicine, no, chemist'
impossibility	→	'perhaps, not'
protocol	→	'high person, NATO, queen'
legitimate	→	'solicitors, near'
perjury	→	'jury or uh bad, naughty'
legality	→	'solicitors or uh, jury, no, parliament'
receptive	→	'wedding, service'
grant	→	'lend, house'
ornament	→	'jewels, no; Vaseline'

*Note: This is a small subset of reading responses of this type by P.W., included in this corpus of single-word paralexic errors merely to give a fuller picture of the patient's reading behaviour.

Corpus of paralexic errors for D.E.

Semantic paralexias

blowing	→	'wind'	projector	→	'camera'
shining	→	'sun'	lecturer	→	'tutor'
lecturer	→	'student'	excavate	→	'hole'
view	→	'scene'	assaulting	→	'climbing'
guide	→	'tour'	destruction	→	'demolish'
admit	→	'event'	tartan	→	'kilt'
competitor	→	'event'	colonel	→	'uniform'
employ	→	'occupy'	little	→	'small'
lecture	→	'school'	disposal	→	'dustbins'
reality	→	'belief'	thirsty	→	'drink'
scene	→	'tely'	colonel	→	'general'
emergency	→	'ambulance'	applaud	→	'clapping'
jury	→	'judge'	twisted	→	'turning'
admiral	→	'ship'	primary	→	'infant'
product	→	'work'	excavations	→	'digging'
cone	→	'ice cream'	accident	→	'ambulance'
night	→	'sleep'	present	→	'past'
beet	→	'sugar'	painting	→	'pictures'
dream	→	'sleep'	provisions	→	'groceries'
nephew	→	'auntie'	gone	→	'lost'
paddock	→	'kennel'	navy	→	'sailor'
girl	→	'boy'	act	→	'scene'
whip	→	'slash'	lead	→	'steel'
shining	→	'sunny'	sabre	→	'sword'
thermos	→	'flask'			

Derivational paralexias

counter	→ 'counting'		*cloth*	→ 'clothes'
directing	→ 'directions'		*courage*	→ 'courageous'
excavate	→ 'excavations'		*parting*	→ 'apart'
amphibian	→ 'amphibious'		*building*	→ 'builder'
bit	→ 'bite'		*signal*	→ 'sign'
rule	→ 'ruler'		*transportation*	→ 'transport'
arched	→ 'arch'		*directing*	→ 'direct'
calculate	→ 'calculator'		*coil*	→ 'coiled'
classify	→ 'class'		*hovering*	→ 'hover'
contain	→ 'container'		*applaud*	→ 'applause'
employ	→ 'employers'		*soloist*	→ 'solo'
mysterious	→ 'mystery'		*diseased*	→ 'disease'
hire	→ 'hired'		*heroic*	→ 'hero'
agony	→ 'agonise'		*typing*	→ 'typist'
edition	→ 'editor'		*batting*	→ 'bat'
excuse	→ 'excused'		*projection*	→ 'projector'
fact	→ 'facts'		*electricity*	→ 'electric'
grown	→ 'growth'		*beautiful*	→ 'beauty'
lovely	→ 'love'		*heroine*	→ 'hero'
slavery	→ 'slaves'		*directions*	→ 'directors'
slavery	→ 'slaving'		*buy*	→ 'bought'
warmth	→ 'warm'		*cowardly*	→ 'coward'
artist	→ 'art'		*chemical*	→ 'chemist'
owner	→ 'own'		*praying*	→ 'prays'
charter	→ 'chart'		*apart*	→ 'part'
goddess	→ 'god'		*occupied*	→ 'occupation'
marriage	→ 'married'		*truth*	→ 'true'
management	→ 'manager'		*murdered*	→ 'murder'
admiral	→ 'admiralty'		*acknowledge*	→ 'knowledge'
product	→ 'production'		*productive*	→ 'production'
prayer	→ 'praying'		*cowardice*	→ 'coward'
death	→ 'dead'		*stuff*	→ 'stuffed'
cough	→ 'coughing'		*burn*	→ 'burnt'
pour	→ 'pouring'		*heartless*	→ 'heart'
pays	→ 'paid'		*restore*	→ 'store'

Visual paralexias

tying	→ 'tyre'		*crag*	→ 'crab'
arrow	→ 'narrow'		*tantrum*	→ 'tandem'
ceremony	→ 'cemetery'		*probing*	→ 'problem'
funnel	→ 'tunnel'		*gable*	→ 'cable'
appliance	→ 'applied'		*while*	→ 'white'
furrow	→ 'furlong'		*idiot*	→ 'idol'
hovering	→ 'Hoover'		*such*	→ 'touch'
confining	→ 'confess'		*shape*	→ 'sharp'
nest	→ 'net'		*arrest*	→ 'rest'

due	→ 'deuce'	*badge*	→ 'bandage'
gratefully	→ 'grape'	*tumble*	→ 'tummy'
imitate	→ 'image'	*counter*	→ 'accountant'
merely	→ 'merry'	*pod*	→ 'pot'
organize	→ 'organ'	*wailing*	→ 'waiting'
recommend	→ 'comrades'	*smoulder*	→ 'shoulder'
quarrel	→ 'squirrel'	*systematic*	→ 'automatic'
favour	→ 'flavour'	*pivot*	→ 'pilot'
agony	→ 'angry'	*postage*	→ 'poster'
decree	→ 'crease'	*appeared*	→ 'applaud'
decree	→ 'degrees'	*bibliography*	→ 'bible'
hint	→ 'hide'	*gradually*	→ 'graduate'
origin	→ 'organ'	*cockerel*	→ 'cockles'
patent	→ 'patient'	*sparkle*	→ 'sparking'
phase	→ 'psalm'	*ornament*	→ 'organ'
phase	→ 'praise'	*applied*	→ 'applaud'
profit	→ 'proof'	*opposite*	→ 'site'
revolt	→ 'revolver'	*own*	→ 'now'
wealth	→ 'well'	*triviality*	→ 'tribute'
wealth	→ 'health'	*carbon*	→ 'car'
tribute	→ 'triviality'	*excise*	→ 'excused'
spray	→ 'sprain'	*cause*	→ 'caution'
poverty	→ 'pottery'	*appear*	→ 'applaud'
evidence	→ 'evict'	*keep*	→ 'kerb'
attribute	→ 'tribute'	*must*	→ 'just'
inhabitant	→ 'hibernation'	*task*	→ 'flask'
fault	→ 'false'	*sake*	→ 'take'
flown	→ 'drowned'	*self*	→ 'sell'
drove	→ 'dove'	*accord*	→ 'account'
bough	→ 'bought'	*combine*	→ 'comb'
beet	→ 'beef'	*deceit*	→ 'descent'
moment	→ 'monument'	*polite*	→ 'politics'
occurrence	→ 'occupied'	*bursting*	→ 'burnt'
scandal	→ 'sandals'	*nourished*	→ 'noxious'

Visual and/or semantic paralexias

edge	→ 'end'	*graduate*	→ 'grade'
amount	→ 'account'	*screen*	→ 'scene'
amount	→ 'accountant'	*judge*	→ 'jury'
incident	→ 'accident'	*terrible*	→ 'trouble'
grown	→ 'ground'	*rate*	→ 'rent'
opponent	→ 'opposite'	*shade*	→ 'shadow'
fragment	→ 'fracture'	*raise*	→ 'rise'
embossed	→ 'embroider'	*newspaper*	→ 'paper'

Visual then semantic paralexias

charter	→ 'map'	*pivot*	→ 'airplane'
favour	→ 'taste'		

Function-word paralexias

(a) SUBSTITUTION OF OTHER FUNCTION WORD

off	→ 'from'		*not*	→ 'no'
was	→ 'and'		*or*	→ 'for'
where	→ 'now'		*by*	→ 'my'
both	→ 'another'		*have*	→ 'has'
your	→ 'you'		*had*	→ 'as'
me	→ 'my'		*her*	→ 'she'
here	→ 'where'		*this*	→ 'is'
his	→ 'he'		*are*	→ 'and'
they	→ 'the'			

(b) SUBSTITUTION OF CONTENT WORD

on	→ 'top'
what	→ 'hat'
that	→ 'hat'

? Paralexias

decay	→ 'ruler'		*crag*	→ 'clock'
wealth	→ 'warm'		*figment*	→ 'fragile'
history	→ 'art'			

Circumlocutions

			freight	→ 'cargo, airport'
debt	→ 'buy, the same'		*sabre*	→ 'sword uh long,
oxide	→ 'chemical, oxygen'			sceptre'
product	→ 'production, work'		*colonel*	→ 'uniform, but which
poster	→ 'postman, post'			one?'
edition	→ 'London, paper,		*fleece*	→ 'flee but no, like sheep'
	editor'		*resist*	→ 'mixed-up sister'

Reading responses of K.F.
Tim Shallice and Elizabeth K. Warrington

The reading performance of K.F. is analysed in detail in Shallice and Warrington (1975). Other aspects of his performance in psychological experiments are reviewed in Shallice and Warrington (1977); clinical details are available in Warrington and Shallice (1969) and Warrington, Logue and Pratt (1971). This appendix provides further details of his reading responses.

The reading corpus

The corpus of responses used for the analysis reported in Shallice and Warrington (1975) was based on K.F.'s performance reading five sets of words. The actual responses he gave for two of those sets are given below.

The words were typed in columns and in alphabetical order (normally reading across the page). He read down the columns. We have divided his responses into four categories for convenience of presentation – one-word correct responses, omissions (no response), one-word error responses and multiple-word responses. Asterisked words were presented twice.

The 'multiple-word response' category includes all responses which are difficult to classify; it contains not only the responses classified as paraphasic (i.e. circumlocutory) in our original analysis, but also ones allocated on a somewhat arbitrary basis to the other three categories, corrects, omissions and errors. In this 'multiple-word response' category, the placing of his response within single brackets e.g. family → (a lot of people, brothers and sisters) means that it was clear that his response was not intended as the word itself but as a comment on the word; square brackets e.g. tangle → [described tattoo] indicates our interpretation of his response. This corpus also contains certain stimuli deleted from the earlier analysis e.g. I'd, I'm, boy friend.

One-word correct responses (AA frequency from Thorndike-Lorge list)

as, at, by, go, it, me, Mr., up, act, add, ago, are, arm, art, bad, bag, bed, big, bit, box, boy, but, buy, can, car, cry, cup, cut, day, die, dog, dry, ear, eat, egg, end, eye, fat, few, fit, fly, god, hat, hot, ice, ill, job, joy*, joy, law, lay, leg, lip, man, may, men, Mrs., new, oil, old, one, out, pay, red, run, sat, saw, sea, see, she, sir, six, sky, son, sun, ten, the, tie, top, two, war, way, win, yes, army, away, baby, back, ball, bank, bear, bill, bird, blow, blue, body, book, born, burn, camp, case, cash, cent, city, club, coal, coat, cold, cook, dark, date, dead, door, drop, edge, face, fair, farm, fast, feet, fire, fish, five, food, fool, foot, four, free, full, game, gate, girl, gold, good, gray, hair, half, hall, hang, head, heat, help, high, hill, hole, home, hour, iron, John, join, just, kill, king, kiss, knee, knew, lady, lake, land, late, left, life, lift, line, long, look, lord, lost, love, make, mark, meat, meet, mile, milk, mine, miss, moon, name, neck, news, nice, nine, nose, note, open, page, pain, pair, part, pass, past, poor, post, race, rain, read, rich, ride, ring, rise, road, rock, roll, roof, room, rose, rule, safe, sail, salt, seat, sell, ship, shoe, shop, shot, sick, side, sing, skin, snow, song, spot, star, stop, suit, tall, thee, time, town, tree, turn, view, vote, wait, walk, wall, warm, wash, wave, week, west, wife, wild, wind, wood, work*, work, yard*, yard, year, black, blood, brown, catch, chair, chick, child, class, claim, clean, close, cloud, cover, cross, crowd, daily, dance, dream, dress, drink, drive, earth, eight, enemy, field, floor, fresh, fruit, glass, going, grass, great, green, guard, guess, guide, happy, Henry, horse, house, hurry, judge, large, leave, light, march, money, mount, mouth, music, night, ocean, paint, paper, piece, place*, place, point, pound, power, press, price, queen, river, scene, seven, sleep, small, smile, smoke, sound, south, space, state, stick, stone, store, story, sugar, sweet, table, today, train, truth, uncle, under, voice, watch, water, white, whole, woman, women, world, wrong, young, animal, Arthur, battle, bridge, bright, butter, church, circle, colour, common, cotton, danger, dinner, doctor, dollar, double, escape, family, father, finger, finish, flower, forest, France, French, garden, George, ground, health, heaven, island, knight, leader, letter, London, market, master, member, mother, nature, number, people, please, pretty, public, record, report, school, second, silver, single, sister, spirit, square, street, strong, summer, travel, twelve, valley, weight, window, winter*, winter, yellow, America, brother, captain, century, clothes, college, England, evening, express, foreign, Germany, hundred, kitchen, machine, million, morning, New York, picture, quarter, soldier, station, teacher, village, weather.

Omissions (AA frequency from Thorndike-Lorge list)

an, do, I'd, I'm, in, is, no, of, oh, or, so, St., to, we, all, and, ask, did, for, get, got, has, his, how, I'll, its, it's, let, nor, not, now, off, our, own, put, too, use, who, why, you, also, base, beat*, beat, been, call, came, care, dare, deal, does, don't, down, draw, each, east, easy, else, fail, fall, fear, feel, felt, fill, find, flow, form, from, give, hand, hard, have, hear, heir, hers, hold, inch, into, isn't, know, laid, lead, less, like, live, many, mind, more, move, need, next, only, over, pick, plan, play, pull, real, rest, rush, said, seem, seen, send, sent, show, size, soil, sold, some, soon, sort, soul, stay, such, sure, take, talk, tell, than, that, them, then, they, this, thou, thus, till, took, type, very, want, wear, well, went, were, what, when, whom, will, wise, wish, with, won't, your, about, above, admit, again, agree, allow, alone, along, among, began, begin, being, below, bring, carry, cause, court, didn't, doubt, early, enjoy, every, fight, given, heard, heart, heavy, issue, laugh, learn, least, marry, never, often, order*, order, other, ought, peace, plain, prove, reach, ready, reply, right, sense, serve, shade, shape, short, since, spend, spoke, stand, start, stern, still, stood, taken, that's, their, these, thing, third, those*, those, three, tried, union, until, value, wasn't, waste, where, which, while, whose, worth, would, you're, accept, across, action, affair, afraid, almost, always, amount, answer, appear, around, arrive, became, become, before, behind, belong, beside, better, beyond, branch, cannot, caught, chance, change, charge, coming, course, decide, degree, demand, direct, divide, doesn't, during, effort, either, enough, famous, figure, follow, forget, friend, future, gather, indeed, itself, matter, method, moment, myself, nation, nearly, object, obtain, period, proper, rather, really, reason, regard, remain, result, settle, should, simple, spread, strike, sudden, supply, system, thirty, though, unless, within, wonder, account, advance, already, against, another, article, attempt, because, believe, between, brought, certain, command, company, contain, control, couldn't, declare, destiny, example, explain, finally, forward, general, herself, himself, however, include, instead, journal, measure, meeting, mention, neither, nothing, opinion, outside, perhaps, prepare, present, problem, produce, promise, provide, purpose, quickly, realize, require, society, special, strange, subject, success, suggest, support, suppose, thought, through, trouble, usually, various, whether, without, wouldn't.

One-word error responses (AA frequency from Thorndike-Lorge list)

am → 'be'	last → 'late'	party → 'part'
be → 'by'	lose → 'stole'	plant → 'level'
he → 'his'	loss → 'lost'	quite → 'quiet'
if → 'it'	Mary → 'May'	raise → 'rise'
my → 'by'	mean → 'meat'	shall → 'shell'
on → 'go'	most → 'lost'	share → 'shark'
us → 'just'	much → 'chum'	shore → 'shoe'
air → 'fly'	none → 'lost'	shout → 'shot'
any → 'you'	once → 'one'	sight → 'signal'
far → 'fair'	paid → 'pay'	stock → 'sock'
had → 'hat'	path → 'Pathe'	study → 'student'
her → 'she'	rate → 'rat'	taste → 'paste'
he's → 'his'	same → 'name'	think → 'thinking'
him → 'his'	save → 'raise'	touch → 'torch'
led → 'leg'	seek → 'see'	trade → 'tract'
lie → 'die'	soft → 'stole'	trust → 'truth'
low → 'lost'	sold → 'stole'	visit → 'wait'
met → 'meet'	step → 'lane'	write → 'writing'
ran → 'rat'	tear → 'crying'	broken → 'broke'
say → 'as'	thin → 'tall'	corner → 'corn'
set → 'sat'	tire → 'tie'	desire → 'desert'
sit → 'sat'	told → 'lost'	except → 'exit'
was → 'saw'	true → 'truth'	expect → 'exit'
yet → 'yes'	upon → 'up'	farmer → 'farm'
able → 'table'	wing → 'wind'	fellow → 'falling'
best → 'bless'	word → 'world'	former → 'farmer'
busy → 'buying'	board → 'broad'	gentle → 'gentleman'
can't → 'can'	break → 'breaking'	German → 'Germany'
come → 'comb'	build → 'building'	golden → 'gold'
cost → 'coast'	built → 'building'	happen → 'happy'
deep → 'deer'	chest → 'chess'	honour → 'horror'
done → 'lost'	count → 'county'	Indian → 'India'
duty → 'deputy'	crowd → 'crown'	length → 'lean'
ever → 'even'	death → 'dying'	middle → 'muddle'
fact → 'act'	enter → 'exit'	modern → 'model'
fine → 'five'	fifty → 'five'	narrow → 'sparrow'
gain → 'grain'	force → 'foreign'	native → 'nation'
gave → 'grave'	forth → 'fault'	person → 'parson'
glad → 'great'	front → 'fort'	refuse → 'suffer'
gone → 'none'	grant → 'gran'	return → 'truth'
grew → 'green'	group → 'gross'	speech → 'speak'
grow → 'gross'	known → 'gone'	stream → 'steam'
hope → 'hop'	lower → 'slower'	suffer → 'snuff'
hurt → 'injure'	might → 'night'	toward → 'town'
keep → 'left'	month → 'mouth'	British → 'Britain'
kind → 'king'	offer → 'before'	country → 'county'

English →	'England'	*officer* →	'office'	*several* →	'seven'
further →	'fortune'	*passage* →	'passport'	*silence* →	'silent'
natural →	'nature'	*service* →	'forces'		

Multiple-word responses (AA frequency from Thorndike-Lorge list)

age	→ 'old . . . no . . . age'	round	→ '(not ground)'
bay	→ 'baby . . . no . . . bay'	speak	→ '(someone talks)'
		teach	→ 'class . . . no . . . teacher'
due	→ '(play snooker) . . . cue'	there	→ 'begin . . . no'
lot	→ 'lost . . . lot'	wrote	→ 'wrong . . . no . . . write'
cool	→ 'cold . . . cool'		
dear	→ '(say when writing letter)'	beauty	→ 'daughter or beautiful'
		Europe	→ '(like in Germany)'
even	→ 'ever . . . no'	favour	→ '(you can eat)'
fell	→ '(name of oil) shell'	height	→ 'high . . . higher'
held	→ 'left or right'	labour	→ '(government) ((correct in 1969))'
idea	→ 'good idea'		
kept	→ 'left (or is it right)'	listen	→ 'quiet . . . ssh'
made	→ 'make . . . no'	little	→ 'small . . . letter'
must	→ 'must (got it from mustard)'	minute	→ 'time . . . minute'
		notice	→ '(not note)'
near	→ '(ear is part of it)'	prince	→ '(not a king)'
sign	→ 'single . . . no'	season	→ '(sea and son)'
trip	→ 'type . . . no . . . tight (as in tightrope)'	spring	→ '(not ring)'
		Chicago	→ '(in US) Chi. . . .'
after	→ '(in afternoon)'	history	→ '(not now . . . the past)'
first	→ 'finish or start'		
found	→ 'lost or lose'	husband	→ '(not brother)'
human	→ '(alive)'	written	→ 'writing . . . no . . . writer'

One-word correct responses (Brown and Ure list, 1969)

acorn, ambulance, anger, aquarium, army, art, baby, bad, bag, bandage,
barber, bath, battle, bed, beef, beggar, bible, big, bird, black, blossom,
blue, bomb, book, box, boy, boyfriend, brave, bread, bride, broad,
brother, butter, butterfly, cabbage, carpet, carrot, cemetery, chair,
cheese, child, church, city, class, clean, clothing, cold, colour, cook, cow,
cripple, cry, curtains, cushion, cut, daddy, dance, danger, dark,
daughter, dead, die, dirt, doctor, dog, door, dream, dress, drink, dwarf,
eagle, earth, eating, engine, fairy, faith, farm, farmhouse, father, female,
finger, fire, flower, foot, friend, friendly, frog, fruit, fur, garage, ginger, girl,
girl-friend, glass, go, good, gray, green, hand, happy, hard, hat, hay,
head, health, heart, hide, history, home, horse, hospital, house, hungry,
ink, island, jelly, joy, key, king, kiss, kitchen, lamp, lawyer, light,

lighthouse, lion, little, long, love, make, man, mental, milk, money, moon, mother, motor, mountain, music, name, nation, nature, needle, new, ocean, odd, office, old, paper, perch, phone, pirate, police, pond, power, puppy, race, red, ring, rip, salad, salt, scent, school, scissors, screen, seat, shadow, ship, shut, sick, sleeping, slow, small, smash, smoking, soldier, son, spider, spring, star, state, stomach, stove, street, suck, sweet, taxi, time, toilet, train, treasure, trumpet, trunk, uncle, voyage, walk, war, water, whiskey, white, wild, window, wink, woman, women, work, working, world.

Omissions (Brown and Ure list, 1969)

absorption, afraid, agility, alert, anxiety, applaud, applause, argon, ascend, autumn, baronet, barracks, beating, beautiful, beauty, bowl, bully, bust, caress, caring for, carry, caught, caution, census, change, choose, choosing, chore, citizen, client, climb, clumsy, coarse, column, comedy, comfort, command, comparison, compete, conduct, conscience, contents, context, corpse, corridor, corrupt, courage, crutch, dancer, darn, death, debate, decade, decent, deep, defeat, defect, definition, depressed, deputy, description, despise, detail, dimension, direct, disgust, dismal, distribution, divorce, eldest, employ, erosion, esteem, excuse, faithless, false, famous, fasten, fearing, forbid, frame, fringe, froth, fuss, garment, glisten, gossip, grief, grudge, habit, hatred, heavy, hinder, humour, income, indignation, industry, inferior, insomnia, insult, journey, jump, kerosene, kindness, kneel, lake, legend, leisure, levity, lick, limp, lose, loud, luck, maintenance, malice, mallet, mane, mature, measurement, medley, melody, memory, menace, mitten, modification, moment, movies, muddy, mural, mutton, narrow, nature, nectar, nice, nitrogen, normal, notice, obtain, occurrence, offend, opinion, option, pamphlet, part, parting, party, patent, patriotism, peace, perfume, person, pinch, plenty, ploughing, plum, prairie, pray, preach, prick, priest, priority, prosper, proud, punch, pure, purpose, qualm, quarrelling, quart, quick, quiet, quota, radiator, ram, rattle, religion, removal, revolt, rich, riddle, ridicule, river, rotation, rough, rude, rug, rustle, sad, salute, sap, scar, scold, scrub, secret, secure, seed, seen, sequel, sheep, short, should, shove, shy, sickness, silly, sin, sister, slap, sleep, slime, smooth, sneak, sneer, sniff, social, socialism, soft, soothe, sour, speak, sphere, spill, spit, splash, square, squeeze, stammer, steady, steeple, stem, stern, stolen, stool, stork, strict, stripes, strong, stumble, stupid, success, suicide, supplicate, swear, swift, table, tame, tattoo, tease, temper, tempt, theory, thief, thigh, think, thirsty, threat, tickle, timid, tired, torture, travel, truth, try, unjust, upset, valentine, valour, vanity, vehicle, veneer, vigorous, violation, vision, wagon, wait, warmth, weak, wealth, whine, whistle, wicked, windmill, wine, wish, woo, worry, wound, wretch, wrinkles, zero.

One-word errors (Brown and Ure list, 1969)

abusing	→ 'business'		*hoist*	→ 'host'
accent	→ 'accident'		*hunger*	→ 'hungry'
action	→ 'actor'		*injure*	→ 'juggler'
agency	→ 'agerm'		*insane*	→ 'name'
alone	→ 'alost'		*instep*	→ 'stepping'
ask	→ 'asked'		*iodine*	→ 'idle'
attack	→ 'attacked'		*ivory*	→ 'Ivor'
bake	→ 'baker'		*jerk*	→ 'jeep'
baker	→ 'bakery'		*jolly*	→ 'joy'
beat	→ 'meat'		*justice*	→ 'judging'
behind	→ 'begin'		*kissing*	→ 'beginning'
bite	→ 'beaten'		*kite*	→ 'Kate'
bleed	→ 'bleeding'		*laugh*	→ 'laughing'
bowel	→ 'towel'		*lie*	→ 'life'
branch	→ 'ranch'		*loveliness*	→ 'lovely'
bright	→ 'bridge'		*manner*	→ 'making'
bury	→ 'burn'		*marry*	→ 'Harry'
centre	→ 'circle'		*modest*	→ 'model'
choice	→ 'choir'		*month*	→ 'moth'
cooking	→ 'cookery'		*museum*	→ 'music'
cork	→ 'core'		*painting*	→ 'painter'
custom	→ 'usherette'		*passage*	→ 'passport'
damage	→ 'danger'		*penalty*	→ 'penny'
dear	→ 'hearing'		*pencil*	→ 'biro'
dirty	→ 'dirt'		*phase*	→ 'prayer'
dump	→ 'bluff'		*pity*	→ 'pit'
elevator	→ 'electric'		*poetry*	→ 'pottery'
errand	→ 'error'		*pride*	→ 'bride'
evil	→ 'devil'		*scandal*	→ 'scared'
excel	→ 'exit'		*sing*	→ 'song'
fail	→ 'faith'		*smell*	→ 'small'
fall	→ 'wall'		*sprinkle*	→ 'sprinkler'
fear	→ 'faith'		*squeak*	→ 'squeaking'
fiction	→ 'acting'		*statue*	→ 'states'
flush	→ 'bluff'		*sweat*	→ 'sweet'
foolish	→ 'falling'		*swim*	→ 'swing'
future	→ 'fortune'		*swing*	→ 'singing'
gamble	→ 'game'		*tackle*	→ 'sticky'
give	→ 'going'		*thirst*	→ 'wrist'
glacier	→ 'glass'		*trouble*	→ 'travel'
grease	→ 'greaser'		*village*	→ 'valley'
hammer	→ 'hamster'		*virtue*	→ 'vintage'
hate	→ 'hat'		*wishing*	→ 'luck'
healthy	→ 'health'		*writer*	→ 'writing'
high	→ 'tall'		*youth*	→ 'young'

Multiple-word responses (Brown and Ure List, 1969)

accordance	→	(. . . dance)
altar	→	(different country)
angel	→	[recognized Tube Station i.e., Angel]
angry	→	(like anger)
antelope	→	(animal)
bitter	→	(like butter)
bodice	→	(dice at end)
bring	→	(B with ring)
camera	→	(I've got one)
candy	→	(American children eat a lot . . . candy)
career	→	(car part of it)
chapter	→	(name of person . . . Chaplin)
clay	→	(Boxer's name . . . Clay)
cottage	→	(not a house)
coward	→	(place in the Isle of Wight) [i.e., Cowes]
deceive	→	(to do with police force . . . detective)
dentist	→	(have your teeth done . . . dentist)
enter	→	(exit . . . no . . . ending)
estate	→	(different places in U.S.A.)
family	→	(a lot of people, brothers and sisters)
fight	→	(to do with pilot)
foster	→	(name Frosty)
free	→	(tree . . . no . . . free)
grime	→	(against everyone)
guilty	→	(cuts)
hostage	→	(not hospital)
hug	→	(not few)
lantern	→	(light)
misfortune	→	(fortune plus a little bit)
monkey	→	(man . . . key)
nasty	→	(in Germany in war) [Nazi??]
navigation	→	(begins like navy)
orchestra	→	(not a band . . . orch . . .)
paddock	→	(station) [Paddington??]
plant	→	(part of it island)
quarrel	→	(qua . . .)
rally	→	(name of car)
ratio	→	(looks like wireless)
sponge	→	(not a jelly)
stalk	→	(tall . . . or short)
story	→	(not Labour the other)
tangle	→	[described a tattoo]
taxes	→	(not tax)
thermometer	→	(weather . . . thing going up or down . . . or under arm)
tobacco	→	(in a cigarette)

tree	→	[pointed out of window at a tree]
wrinkle	→	(can eat winkles)
yellow	→	(colour) [pointed at it]

References

Brown, W. P. and Ure, D. M. N. (1969) Five rated characteristics of 650 word association stimuli. *British Journal of Psychology, 60,* 223–50.

Kapur, N. and Perl, N. T. (1978) Recognition reading in paralexia. *Cortex, 14,* 439–43.

Patterson, K. E. and Marcel, A. J. (1977) Aphasia, dyslexia and phonological coding of written words. *Quarterly Journal of Experimental Psychology, 29,* 307–18.

Shallice, T. and Warrington, E. K. (1975) Word recognition in a phonemic dyslexic patient. *Quarterly Journal of Experimental Psychology, 27,* 187–99.

Shallice, T. and Warrington, E. K. (1977) Auditory-verbal short-term memory and conduction aphasia. *Brain and Language, 4,* 479–91.

Thorndike, E. and Lorge, I. (1944) *The Teachers' Oral Book of 30,000 Words.* New York: Teachers' College, Columbia University Press.

Warrington, E. K., Logue, V. and Pratt, R. T. C. (1971) The anatomical localisation of selective impairment of auditory short-term memory. *Neuropsychologia, 9,* 377–87.

Warrington, E. K. and Shallice, T. (1969) The selective impairment of auditory verbal short-term memory. *Brain, 92,* 885–96.

Index